Controversies in the Description of Congenitally Malformed Hearts

Cardiopulmonary Medicine from Imperial College Press

Controversies in the Description of Congenitally Malformed Hearts

R. H. Anderson
Imperial College School of Medicine

A. E. Becker
Academic Medical Centre, University of Amsterdam

ICP

Imperial College Press

Published by

Imperial College Press
516 Sherfield Building
Imperial College
London SW7 2AZ

Distributed by

World Scientific Publishing Co. Pte. Ltd.
P O Box 128, Farrer Road, Singapore 912805
USA office: Suite 1B, 1060 Main Street, River Edge, NJ 07661
UK office: 57 Shelton Street, Covent Garden, London WC2H 9HE

British Library Cataloguing-in-Publication Data
A catalogue record for this book is available from the British Library.

CONTROVERSIES IN THE DESCRIPTION OF CONGENITALLY MALFORMED HEARTS

ISBN 1-86094-067-6

Printed in Singapore.

Foreword

The morphologic examination of congenitally malformed hearts has moved a long way. Initially, the anomalous organs were described very much as what they were — pathological curiosities. Indeed, in early times the birth of an infant with a congenital malformation was considered an ill-omen. With increasing experience, physicians began to collect and categorize the cases. An excellent example of the art of description was provided by Peacock, working in London in the middle of the nineteenth century. Von Rokitansky, practising in Vienna about twenty years later, demonstrated the potential value of cardiac anomalies as a proving ground for theories of embryogenesis. It was Fallot, however, working all his life in Marseilles, who showed the value of clinico-pathological correlation, clarifying the cause of "la maladie bleue". Other giants then left their footprints during the first half of the twentieth century, notably Maud Abbott working in Montreal, Canada. This marked the shift of innovative morphologic thinking to the America's and, during the 1960's and early 1970's, two morphologists developed, in parallel, the segmental approach to diagnosis of congenital heart malformations. They were Richard van Praagh, working in sequence in Toronto, Rochester (Minnesota), and Boston, and Maria Victoria de la Cruz from Mexico City. Along with other notable pathologists, particularly Jesse Edwards and Maurice Lev, these investigators laid the foundations of our present-day understanding of congenital cardiac anomalies. But, despite the considerable steps made, controversies remain, particularly with respect to the best, and the most accurate, way to describe and categorize some of the more complex malformations. We have been involved in many of these controversies.

It is these persisting differences which will provide the focus for this book, and the videodemonstrations it accompanies. Richard Van Praagh once commented that the wine of understanding may, on occasion, need to be poured into new bottles, but the old bottles should not be smashed. We agree totally with this philosophy. Another saying is that good wine needs no bush. So it is with cardiac anatomy, which is immediately apparent to all who seek to observe it. It is the interpretations of the observed anatomy which vary. In this book, and the accompanying videotapes, therefore, we have attempted to demonstrate the good wine, needing no bush. We then discuss the old, and the new, bottles in which it has matured. Obviously, we have, and recognize, our biases. Notwithstanding this, we have tried to present the controversies, as best we can, in balanced fashion.

As with so many of our works, the current project would not have been completed without the support of our clinical colleagues, and those with whom we have collaborated with in the past. With this particular undertaking, we owe a particular debt to Siew Yen Ho, Christine Anderson, and Karen McCarthy, who worked over and above the call of duty to produce the manuscript and illustrations. The videotapes could not have been completed without the tireless help and support of Jeremy Weaver and Andrew Williamson. Finally, it is a pleasure to acknowledge our indebtedness to Nancy Vaughan, of Imperial College Press, who is everything an Editor should be.

RHA
AEB
London and Amsterdam
April 1997

Contents

Chapter 1
Introduction

In this short book, we will review some of the controversies which persist concerning the most appropriate means of describing congenitally malformed hearts. Although many lesions could be cited as continuing to produce problems of nomenclature, for the purposes of our discussion, we will limit ourselves to four malformations. The first is the one in which concepts derived from development have, perhaps, produced the most confusion. This is the variant of atrioventricular septal defect which exists in tandem with a common atrioventricular junction. In our approach to this lesion, as with the subsequent malformations, we will show how concepts derived from presumed, albeit unproven, morphogenetic mechanisms have produced markedly inappropriate accounts of the underlying anatomy. The other lesions we will then address are those hearts which are found in the setting of isomeric atrial appendages, the time-honoured malformation of tetralogy of Fallot, where we will discuss its vexed relationship with double outlet right ventricle, and the hearts which are unified because they possess a univentricular atrioventricular connection. In our approach to all these lesions, we will make continued reference to certain common philosophic principles. In this introduction, therefore, we will chart the anatomic background to these principles which guide our analysis, discussing specifically the morphologic method and the sequential segmental approach.

THE MORPHOLOGIC METHOD

When describing any malformed heart, it is necessary to have reliable means of identifying the morphologic nature of the cardiac chambers within the heart, no matter how deformed they may be. These means are provided by what has become known as the "Morphologic Method". The philosophy underscoring this principle was first suggested by Lev,[1] and then developed as a practical tool by Van Praagh and his colleagues.[2] In their earlier writings, Van Praagh and his colleagues had followed accepted wisdom and used the term "single ventricle" to describe hearts in which both atriums drained to the same ventricle, irrespective of the fact that, when that chamber had left ventricular characteristics, another small chamber was to be found within the ventricular mass.[3] This additional chamber was considered to be the "conus", although no specific name was provided for it. We felt uncomfortable with this particular approach, and tried to provide logic in the use of "single ventricle", or "univentricular heart", by introducing criterions which denied

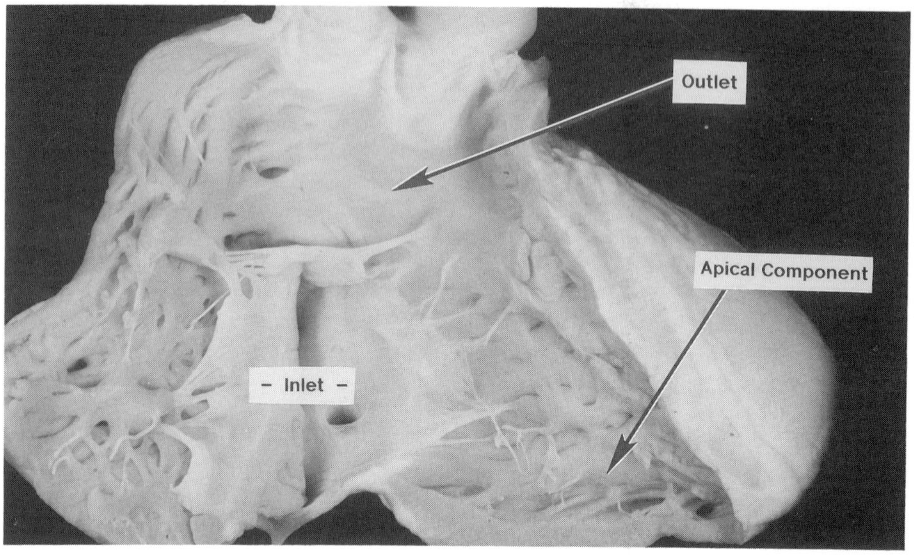

Fig. 1 The normal morphologically right ventricle has three clearly defined anatomic components — the inlet, apical trabecular, and outlet parts. The latter is completely muscular, while the apex is coarsely trabeculated.

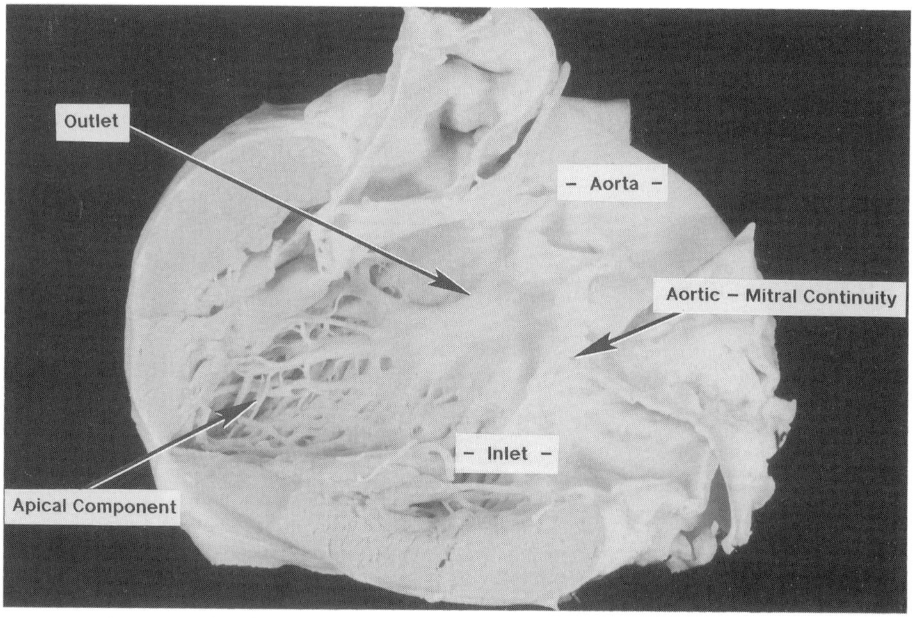

Fig. 2 The normal morphologically left ventricle also has inlet, apical trabecular, and outlet parts, although the outlet part is abbreviated because of the fibrous continuity between the leaflets of the aortic and mitral valves. The apex is finely trabeculated.

ventricular status to the smaller chamber in such hearts. For this purpose, we adopted the approach of Goor and Lillehei,[4] and analyzed normal ventricles in terms of three basic components, an inlet portion, an apical trabeculated part, and an outlet component (Figs. 1 and 2). When a ventricular chamber did not possess an inlet component, we suggested that the chamber be considered a "non-ventricle", thus permitting the heart containing it logically to be described as being "univentricular".[5] This attempt to provide logic, particularly when applied to hearts with double inlet right ventricle,[6] was then criticized by Van Praagh and his associates as they emphasized the importance of the morphologic method.[2] They pointed to a fundamental flaw in our approach, namely the attempt to define one variable, in this case the nature of a chamber within the ventricular mass, in terms of another variable, the presence or absence of an inlet component. They argued, quite rightly, that it is much better to define the structure in question on the basis of its own intrinsic myocardial morphology, choosing for the purposes of definition the component which is most constantly present when the chamber is malformed. For the ventricles, this most constant part has proved to be the apical trabecular component. The myocardial characteristics of the apical region are then sufficiently discrete to distinguish the different types of ventricle even when the apical parts exist in isolation (Figs. 3 and 4). Impressed by the logic of this principle, we immediately adopted it in our subsequent analysis of the hearts under discussion.[7,8]

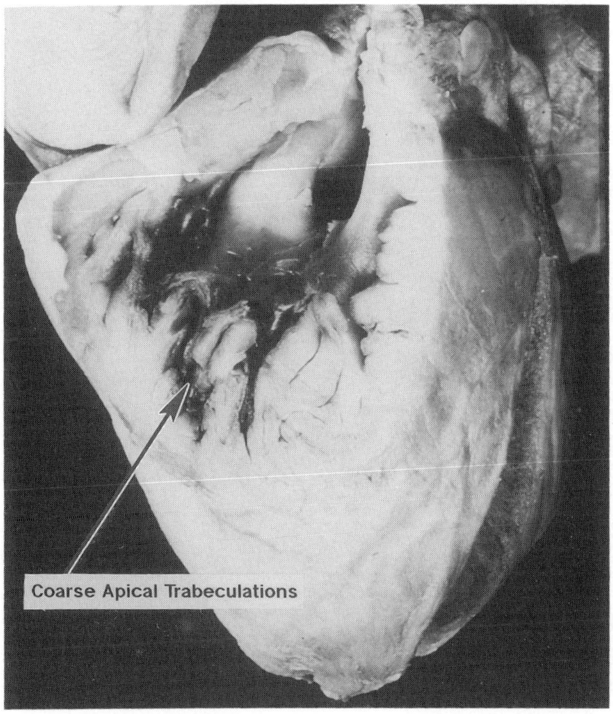

Fig. 3 This right ventricle, made up only of the apical trabecular component, comes from a heart with double inlet to, and double outlet from, a dominant left ventricle. Its right ventricular nature can still be recognized because of the coarse nature of the apical trabeculations.

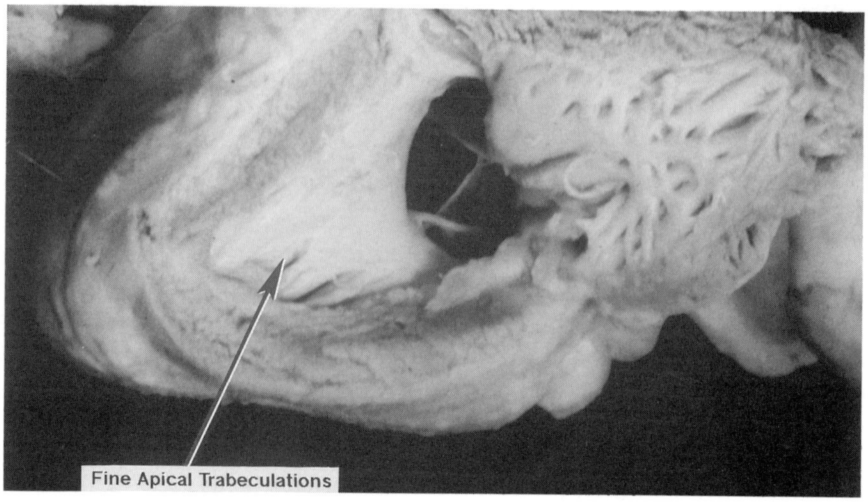

Fig. 4 In this heart, with double inlet to the dominant right ventricle through a common atrioventricular valve, the rudimentary left ventricle made up of only the apical trabecular component is recognized because of its myocardial characteristics.

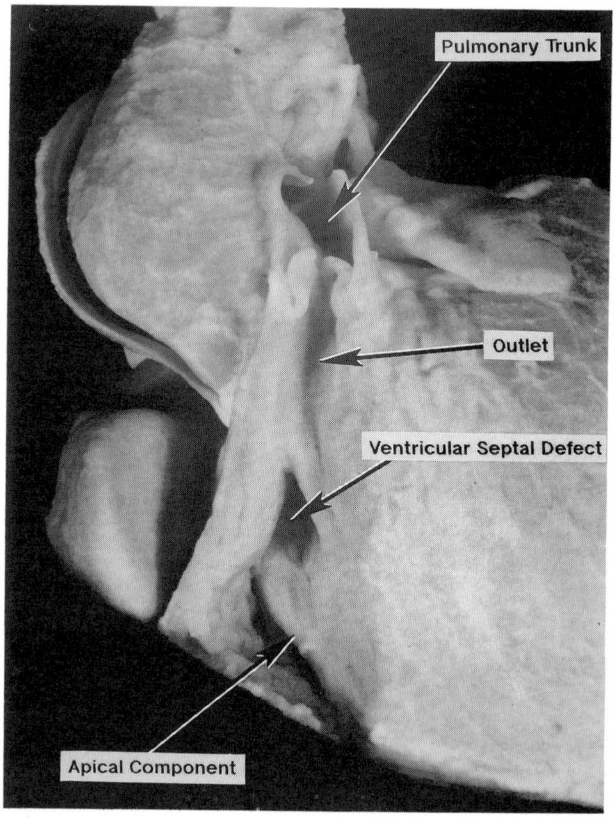

Fig. 5 In this heart with double inlet left ventricle and concordant ventriculo-arterial connections, the apical trabecular component of the rudimentary right ventricle supporting the pulmonary trunk is immediately recognizable on the basis of its myocardial characteristics.

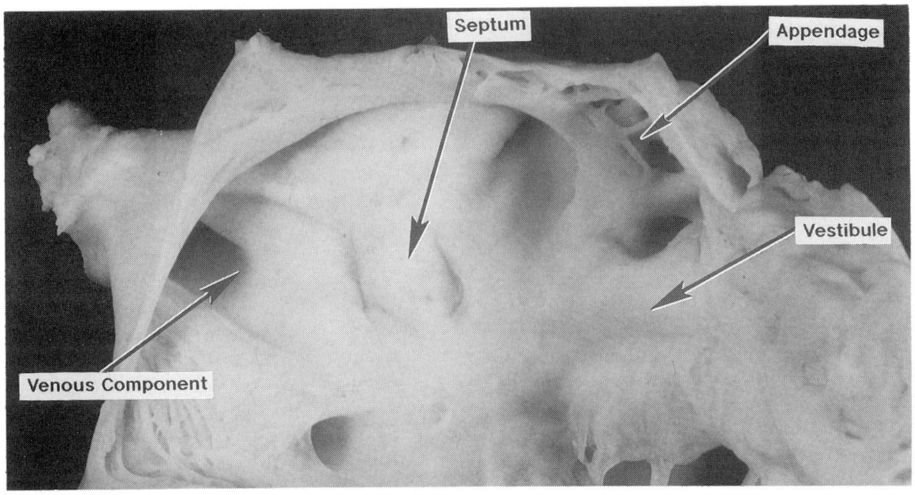

Fig. 6 The normal right atrium possesses an appendage, a vestibule, a venous component, and a septal surface.

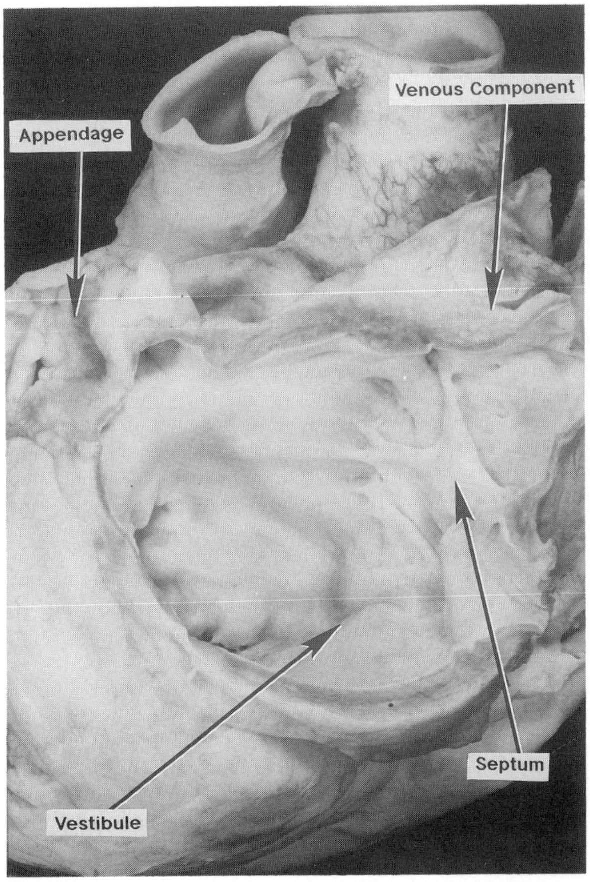

Fig. 7 The normal left atrium, as with the right (see Fig. 6), also possesses an appendage, a vestibule, a venous component and is separated from its partner by the atrial septum.

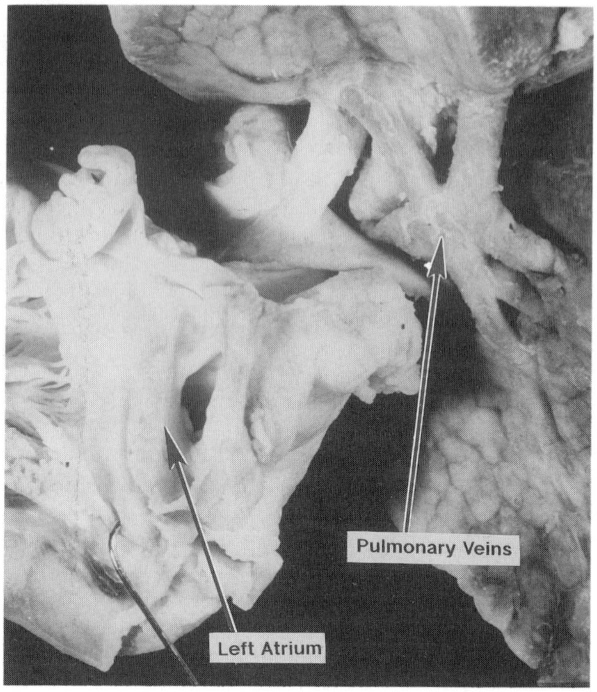

Fig. 8 The left atrium in this heart with totally anomalous pulmonary venous connection is recognizable as being morphologically left on the basis of its myocardial structure, even though it lacks its venous component.

It now surprises us that, although Van Praagh and his colleagues rightly used this method to criticize our earlier definitions,[2] they themselves continue to describe hearts with double inlet left ventricle as "single left ventricle",[9] seemingly ignoring the fact that such hearts possess an additional chamber within the ventricular mass which possesses an apical trabecular component with myocardial characteristics of unequivocal right ventricular pattern (Fig. 5). We will discuss this matter in greater detail in our final chapter. At present, we will demonstrate that the important principle of the morphologic method extends far beyond the analysis of ventricles. It is invaluable in defining the morphologic nature of all chambers of the heart, as well as serving to provide solid and unambiguous definitions for other cardiac components.

Thus, when the atrial chambers are considered in the context of the morphologic method, it is necessary first to establish which is their most constant component part. Each normal atrium possesses four parts, a venous component, a vestibule, a septal surface, and an appendage (Figs. 6 and 7). When these parts are considered in terms of their constancy in malformed hearts, it can readily be shown that the venous component, although an obvious feature of the normal atriums, is ruled out as a defining component, since the venous connections are very frequently absent or abnormal when the atrial chambers are abnormal. This is particularly so in the setting of visceral heterotaxy, when it is, perhaps, most important to be able to identify the specific morphology of the atriums. Similarly, whenever there is a totally

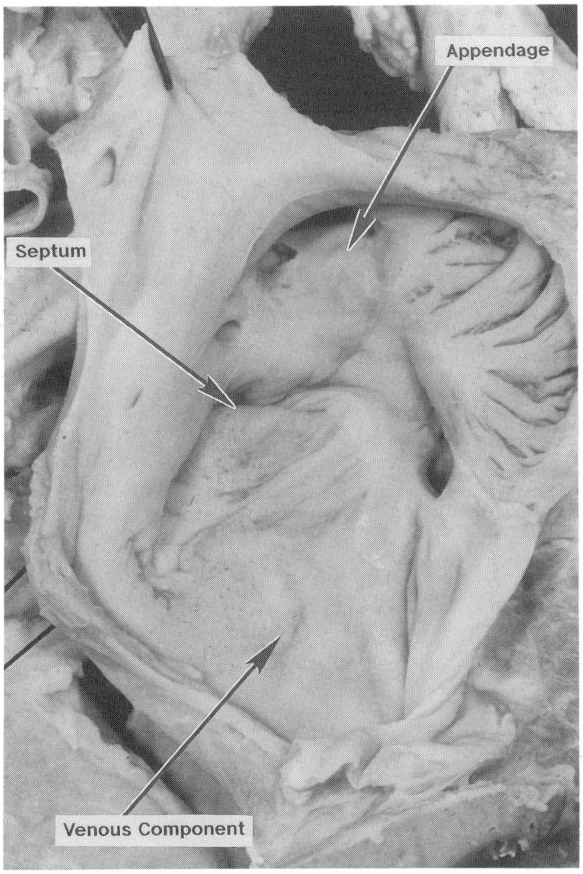

Fig. 9 This chamber is recognizable as the morphologically right atrium although it lacks its vestibule because of absence of the right atrioventricular connection (tricuspid atresia).

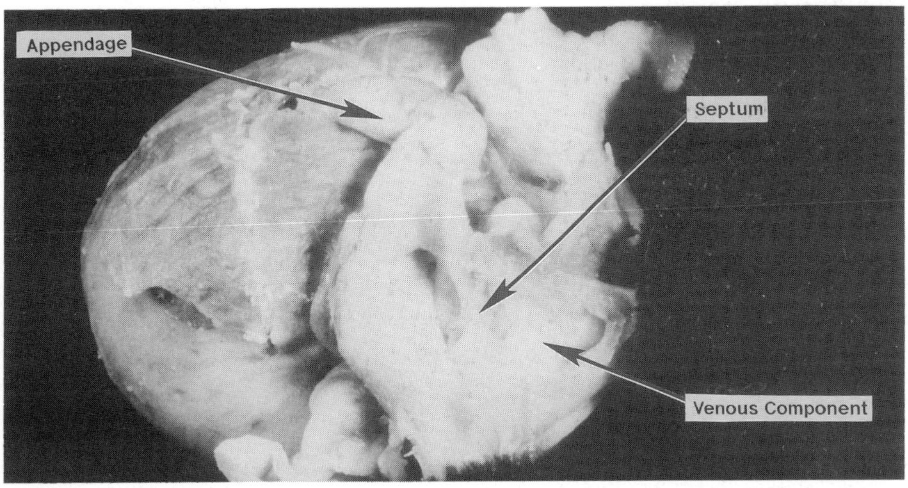

Fig. 10 In this heart with mitral atresia, the atrium is recognized as being morphologically left in the absence of its vestibule.

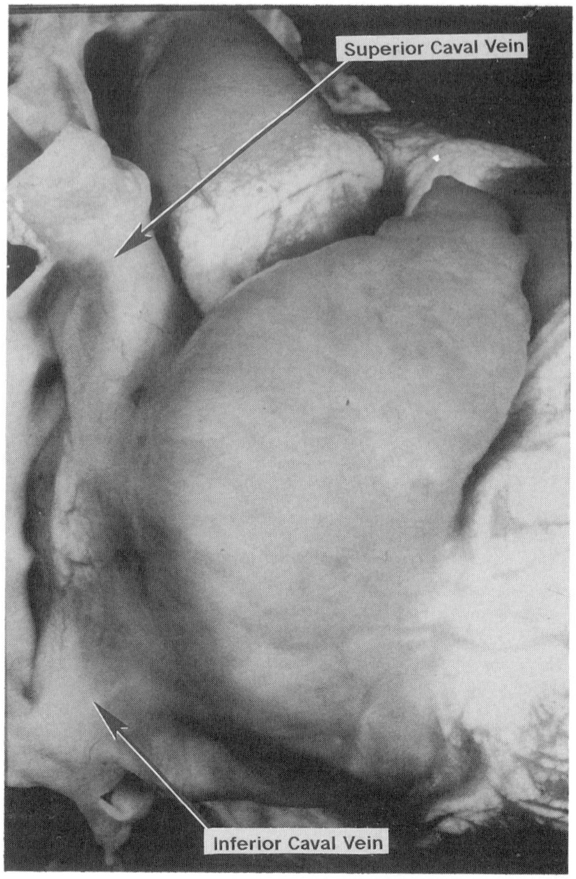

Fig. 11 The morphologically right atrial appendage is triangular in shape, and has a broad junction with the systemic venous component.

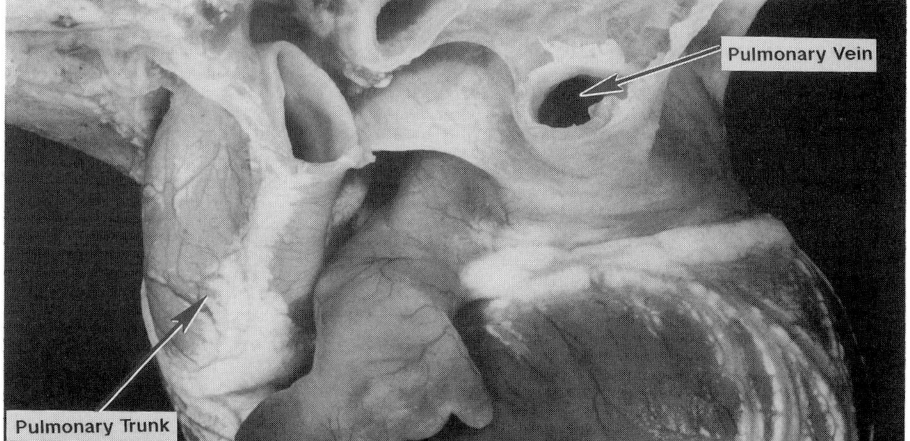

Fig. 12 The morphologically left appendage is narrow and tubular, and has a narrow junction with the pulmonary venous component.

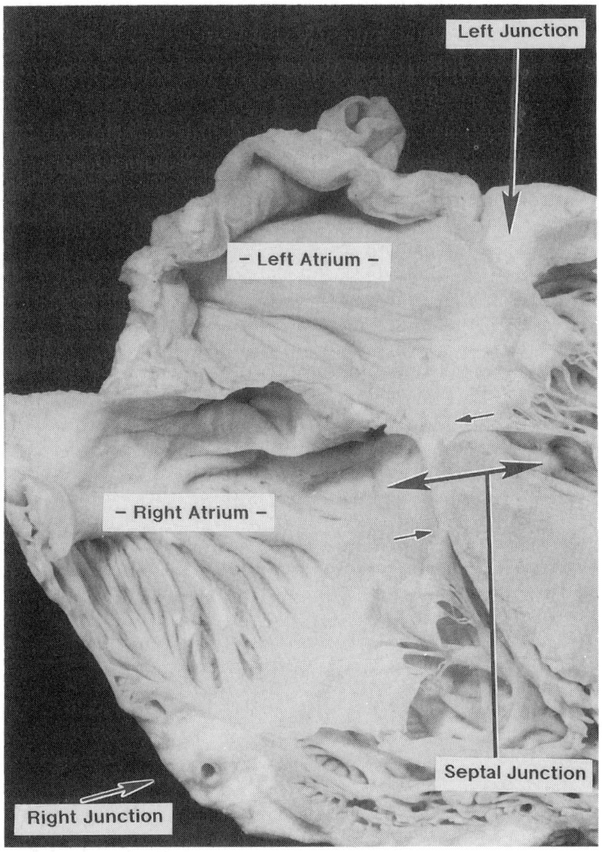

Fig. 13 This four-chamber dissection of the heart shows how the extent of the pectinate muscles relative to the atrioventricular vestibules is a distinguishing myocardial feature between the morphologically right and left appendages.

anomalous pulmonary venous connection in an otherwise normal heart, the left atrium is still readily recognizable even though the pulmonary veins drain to an extracardiac site (Fig. 8). Analysis in this fashion rules out also the vestibule as a defining criterion, since either the right (Fig. 9) or the left (Fig. 10) atrium can be recognized when its atrioventricular connection is lacking totally, as seen in the presence of the commonest variants of atrioventricular valvar atresia. The septal surface of the atriums might seem a better candidate, because it has characteristic features for its morphologically right and left sides. Indeed, this was the criterion chosen by Lev[1] to distinguish between the atriums, but the difference is of little value when the septum itself is absent. The atrial appendage also shows marked differences in its myocardial structure for the morphologically right (Fig. 11) and morphologically left (Fig. 12) chambers, and the appendage is absent only on exceedingly rare occasions. Furthermore, when it is the extent of the pectinate muscles within the appendage which is used as the defining criterion, the myocardial differences between the morphologically right and left appendages can always be recognized (Fig. 13), even when the atriums are most malformed as in visceral heterotaxy[10] (see also Chapter 3). Use of the morphologic method, therefore, dictates that it should be the myocardial structure of the appendage which is the ultimate arbiter in distinguishing morphologically rightness or leftness in the atrial segment of the heart.

As we have indicated, the general principle of the morphologic method can also be applied to components of the heart other than the atrial or ventricular chambers. Consider the nature of the atrioventricular valves. In the past, it has often proven difficult to define with precision the nature and location of commissures between their leaflets. This is why arguments still continue as to whether the mitral valve has two, four or more leaflets.[11–13] As we will see, the precise nature of the mitral valve, and the structure of its leaflets, will be crucial items when we come to discuss the morphology of atrioventricular septal defects (see Chapter 2). Those who have attempted to define commissures in the atrioventricular valves[14,15] have tended to do so on the basis of presence or absence of a so-called fan-shaped commissural cord supporting the space between putative leaflets. But similar fan-shaped cords, at least in the mitral valve, also support the spaces between the so-called scallops in the mural leaflet (compare Figs. 14 and 15). Defining the commissure in this fashion, on the basis of the morphology of its supporting cordal apparatus, unequivocally runs counter to the principle of the morphologic method. The structure of the supporting cord is just as variable as the structure it is supposed to define. It is much simpler, therefore, as well

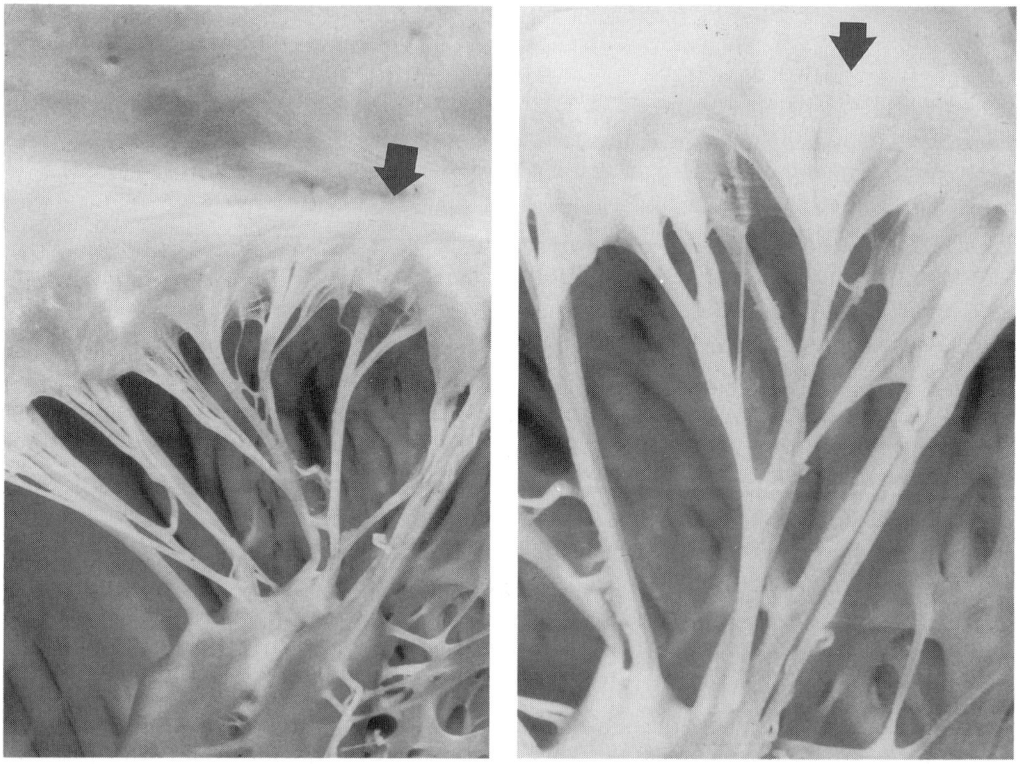

Figs. 14,15 These pictures show (14) a so-called commissural cord (arrow) of the mitral valve compared to the cord (arrow) which supports the division between adjacent scallops of the mural leaflet (15). It is difficult to distinguish between the two.

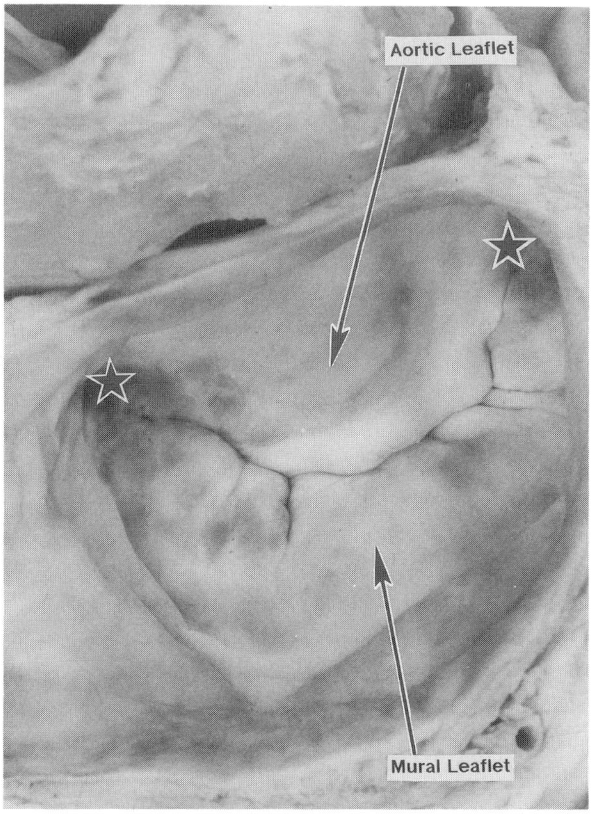

Fig. 16 The view of the mitral valve in closed position shows the solitary zone of apposition (between stars) which separates the two major components of the overall skirt of leaflet tissue.

as more logical, to determine directly the presence or absence of a commissure, since the commissure is no more than the end of the zone of apposition between the components of the overall skirt of valvar tissue. This is done most readily with the valve in its closed position (Fig. 16). The overall principle of the morphologic method, therefore, namely that of defining structures in their own right rather than on the basis of other variables, will be used throughout our analysis of the congenitally malformed hearts to be discussed in the subsequent chapters.

SEQUENTIAL SEGMENTAL ANALYSIS

Although it is now generally accepted that the segmental approach provides the best means of analyzing and describing the so-called complex congenital cardiac malformations, there are marked differences in the way that the system is now used.[16,17] The concept of analyzing the heart in terms of its atrial, ventricular, and arterial segments was introduced initially by Van Praagh and his colleagues,[3,18,19] with a comparable system being developed over the same period by de la Cruz and her associates.[20,21] Both these systems emphasized the importance of the topological arrangement, and the relationships, of the components within the separate segments of the heart. Much less emphasis was placed on the way in which the components of the adjacent segments were or were not joined together across the intervening junctions. Thus, when Van Praagh and his associates introduced the concept of concordance and discordance between adjacent segments, they judged the nature of these features according to the coincidence of segmental topologies rather than on the nature of the anatomic junctions between the chambers or arterial trunks within each segment. For example, using the definitions of Van Praagh as established at that time,[19] atrioventricular concordance was considered to be present whenever a heart possessed the usual atrial arrangement (so-called solitus) in association with a right-hand (d-) ventricular loop. Such concordance was defined irrespective of whether each atrium was connected to its own ventricle, or whether there was double inlet ventricle, or atrioventricular valvar atresia, or visceral heterotaxy. Similarly, within the segmental approach advocated by the Boston group,[19] concordance was also held to exist whenever the mirror-imaged atrial arrangement (so-called situs inversus) co-existed with a left-hand (l-) ventricular loop, again irrespective of whether each atrium was joined to its regular partner, or whether there was double inlet or some other abnormal pattern. Discordance was held to exist, again irrespective of the way the chambers were joined together, whenever solitus co-existed with l-ventricular loop, or mirror-imaged atriums were found along with d-loop ventricles.

Subsequent to this, the European school, of which we were a constituent part,[22,23] extended the segmental approach by promoting the view that the nature of the junctions between the adjacent segments was the most important aspect of sequential analysis. We sought to distinguish between the arrangements we interpreted as concordance and discordance, and those other arrangements of the junctions which were produced in the setting of isomeric atrial appendages, double inlet ventricle, or atrioventricular valvar atresia. Hence, the European school argued that concordance existed only when each of the two atriums was joined across the atrioventricular junction to its morphologically appropriate ventricle. Discordance was defined only when atriums were each joined to morphologically inappropriate ventricles. The other settings mentioned above were considered to represent different arrangements from concordance or disordance. This overall feature, namely the way in which the atrial cavities were joined, or not joined, to the ventricular cavities across the atrioventricular junctions, was described as the "type of connection", with the morphology of the valve or valves guarding the junctions being called the "mode of connection". At that time,[22] we were unable to appreciate why analysis in this fashion gave problems to Van Praagh and his colleagues.[24] We eventually became aware of the fact that the group from Boston were using concordance and discordance defined according to segmental harmony or disharmony, as outlined above. So as to clarify this situation, therefore, we tried to make it plain that our use of concordance and discordance qualified the pattern of the atrioventricular connections. This we did by no longer describing "atrioventricular concordance", or "discordance", in isolation. Instead, we subsequently used the terms "concordant atrioventricular connections" (Fig. 17), or "discordant atrioventricular connections" (Fig. 18) to describe the two junctional arrangements we sought to distinguish from ambiguous connections, double inlet ventricle, and absence of one or other atrioventricular connection. This change was meant to emphasize that our use of these terms describes the nature of the union of atrial and ventricular chambers across the atrioventricular junctions, rather than being concerned with the topologic arrangement of the segments themselves. This is not meant to belittle the importance of segmental topology, since the European school recognizes fully that analysis cannot properly be started without also determining the topological arrangement of the atriums and the ventricular mass. The major departure of the European approach,[23] from that of Van Praagh and his colleagues in Boston,[19,24] was simply to emphasize the nature of the "plumbing" between the atrial and ventricular chambers, and between the ventricles and the arterial trunks. It is this feature, the "plumbing", which determines primarily how the blood flows round the heart, although obviously patterns of flow are then modified by the prevailing haemodynamic circumstances.

The seemingly different definitions proposed by our colleagues and ourselves[23] as compared to those used by the Boston school[16,24] did, however,

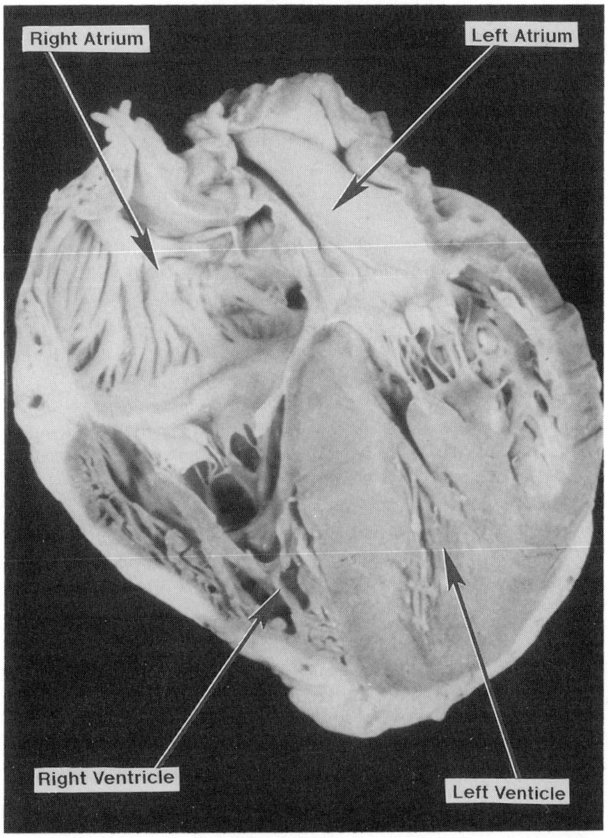

Fig. 17 This four-chamber section shows the normal paired junctions which exist between the atriums and the ventricles, producing concordant atrioventricular connections.

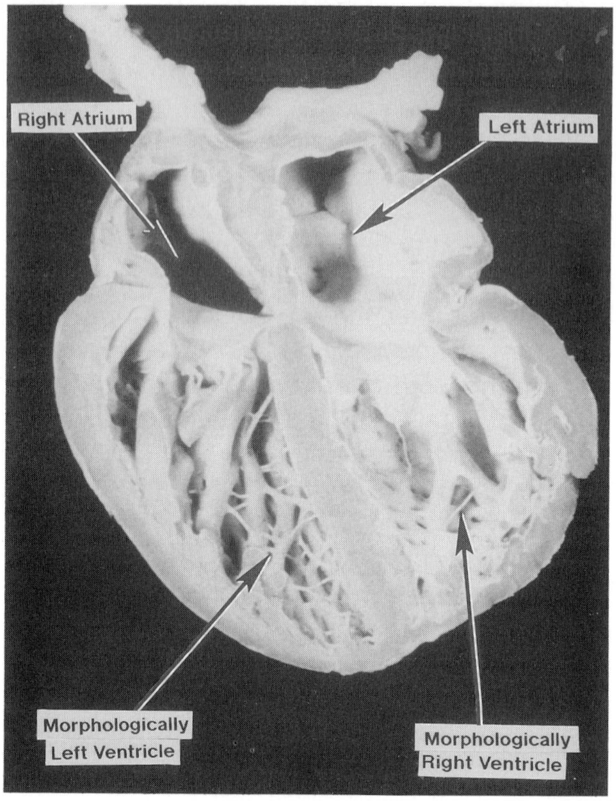

Fig. 18 In this heart, again revealed by a four-chamber section, the atriums are connected to morphologically inappropriate ventricles. The junctional arrangement is described as showing discordant atrioventricular connections, distinguishing it not only from the concordant arrangement (Fig. 17), but also from biventricular and ambiguous connections as seen when the atrial appendages are isomeric, and from the double inlet and absent connections which, collectively, produce univentricular atrioventricular connections (see Chapter 5).

give problems in the recognition of the feature we had chosen to describe as the "type of connection". In making their own revisions of the segmental approach, Van Praagh and his colleagues had first held that the concept proposed by the European school "attempts to finesse the situs of the ventricular part of the heart".[24] This argument, as we have explained, was incorrect since it was based on the presumption that, like the Boston school, the Europeans were defining concordance and discordance in terms of segmental harmonies. As we have emphasized, for the Europeans the "connections" specified the anatomic arrangement at the atrioventricular junctions. Subsequently, Van Praagh and his colleagues shifted ground still further, and argued that the basic atrial, ventricular and arterial segments were not connected together at all, but rather were separated from each other by the atrioventricular canal and the conuses, respectively. According to the arrangement of these intermediate components, the initial three segments were held to be aligned in different fashions.[25] This argument misses the point that, in terms of anatomic boundaries, the heart remains divisible into atrial, ventricular and arterial segments as defined initially by Van Praagh and de la Cruz with their respective co-workers.[18–22] For those who follow the principles established by the European school, the atrioventricular connections are real anatomic entities. It should be noted also that this introduction of the concept of "alignments" rather than "connections" breaks another rule favoured greatly by Van Praagh and his associates. This rule had been emphasized when criticizing the Europeans in stating[24] that "The wine of new understanding should be poured into the old bottles. The old bottles (terms) should not be smashed". Smashing the old bottles was precisely the step advocated by Van Praagh and his colleagues[25] when they suggested that the heart had five rather than three segments, and that "alignments" were necessary to describe the feature then recognized widely as "connections".

ONGOING CONTROVERSIES

Fundamental differences still exist, therefore, in the approach to the description of congenitally malformed hearts advocated by our colleagues and ourselves when compared to the principles currently recommended by Van Praagh and his associates. The differences will be addressed specifically in the chapters which will follow. As outlined above, our own system of sequential segmental analysis is now based firmly on the morphologic method established by Van Praagh *et al.*[2] It then emphasizes the structure of the connections between cardiac chambers and arterial trunks established by the existence of the anatomic junctions between these segments. This emphasis has been increased and refined over the years, and has now been made entirely logical by recognition of the importance of univentricular as opposed to biventricular atrioventricular connections.[7,8] This different approach to the cardiac segments is now, perhaps, the major difference between the Bostonian and European philosophies.[16,17] Of the other differences, suffice it to say that, although Van Praagh and his followers have now acknowledged the existence of different junctional arrangements,[26] these are described in terms of "alignments" rather than "connections". Equally importantly, they now define atriums on the basis of their vessel of entry,[27] clearly ignoring in this respect the logic and significance of their own morphologic method based primarily on myocardial characteristics.[28] This also applies when they disqualify chambers within the ventricular mass from ventricular status, again irrespective of their gross morphologic myocardial characteristics.[9] Finally, the Boston group and their followers continue to favour codification of diagnosis, arguing that symbolic representation is preferable to descriptions which may require many words to become unambiguous.[16] Our stance remains that, while brevity may be the soul of wit, clarity is the watchword when describing malformed hearts, no matter how many words are required to achieve the necessary precision.[17]

REFERENCES

1. Lev M. Pathologic diagnosis of positional variations in cardiac chambers in congenital heart disease. *Lab Invest* 1954;**3**:71–82.
2. Van Praagh R, David I, Wright GB, Van Praagh S. Large RV plus small LV is not single RV. *Circulation* 1980;**61**:1057–1058.
3. Van Praagh R, Ongley PA, Swan HJC. Anatomic types of single or common ventricle in man: morphologic and geometric aspects of sixty necropsied cases. *Am J Cardiol* 1964;**13**:367–386.
4. Goor DA, Lillehei CW. The anatomy of the heart. In: *Congenital Malformations of the Heart.* New York: Grune & Stratton. 1975: pp 1–37.
5. Anderson RH, Becker AE, Freedom RM, Quero-Jimenez M, Macartney FJ, Shinebourne EA, Wilkinson JL, Tynan MJ. Problems in the nomenclature of the univentricular heart. *Herz* 1979;**4**:97–106.
6. Keeton BR, Macartney FJ, Hunter S, Mortera C, Rees P, Shinebourne EA, Tynan M, Wilkinson JL, Anderson RH. Univentricular heart of right ventricular type with double or common inlet. *Circulation* 1979;**59**:403–411.
7. Anderson RH, Macartney FJ, Tynan M, Becker AE, Freedom RM, Godman MJ, Hunter S, Quero Jiménez M, Rigby ML, Shinebourne EA, Sutherland GR, Smallhorn JF, Soto B, Thiene G, Wilkinson JL, Wilcox BR, Zuberbuhler JR. Univentricular atrioventricular connection: the single ventricle trap unsprung. *Pediatr Cardiol* 1983;**4**:273–280.
8. Anderson RH, Becker AE, Tynan M, Macartney FJ, Rigby ML, Wilkinson JL. The univentricular atrioventricular connection: getting to the root of a thorny problem. *Am J Cardiol* 1984;**54**:822–828.
9. Bevilacqua M, Sanders SP, Van Praagh S, Colan SD, Parness I. Double-inlet single left ventricle: echocardiographic anatomy with emphasis on the morphology of the atrioventricular valves and ventricular septal defect. *J Am Coll Cardiol* 1991;**18**:559–568.
10. Uemura H, Ho SY, Devine WA, Kilpatrick LL, Anderson RH. Atrial appendages and venoatrial connections in hearts from patients with visceral heterotaxy. *Ann Thorac Surg* 1995;**0**:561–569.
11. Yacoub M. Anatomy of the mitral valve chordae and cusps. In: Kalmanson D (ed). *The Mitral Valve. A Pluridisciplinary Approach.* London: Edward Arnold. 1976: pp 15–20.
12. Victor S, Nayak VM. Definition and function of commissures, slits and scallops of the mitral valve: analysis in 100 hearts. *Asia Pacific J Thorac Cardiovasc Surg* 1994;**3**:10–16.
13. Kumar N, Kumar M, Duran CMG. A revised terminology for recording surgical findings of the mitral valve. *J Heart Valve Dis* 1995;**4**:70–76.
14. Lam JHC, Ranganathan N, Wigle ED, Silver MD. Morphology of the human mitral valve. I. Chordae Tendineae: A new classification. *Circulation* 1970;**41**:449–458.
15. Silver MD, Lam JHC, Ranganathan N, Wigle ED. Morphology of the human tricuspid valve. *Circulation* 1971;**43**:333–348.
16. Van Praagh R. Tetralogy of Fallot {S,D,I}: a recently discovered malformation and its surgical management. *Ann Thorac Surg* 1995;**60**:1163–1165.
17. Anderson RH. How should we optimally describe complex congenitally malformed hearts? *Ann Thorac Surg* 1996;**62**:710–716.
18. Van Praagh R, Van Praagh S, Vlad P, Keith JD. Anatomic types of congenital dextrocardia. Diagnostic and embryologic implications. *Am J Cardiol* 1964;**13**:510–531.
19. Van Praagh R. The segmental approach to diagnosis in congenital heart disease. In: Bergsma D (ed). *Birth Defects: Original Article Series,* Vol. VIII, No. 5. The

National Foundation — March of Dimes. Baltimore: Williams and Wilkins. 1972: pp 4–23.
20. de la Cruz MV, Anselmi G, Munos-Castellanos L, Nadal-Ginard B, Munoz-Armas S. Systematization and embryological and anatomical study of mirror image dextrocardias, dextroversions and laevoversions. *Br Heart J* 1971;**33**:841–853.
21. de la Cruz MV, Nadal-Ginard B. Rules for the diagnosis of visceral situs, truncoconal morphologies and ventricular inversions. *Am Heart J* 1972;**84**:19–32.
22. Tynan MJ, Becker AE, Macartney FJ, Quero-Jimenez M, Shinebourne EA, Anderson RH. Nomenclature and classification of congenital heart disease. *Br Heart J* 1979;**41**:544–553.
23. Anderson RH, Becker AE, Freedom RM, Macartney FJ, Quero-Jimenez M, Shinebourne EA, Wilkinson JL, Tynan MJ. Sequential segmental analysis of congenital heart disease. *Pediatr Cardiol* 1984;**5**:281–288.
24. Van Praagh R, David I, Gordon D, Wright GB, Van Praagh S. Ventricular diagnosis and designation. In: Godman MJ (ed). *Paediatric Cardiology* Vol. 4. Edinburgh: Churchill Livingstone. 1981: pp 153–168.
25. Van Praagh R, Weinberg PM, Smith SD, Foran RB, Van Praagh S. Malpositions of the heart. In: Adams FH, Emmanouilides GC, Riemenschneider TA (eds). *Moss' Heart Disease in Infants, Children, and Adolescents,* 4th ed. Baltimore: Williams & Wilkins. 1989: pp 530–580.
26. Geva T. Segmental approach to the diagnosis of congenital heart disease. In: Braunwald E (Series ed), Freedom RM (ed). *Atlas of Heart Diseases. Congenital Heart Disease,* Vol. XII. Philadelphia: Mosby (Current Medicine). 1997: pp 5.1–5.12.
27. Rubino M, Van Praagh S, Kadoba K, Pessetto R, Van Praagh R. Systemic and pulmonary venous connections in visceral heterotaxy with asplenia: diagnostic and surgical consideraitons based on seventy-two autopsied cases. *J Thorac Cardiovasc Surg* 1995;**110**:641–650.
28. Van Praagh R, Wise JRJr, Dahl BA, Van Praagh S. Single left ventricle with infundibular outlet chamber and tricuspid valve opening only into outlet chamber in 44-year-old man with thoracoabdominal ectopia cordis without diaphragmatic or pericardial defect: importance of myocardial morphologic method of chamber identification in congenital heart disease. In: Van Praagh R, Takao A (eds). *Etiology and Morphogenesis of Congenital Heart Disease.* Mount Kisco, New York: Futura Publishing Company. 1980: p 410.

Chapter 2

Atrioventricular Septal Defects

The group of congenitally malformed hearts to be described in this chapter has unmistakable morphology. It is characterized by deficient atrioventricular septation in the setting of a common atrioventricular junction. When the abnormal junctional morphology (Fig. 1) is contrasted with the normal (Fig. 2), the difference is striking. Why, then, does the lesion, in its various guises, continue to generate conflicts of opinion concerning the basic anatomy,[1,2] and why has there been such difficulty in reaching consensus on the most appropriate terms for description[2]?

The problems apparently still existing are the more difficult to understand when we examine previous accounts. We find that, as long ago as 1846, Thomas Bevill Peacock gave a description upon which it is difficult to improve today. Peacock[3] wrote "The interesting points in the case were, first, a deficiency of the base of the inter-auricular septum, with a perfect closure of

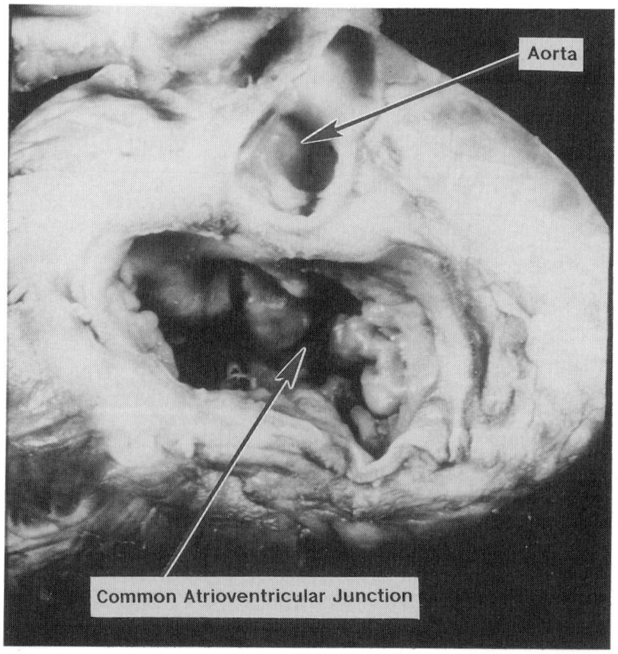

Fig. 1 The pathognomonic morphology of the lesion under discussion in this chapter is a common atrioventricular junction in the setting of deficient atrioventricular septation, seen here with a common atrioventricular valvar orifice. Note the unwedging of the aorta. The morphology has been revealed by removing the atrial musculature and the arterial trunks.

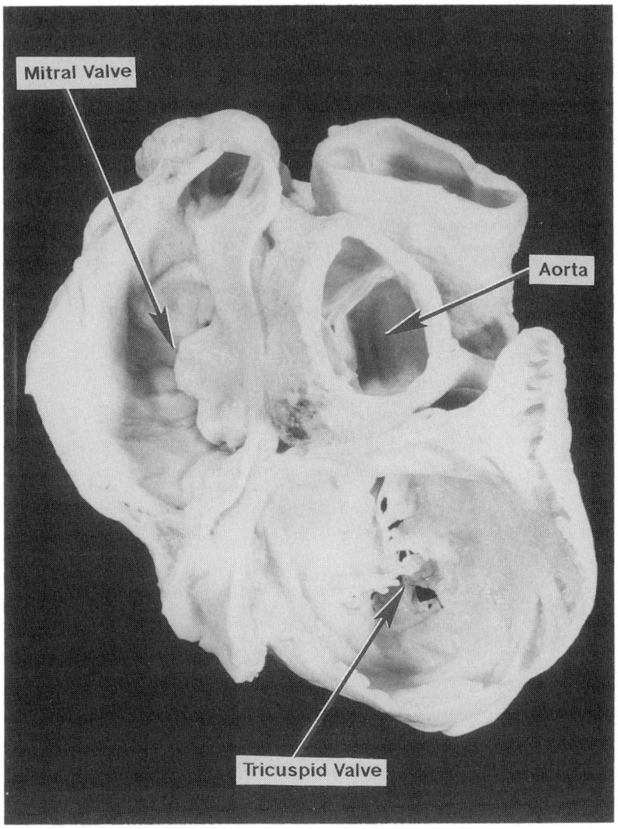

Fig. 2 A normal heart has been dissected in comparable fashion to the heart shown in Fig. 1. Note the separate atrioventricular junctions, and the location of the aorta between the tricuspid and mitral orifices.

the foramen ovale. The deficient space allowed of free communication between the two auricles, so that there could only be said to be one auriculo-ventricular aperture. Secondly, a distinctly tricuspid form of the left auriculo-ventricular valve; and thirdly, a deficiency at the base of the septum of the ventricles, nearly closed by an extension of the anterior fold of the left auriculo-ventricular valve." By 1875, the reason for the problems which still confront us today had become clear. Although making beautiful illustrations of the abnormal hearts (Figs. 3, 4), the Viennese pathologist Rokitansky, having illustrated the common atrioventricular junction emphasized by Peacock, described the left atrioventricular valve, which he labelled as bicuspid, as demonstrating a cleft in its aortic leaflet.[4] Since the so-called "cleft" points directly at the ventricular septum in both hearts illustrated, and has no relationship whatsoever with the aorta, it is difficult to appreciate why Rokitansky should have chosen to consider this leaflet as "aortic", the more so since he avoided the recurring pitfall which has coloured the subsequent literature, namely that of describing the cleft as existing in the anterior leaflet of the mitral valve.

Rokitansky, at the time of constructing his masterpiece,[4] was working in Vienna, so he presumably was well aware of the opinions of Joseph Hyrtl, the

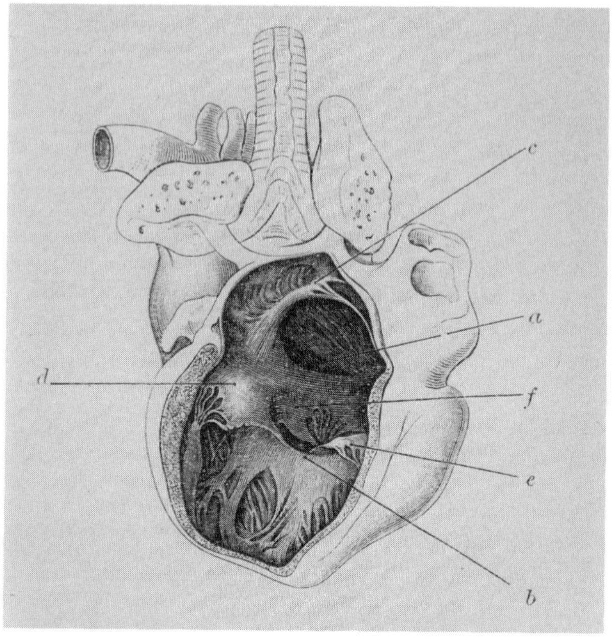

Fig. 3 This illustration from the atlas of Von Rokitansky[4] shows an atrioventricular septal defect with common valvar orifice.

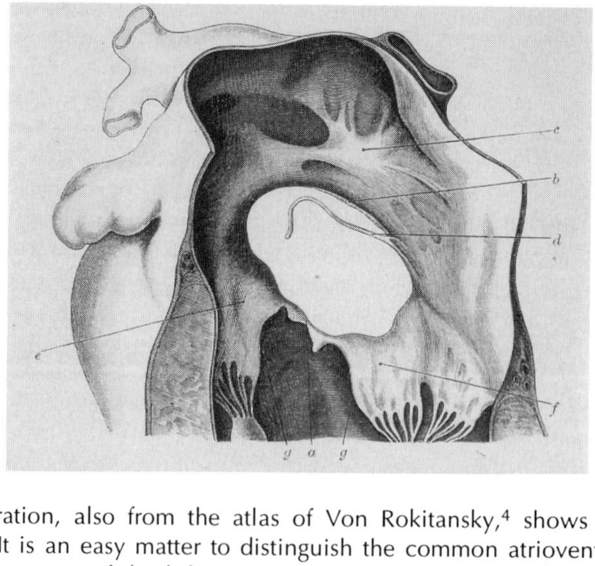

Fig. 4 This illustration, also from the atlas of Von Rokitansky,[4] shows a so-called "ostium primum" defect. It is an easy matter to distinguish the common atrioventricular junction and the trifoliate arrangement of the left atrioventricular valve. Note that two leaflets bridge the ventricular septum, and note also the comparable morphology with the heart having a common valvar orifice (Fig. 3).

foremost Viennese anatomist of the period. Ebels,[5] in his thesis concerned with surgical treatment of atrioventricular septal defect, emphasized how Hyrtl commented that the adjective "mitral", when used for description of the left atrioventricular valve, came into the heart like "the devil into the baptismal font". This is certainly no exaggeration. In our opinion, it is the description of clefts in this purported "mitral" valve which has hindered subsequent appreciation of the appropriate morphology, a morphology which is dominated by the presence of a common atrioventricular junction (Fig. 1). It is this fundamental difference, produced by the presence of common versus separate (Fig. 2) atrioventricular junctions, which we will stress throughout this chapter. So as to set the scene, we will recapitulate the morphology of the normal junctions, particularly the arrangement of the normal mitral valve.

STRUCTURE OF THE NORMAL ATRIOVENTRICULAR JUNCTIONS AND THE MITRAL VALVE

Throughout this chapter, we will emphasize the need to distinguish between the location of the atrioventricular junction and the attachment of the hingepoints of the leaflets of the atrioventricular valve. This distinction is of relatively little importance in the normal heart. This is because the two anatomic features more or less correspond (Fig. 5). Thus, around the greater

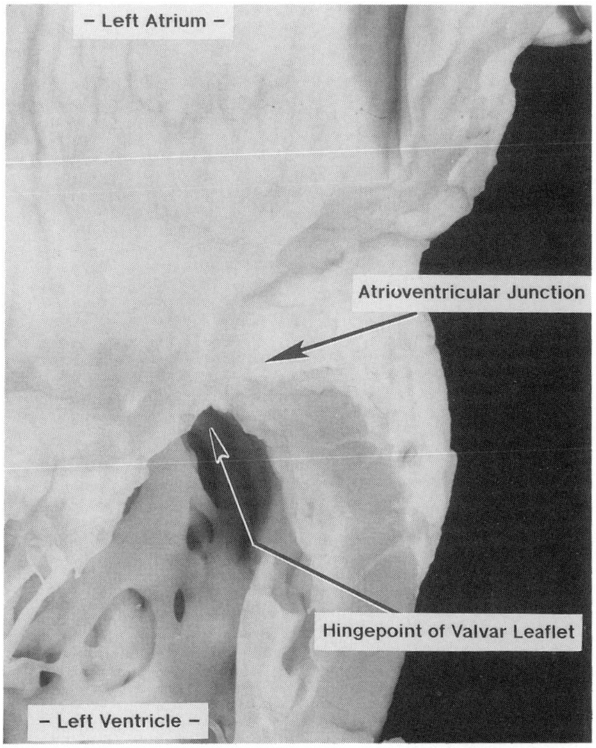

Fig. 5 In the normal left atrioventricular junction, the hingepoint of the leaflet of the mitral valve coincides with the point of insulation between the atrial and ventricular muscle masses.

part of the area in which the distal edge of the atrial musculature abuts against the proximal part of the ventricular muscle mass, the fibrofatty tissue plane which produces insulation between the two muscle masses also becomes continuous with, and supports, the hingepoints of the leaflets of the tricuspid and mitral valves. When the atrial myocardium is cut away, leaving only its most distal segment, and the non-coronary leaflet and sinus of the aortic root are similarly removed, it is possible to establish the precise junctional arrangement which constitutes normality (Fig. 6). It can then be seen that, in the normal heart, there are separate muscular junctions which surround the orifices of the mitral and tricuspid valves. The outlet component of the left ventricle, however, is positioned such that the two junctions are opposite each other over only a very short distance. Anterior to this area, which, by virtue of the off-setting of the hingepoints of the mitral and tricuspid valves produces a muscular atrioventricular septum (Fig. 7), the subaortic outflow tract excavates a deep diverticulum between the mitral valve and the septum. Forming the posterior and lateral wall of this diverticulum is the area of fibrous continuity between the leaflets of the mitral and aortic valves, with the two ends of this area being thickenend to form the right and left fibrous

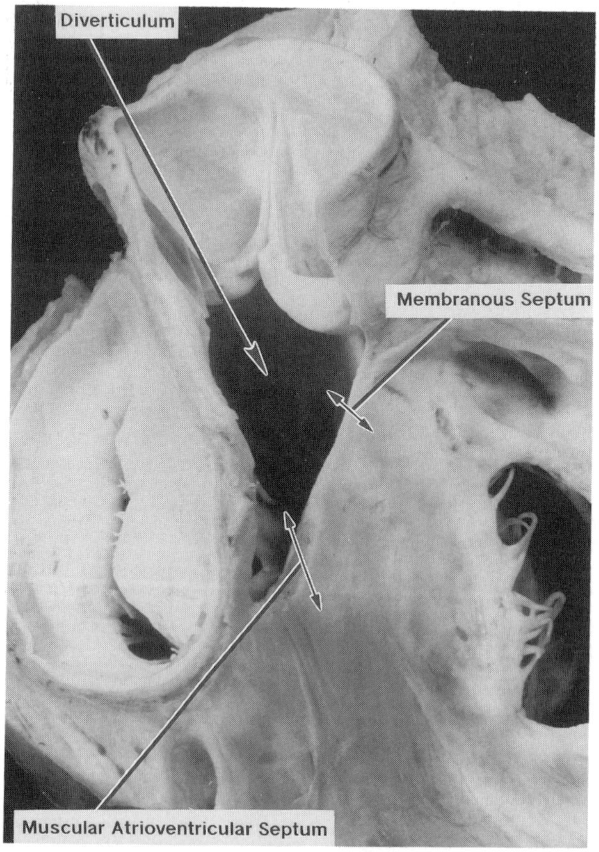

Fig. 6 These normal atrioventricular junctions are displayed by removing the non-coronary sinus and aortic valvar leaflet. Note the deep diverticulum between the mitral valvar orifice and the atrioventricular septal area.

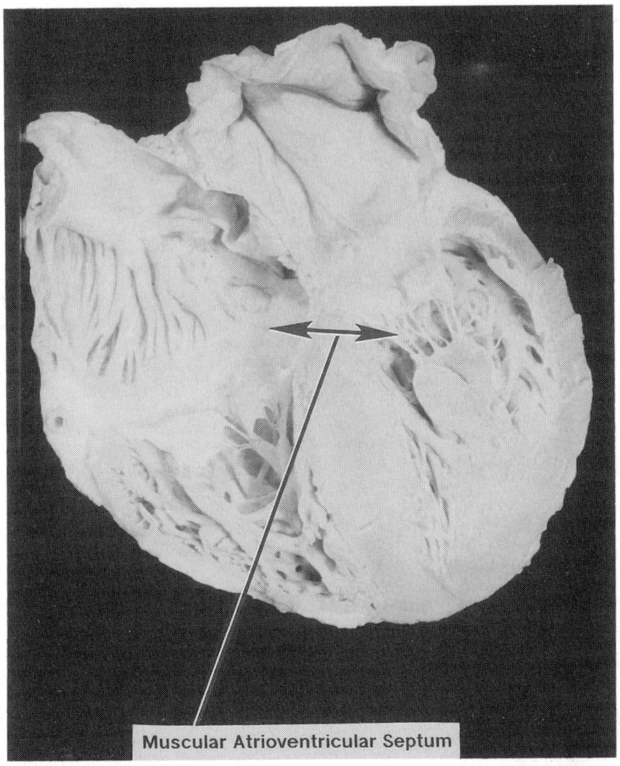

Fig. 7 The normal atrioventricular junctions revealed by a four-chamber section. Note the right, septal and left atrioventricular junctional areas, the muscular septum existing because of the off-setting of the hingepoints of the leaflets of the mitral and tricuspid valves.

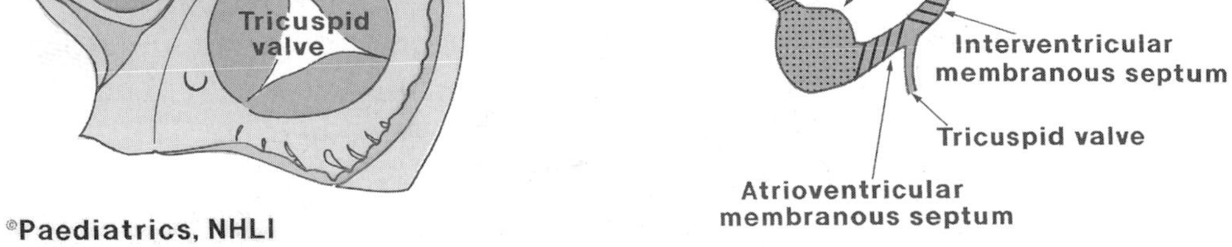

Fig. 8 The location of the area of fibrous continuity between the leaflets of the mitral and aortic valves in the normal heart is shown relative to the overall atrioventricular junctions (left hand diagram). The right hand panel shows the arrangement of the fibrous continuity relative to the membranous part of the septum.

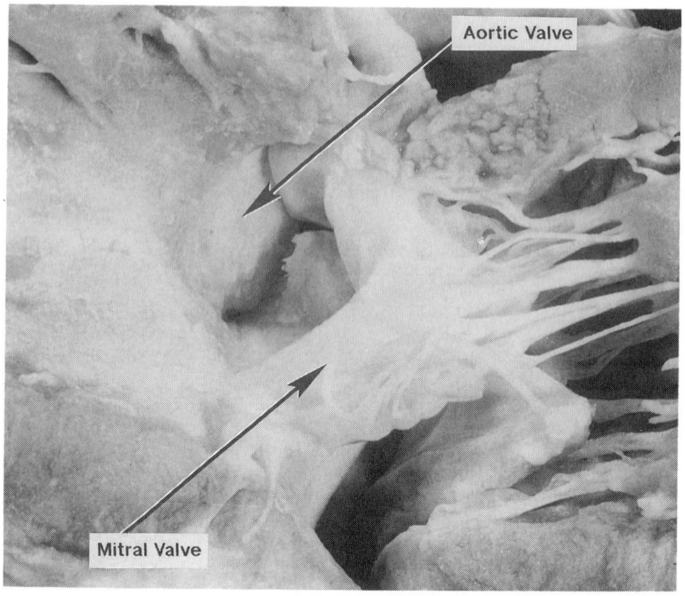

Fig. 9 The normal left ventricular outflow tract has been displayed from beneath, showing how the area of fibrous continuity between the leaflets of the aortic and mitral valves spans the roof of the left ventricle.

trigones, respectively (Fig. 8). The two trigones themselves anchor the area of valvar continuity to the upper edge of the mass of ventricular myocardium, effectively creating a bridge from which is suspended the aortic leaflet of the mitral valve to separate inlet and outlet components of the left ventricle (Fig. 9).

Throughout this area of valvar fibrous continuity, the atrial myocardium inserts into the aortic leaflet of the mitral valve, effectively marking its hingepoint. There is no ventricular myocardium beneath the leaflet at this position; however, the leaflet itself being suspended within the ventricular cavity as a curtain separating inlet and outlet (Fig. 10). Other than in this area of fibrous continuity, the hingepoint of the remainder of the leaflet tissue of the mitral valve is concordant with the area of junctional contiguity between the left atrial and left ventricular muscle masses (Fig. 5). A similar arrangement is then to be found throughout the greater part of the tricuspid valvar orifice (Fig. 11). The only area in which the valvar hingepoint does not correspond also with the line of separation between the right atrial and right ventricular muscle masses is in the region of the membranous septum (Fig. 12). In this area, the hingepoint of the septal leaflet of the tricuspid valve takes its origin from the right side of the fibrous septum, dividing it into atrioventricular and interventricular components (Fig. 13).

The location of the membranous septum itself is such that it also forms part of the wall between the right side of the heart and the subaortic outflow tract. We have already described how the right fibrous trigone, or the rightward end of the zone of aortic-mitral valvar continuity, is attached to the crest of the ventricular septum so as to form the roof and posterior margin of the subaortic outflow tract. It can readily be appreciated, therefore, that the

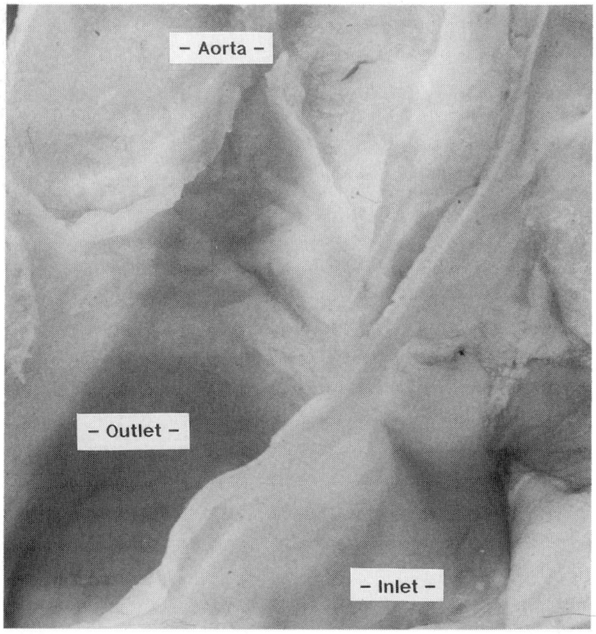

Fig. 10 This cross-section across the long axis of the left ventricle shows how the aortic leaflet of the mitral valve hangs down like a curtain between the ventricular inlet and outlet components.

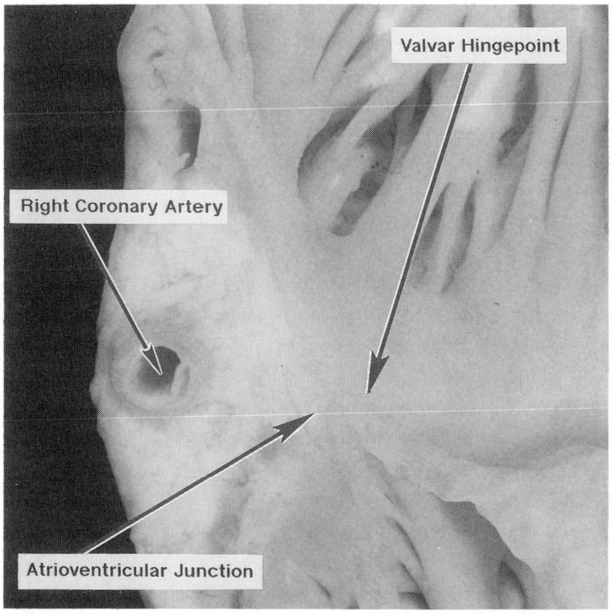

Fig. 11 The hingepoint of the leaflet of the tricuspid valve also corresponds with the anatomic atrioventricular junction at the parietal margin of the tricuspid valvar orifice (compare with Figs. 4 and 6).

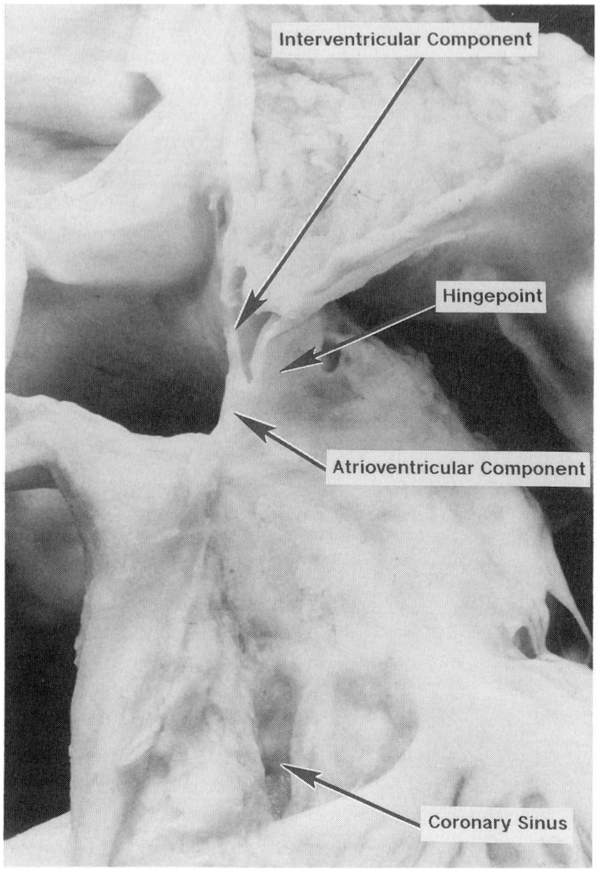

Fig. 12 In the normal heart, in the area of the membranous septum, revealed by removing the non-coronary aortic sinus and valvar leaflet, the hingepoint of the tricuspid valve is no longer coincident with the atrioventricular junction.

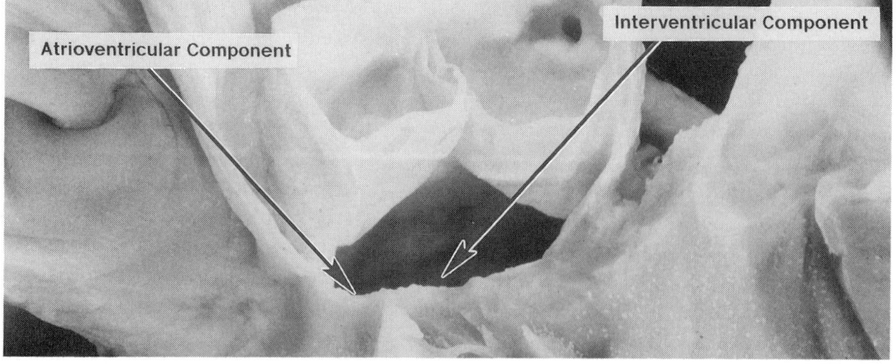

Fig. 13 This dissection of a normal heart is made by removing the right coronary aortic sinus and valvar leaflet (compare with Fig. 12). It shows how the hingepoint of the tricuspid valvar leaflets divides the membranous septum into atrioventricular and interventricular components.

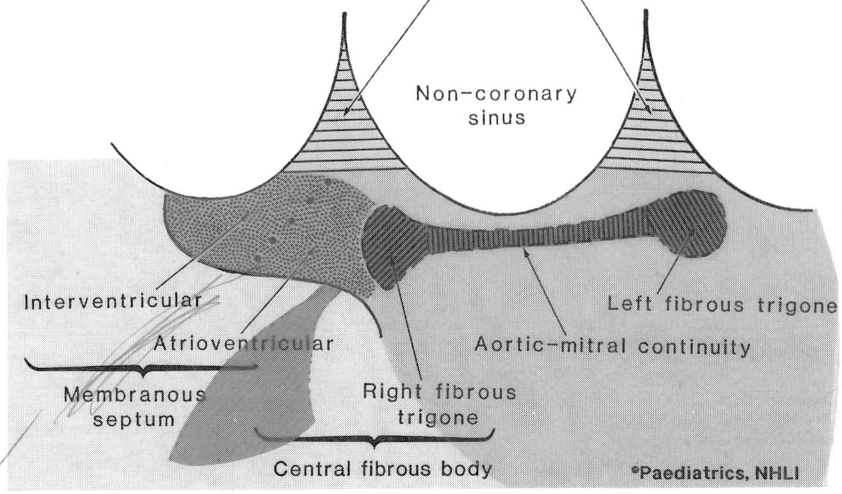

Fig. 14 This diagram shows how, in the normal heart, the central fibrous body is formed by union of the membranous septum with the right fibrous trigone (see also Fig. 9). The structures are shown as they would be seen from the left ventricular aspect.

right fibrous trigone is itself continuous in the normal heart with the membranous septum, the fusion of the two fibrous structures forming the so-called central fibrous body (Fig. 14).

The normal atrioventricular junction, therefore, is divided into discrete right and left components which surround the orifices of the tricuspid and mitral valves, respectively. The two junctions are themselves contiguous over a very short area, that of the muscular atrioventricular septum. Anterior and superior to this septal area, the deep and extensive subaortic outflow tract interposes between the mitral valve and the muscular ventricular septum, the superior and rightward wall of this diverticulum being formed by the fibrous membranous septum. It is through this septum that the atrioventricular bundle (of His) penetrates to produce electrical continuity between the atrial and ventricular muscle masses. At all other points around the atrioventricular junctions, the fibrofatty tissues of the atrioventricular grooves extend inward between the two musculatures and become continuous with the fibrous leaflets of the atrioventricular valves.

The arrangement of the right and left atrioventricular junctions conditions also the patterns of closure of the skirts of leaflet tissue which form the major functional components of the two atrioventricular valves. The orifice of the tricuspid valve is more or less circular, although the obvious acute margin of the ventricular mass confers a triangular configuration on the circle. This then dictates that the overall skirt of tricuspid leaflet tissue closes in trifoliate fashion (Fig. 15), with the three leaflets thus delineated occupying septal, antero-superior and inferior (or mural) positions relative to the atrioventricular junction. In the mitral valve, the situation is markedly different. The fact that the mitral valve itself, as well as the aortic orifice, are contained within the circular profile of the conical left ventricle means that the atrioventricular

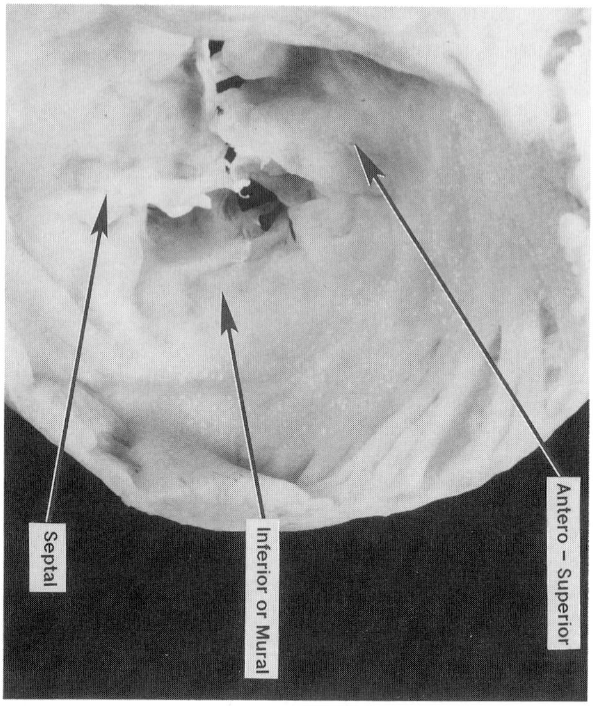

Fig. 15 The tricuspid valve in the normal heart, viewed here from above having removed the right atrial dome, closes in trifoliate fashion and guards the relatively circular right atrioventricular junction.

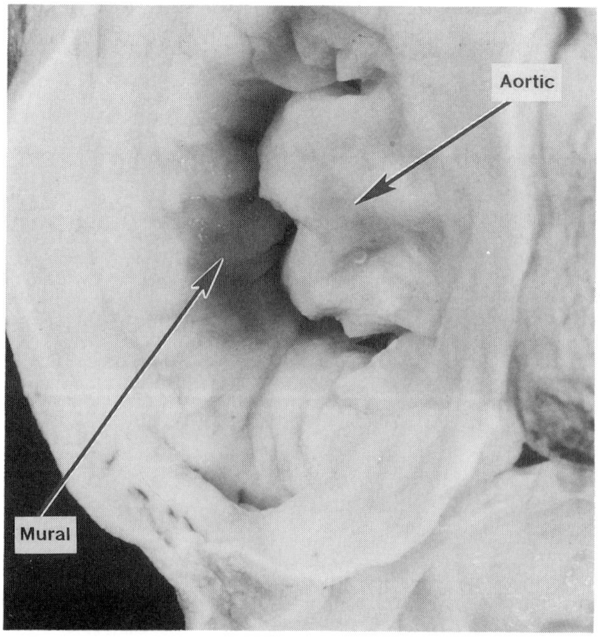

Fig. 16 The mitral valve in the normal heart, guards the kidney-shaped left atrioventricular junction. It has two leaflets guarding grossly unequal components of the junction, and closing together over a solitary zone of apposition. It is the two ends of this zone of apposition which, traditionally, are identified as the valvar commissures.

valvar orifice has a kidney-shaped configuration. Within this orifice, the overall skirt of leaflet tissue closes along a solitary zone of apposition, with the leaflets thus delineated guarding markedly dissimilar segments of the valvar circumference. One of the leaflets, best described as the aortic leaflet, although more frequently termed the anterior leaflet, guards one-third of this circumference. The other leaflet, obviously guarding two-thirds of the circumference, is hinged from the area of muscular contiguity between the left atrial myocardium and the ventricular musculature. It is usually called the posterior leaflet but, because of its oblique position within the body, it is best described as the mural leaflet. It has several slits along its length, most frequently two, which enable it to fit snugly against its aortic counterpart. The overall result is to produce a valve having two leaflets which meet over a solitary zone of apposition (Fig. 16). It is the ends of this zone of apposition which, typically, are said to represent the valvar "commissures". The term "commissure", however, produces problems, not only in description of the mitral valve, but even more so in the context of the lesion which is the subject of this chapter. For this reason, therefore, we prefer to describe zones of apposition of leaflets when seen in their closed position, and to avoid the use of the contentious term "commissure".

Before moving on to discuss the abnormal lesion, nonetheless, we will make one more observation which bears on controversies concerning "commissures". When an artificial cleft is made in the aortic leaflet of the normal mitral valve, the cut leads, as might be expected,[1] directly into the subaortic outflow tract (Fig. 17). The same situation is produced by a congenital cleft in an otherwise normally structured mitral valve. This naturally occurring division also "points" into the subaortic outflow tract or, when found in the setting of double outlet right ventricle, into the outlet component of the right ventricle (Fig. 18).

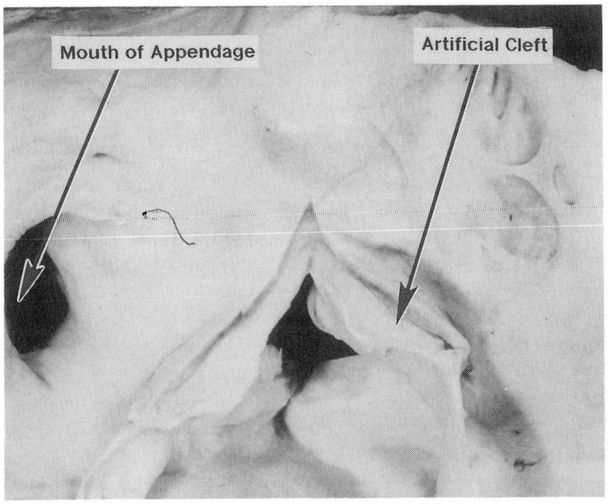

Fig. 17 This normal mitral valve has been opened by making a longitudinal cut in the aortic leaflet, replicating a so-called "cleft". Note that the division leads directly to the subaortic outflow tract.

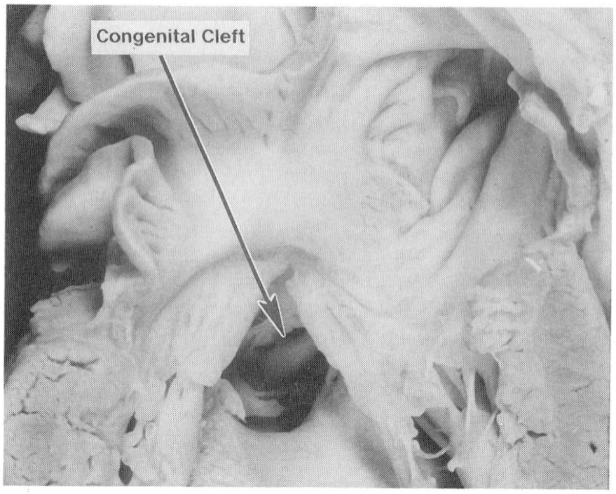

Fig. 18 This heart had double outlet from the right ventricle, with a ventricular septal defect in subpulmonary position. It is viewed from the left atrium, showing a congenital cleft in the anterior leaflet of the mitral valve. The cleft points towards the ventricular septal defect, and has no relationship to the atrial septum (compare with Fig. 4).

THE ESSENTIAL FEATURES OF ATRIOVENTRICULAR SEPTAL DEFECT WITH COMMON JUNCTION

As the name suggests, the cardinal anatomic feature of the abnormal hearts is a complete absence of the normal muscular and fibrous atrioventricular septal structures (Fig. 19). This deficiency in septation, however, does not simply produce a hole between the right side of the heart and the deep diverticulum produced by the subaortic outflow tract, as would be the case if the heart had retained its otherwise normal anatomic structure (Fig. 20). Instead, the septal deficiency exists in the setting of a heart which has grossly abnormal atrioventricular junctional morphology, and in which the subaortic outflow tract no longer interposes between the left and right sides of the junction (Fig. 21). In fact, there is a common atrioventricular junction (Fig. 1), with the septal deficiency effectively producing a midline space between the superior and inferior margins of the persisting septums (Fig. 22). When compared with the normal heart (Fig. 2), it is as if the overall junction has "sprung apart", trapping the subaortic outflow tract between the superior margin of the common junction and the superior wall of the left ventricle. As may be anticipated, this "springing apart" of the junction distorts markedly the fibrous skeleton. The area of fibrous continuity between the aortic and atrioventricular valves is at right angles to the ventricular septum in the abnormal hearts, and the anterosuperior right fibrous trigone is distant from the posteroinferior point of penetration of the atrioventricular conduction axis. The entire space of the septal deficiency, therefore, separates the two fibrous components which, in the normal heart, combine to form the central fibrous body (Fig. 23).

The skirt of valvar tissue which then guards the common junction is arranged with an oval hingepoint confluent with the junction. The

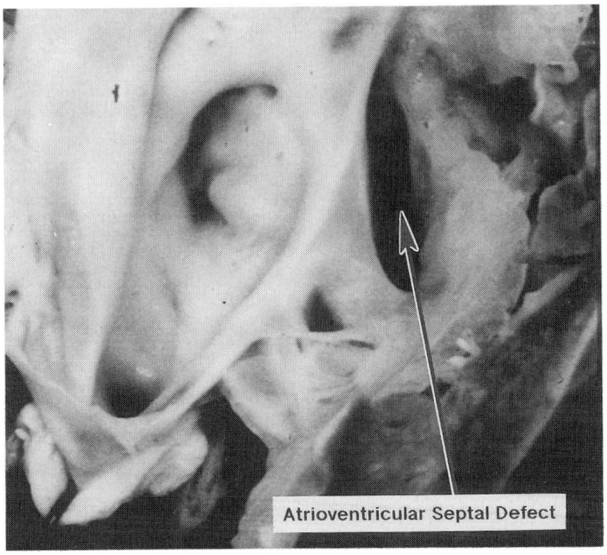

Fig. 19 This heart has a so-called "ostium primum atrial septal defect". Comparison with Fig. 6 shows that the septal deficiency is at the site of the normal atrioventricular septal structures. It can also be seen that the atrial septum itself in this heart is well-formed, and extends down to the level of the atrioventricular junction. In fact, the heart shows an atrioventricular septal defect in the setting of a common atrioventricular junction, but with separate valvar orifices for the right and left ventricles.

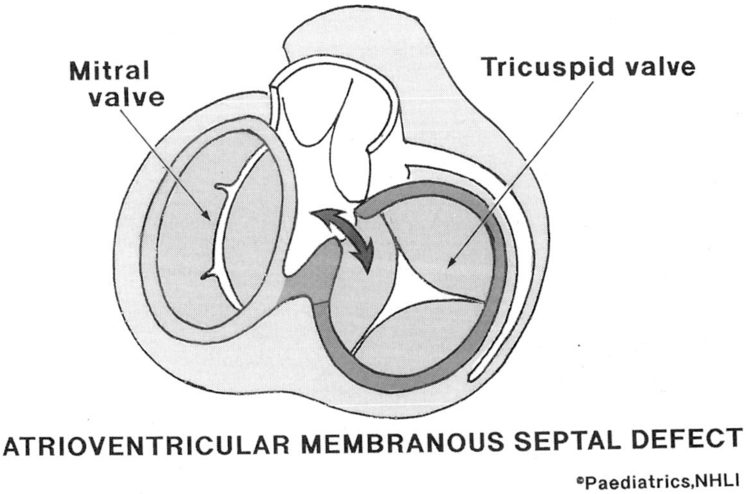

Fig. 20 This diagram, based on the junctional anatomy of the normal heart as revealed in Fig. 6, shows how a defect at the site of the normal atrioventricular membranous septum (purple arrow) would lead to the left ventricular outflow tract, but in the presence of separate right (green) and left (yellow) atrioventricular junctions. The muscular atrioventricular septum is intact, and is shown in orange.

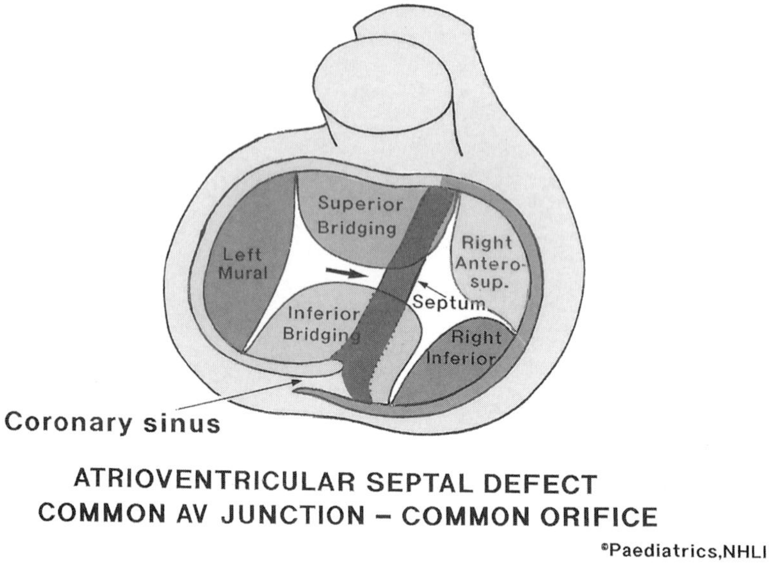

Fig. 21 This diagram, based on the dissection shown in Fig. 1, illustrates the junctional arrangement in hearts with deficient atrioventricular septation and a common atrioventricular junction guarded by a common valve. Note the five leaflets of the valve, and the direction of the zone of apposition between the two bridging leaflets (arrow).

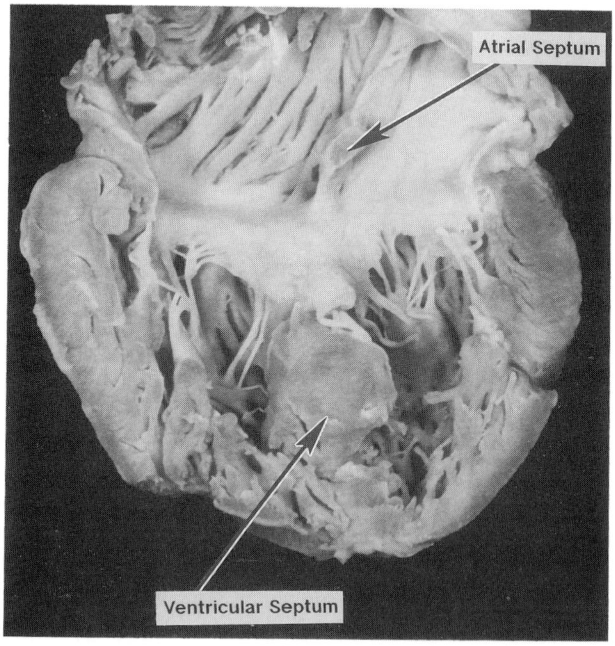

Fig. 22 The heart with deficient atrioventricular septation has been sectioned in four-chamber fashion, showing the pathognomonic common atrioventricular junction, guarded in this heart by a common valve.

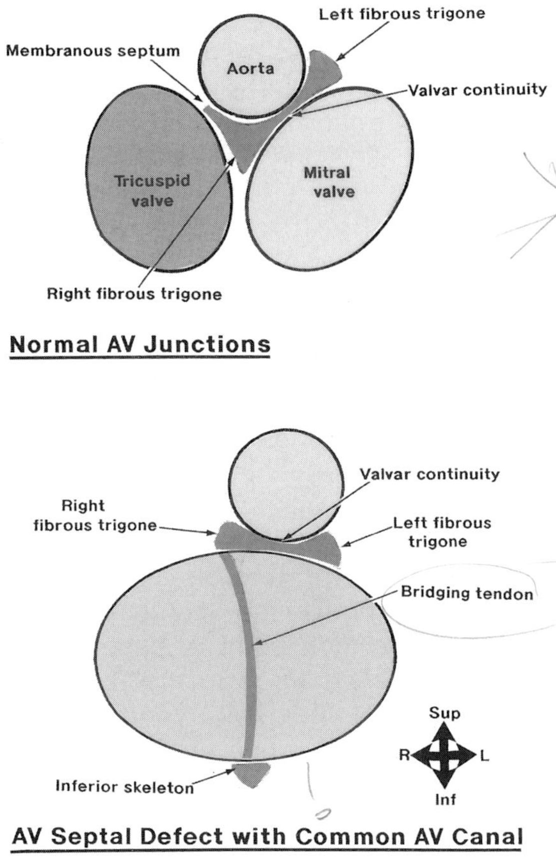

Fig. 23 In this diagram, which is orientated as if the ventricular mass is viewed from beneath (see orientation axis), the arrangement of the normal fibrous skeleton (upper) is compared with the grossly abnormal arrangement found in all hearts with deficient atrioventricular septation and a common atrioventricular junction (lower panel). AV – atrioventricular.

components of this effectively common valve, however, can be arranged so as to produce a common valvar orifice, or to produce two, or even more, valvar orifices within the common junction. This variability reflects the way in which the component parts of the skirt are, or are not, joined to each other.

In the most common pattern, the components are arranged so as to produce a common valvar orifice (Fig. 22). Within this pattern, the zones of apposition seen when the valve is closed delimit five discrete leaflets. One of these leaflets is confined to the left ventricle, where it occupies a mural location. Two of the leaflets are contained exclusively in the right ventricle, and occupy antero-superior and inferior positions. The other two leaflets, located superiorly and inferiorly within the common atrioventricular junction, have no counterpart in the normally structured heart. This is because they extend from right into left ventricle, and bridge the crest of the ventricular septum (Fig. 22). In the setting of common atrioventricular valvar orifice, these two bridging leaflets meet along a zone of apposition which is at right angles to the axis of the ventricular septum and, when closed, the zone of apposition also extends from right to left ventricle (Fig. 24). When examined in its closed position, it can be seen that the part of the valve which guards the left half of the common atrioventricular junction has three leaflets: the mural leaflet and the left ventricular components of the two bridging leaflets. There are, therefore, three zones of apposition to be seen in the closed valve: one each between the two bridging leaflets and the mural leaflet, and one between the bridging leaflets themselves (Fig. 25). The structure of this valve has no resemblance to the normally-structured mitral valve, and even less resemblance to the mitral valve with a congenital cleft in its aortic leaflet (Fig. 26). Analysis of the closed common valve then shows that its right component has four leaflets, with four zones of apposition between them (Fig. 22).

This basic arrangement of the valvar leaflets is to be seen in all hearts having atrioventricular septal defect in the setting of a common atrioventricular junction, but is subtly different in the variant of the malformation which seems to cause most confusion. This is the so-called "partial" variant, or the "ostium primum" defect. Confusion arises in the description of this anomaly because, most frequently, the leaflets of the effectively common atrioventricular valve which bridge the ventricular septum are additionally firmly fused to the septum at their point of bridging (Fig. 27). Furthermore, not only are the bridging leaflets fused to the ventricular septal crest, they are connected also to each other by a tongue of valvar leaflet tissue (Figs. 28, 29). The presence of this connecting tongue, and the fact that it, and the two bridging leaflets, are fused to the ventricular septum, means that the effectively common valve is partitioned into separate valvar orifices for the

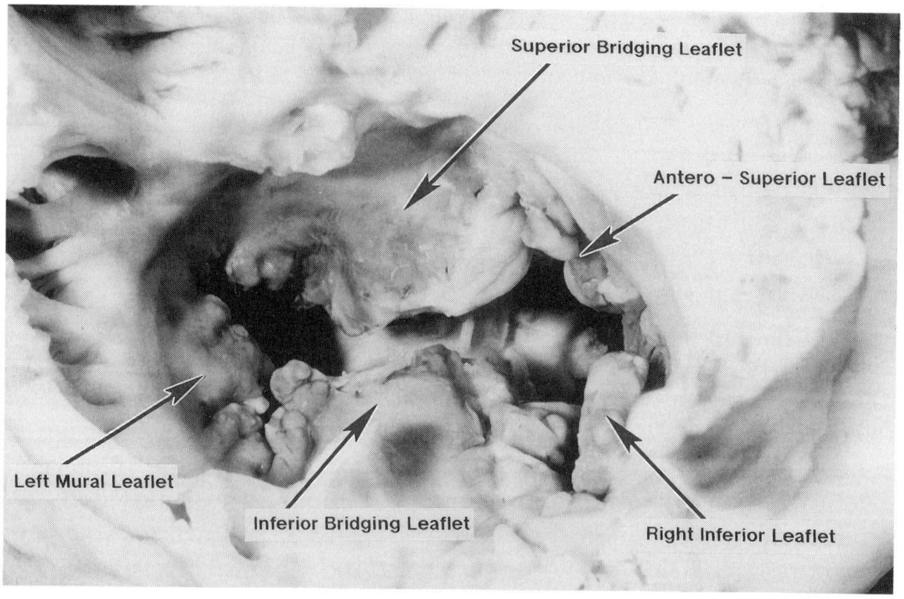

Fig. 24 This heart has isomerism of the right atrial appendages, deficient atrioventricular septation and a common atrioventricular junction guarded by a common valve. The dome of the effectively common atrium has been reflected to show the configuration of the common valve, which has five leaflets (compare with Fig. 21). Note the orientation of the zone of apposition between the bridging leaflets.

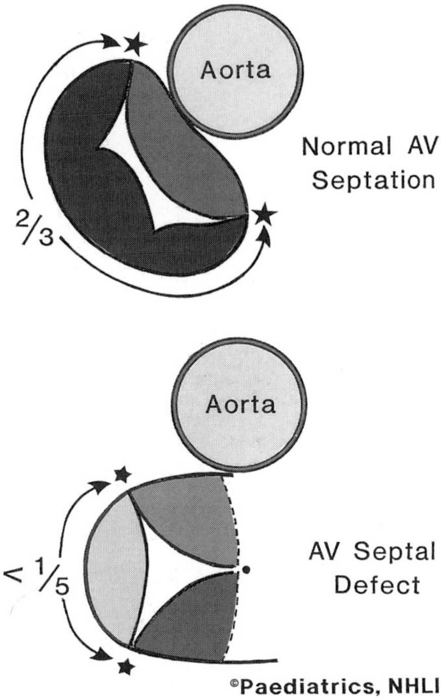

Fig. 25 This diagram compares the structure of the normal mitral valve (upper panel – compare with Fig. 16) and the left component of the common atrioventricular valve in hearts with deficient atrioventricular septation and common atrioventricular junction (lower panel – see Fig. 24). The valves are illustrated as if viewed from above. The fractions show the proportion of the left atrioventricular junction guarded by the mural leaflets.

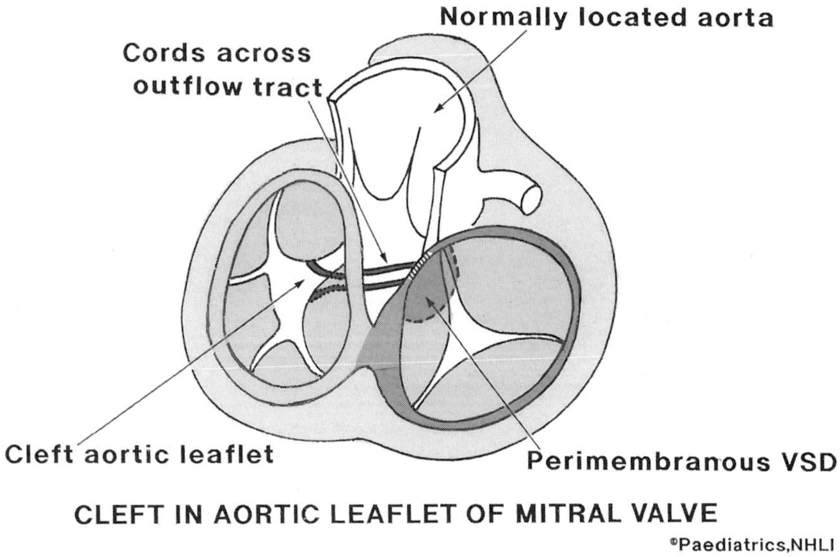

Fig. 26 The arrangement of the atrioventricular junctions as seen in hearts with an "isolated" cleft of the normal mitral valve or, as shown here, a cleft valve co-existing with a perimembranous ventricular septal defect. The morphology is dictated by the separate right and left atrioventricular junctions (compare with Figs. 20 and 21). Note also that the cleft points to the subaortic outflow tract (see Fig. 17).

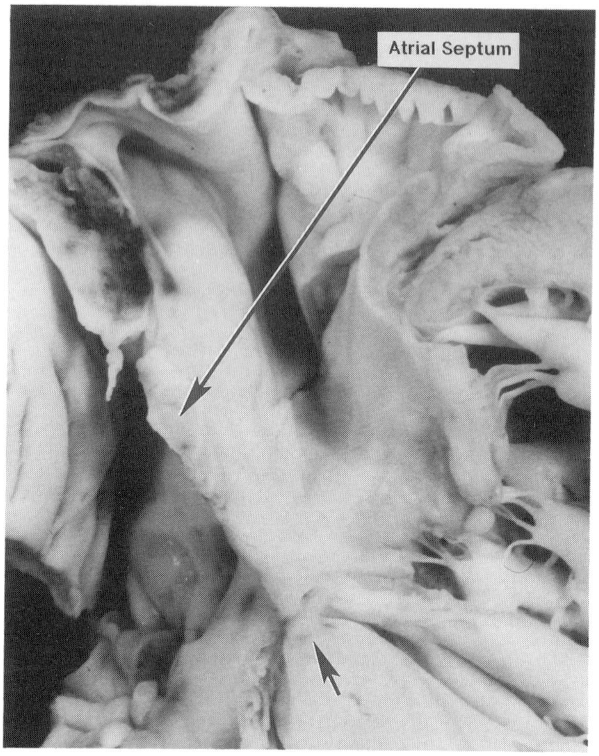

Fig. 27 This four-chamber section is from a heart with a so-called "ostium primum" defect. As can be seen, there is deficient atrioventricular septation with a common atrioventricular junction, but the bridging leaflets are firmly attached (arrow) to the crest of the ventricular septum (compare with Fig. 22).

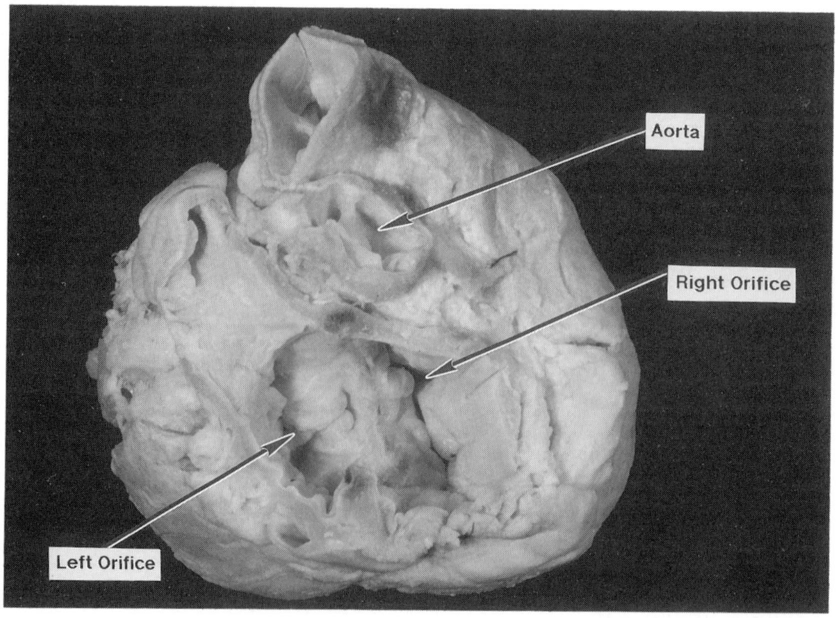

Fig. 28 This dissection, made in the same fashion as for the heart shown in Fig. 1, illustrates the atrioventricular junctional morphology of the so-called "ostium primum" defect. There is a common atrioventricular junction, and unwedging of the subaortic outlet.

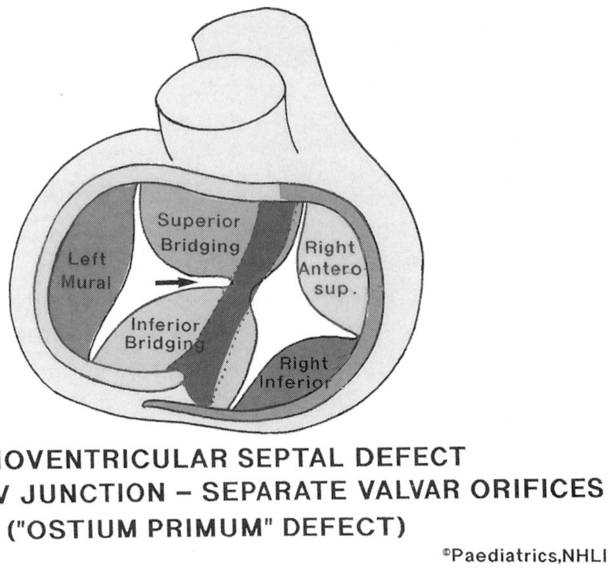

Fig. 29 The anatomy as seen in Fig. 28 is displayed diagrammatically (compare with Fig. 21). There is a common atrioventricular junction guarded by separate right and left atrioventricular valves. Note that the so-called cleft is the zone of apposition between the two leaflets which bridge the ventricular septum (compare with Fig. 4).

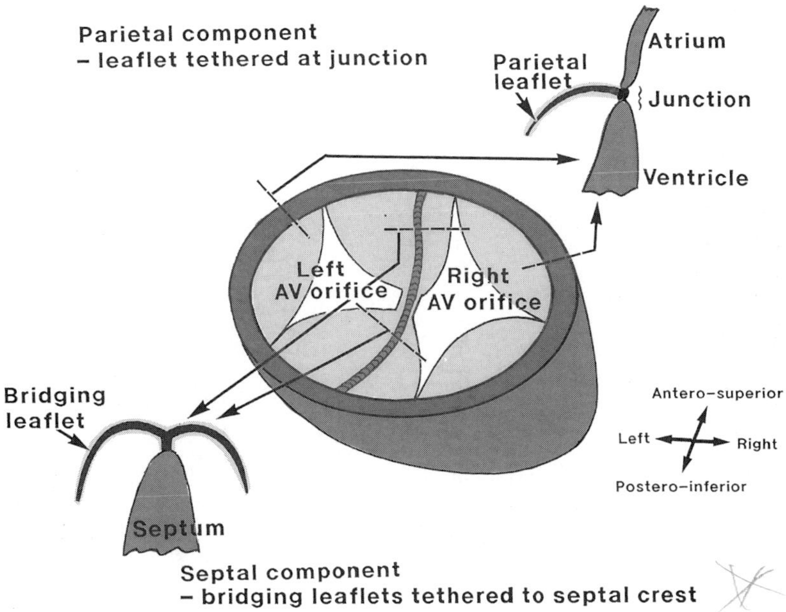

Fig. 30 This diagram, also based on the dissection of the heart as seen in Fig. 28, shows the arrangement of the valvar leaflets in the so-called "ostium primum" defect. The attachment of the bridging leaflets to the ventricular septal crest, and also to each other, produces separate valvar orifices for the right and left ventricles. Note, however, that the so-called "annulus" along the crest of the ventricular septum does not coincide with the atrioventricular junction, as it does round the parietal ventricular walls (see also Fig. 27).

right and left ventricles (Figs. 28, 29). The presence of these two orifices, nonetheless, does not alter the basic atrioventricular junctional arrangement, which is still common to all four cardiac chambers (Fig. 27). When analyzing this anatomy, it can be seen that the hingepoints of the valvar leaflets which are coincident with the muscular atrioventricular junction continue to have a common morphology. The points along which the leaflets, and the connecting tongue, are fused to the ventricular septum also produce hingepoints for both the right and left atrioventricular valves. These hinges, in contrast, are related to the ventricular margin of the atrioventricular septal defect rather than to the atrioventricular junctions, since they have no relationship with the junction (Fig. 30). It is incorrect, therefore, to suggest that the arrangement in the "ostium primum" defect is not "in common".[2] The overall atrioventricular junctional arrangement in the "ostium primum" variant is just as common as in those with common valvar orifice. The identical junctional morphology gives no justification for labelling the two types as being "partial" as opposed to "complete" (compare Figs. 1, 28).

The arrangements in which its common orifice is compartmented by the joining together of adjacent leaflets is seen in situations other than the "ostium primum" variant. Thus, the well-recognized associated anomaly of the valves themselves, known as "dual orifice", is also the consequence of joining together of those valvar leaflets which, in normal circumstances, are discrete structures. Seen most frequently in the left atrioventricular valve (Fig. 31), the anomalous pattern can also be seen in the right valve. It would be possible, theoretically, for a common valve to exist with seven orifices, were all the leaflets joined together by accessory tongues.

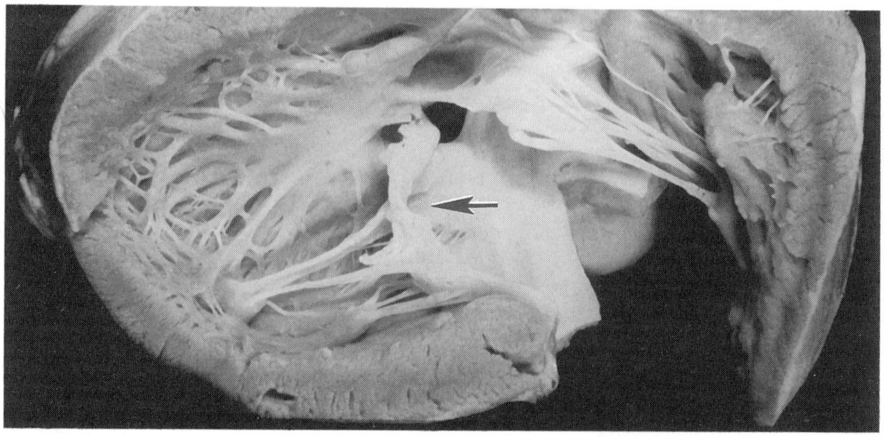

Fig. 31 There is a dual orifice in this left atrioventricular valve from a heart with deficient atrioventricular septation and a common atrioventricular junction because a tongue of leaflet tissue (arrowed) joins together the mural and inferior bridging leaflets within the left ventricle.

Thus far, we have concentrated only upon the common atrioventricular valve and junction in emphasizing the anatomic hallmarks of the hearts with deficient atrioventricular septation. Of the features discussed, the trifoliate arrangement of the left atrioventricular valve is the most distinctive, and is matched by an equally distinctive arrangement of the left ventricular papillary muscles. The pattern of closure of the valve is not oblique, as in the normal mitral valve, nor are the papillary muscles disposed in an oblique fashion. Instead, the paired muscles are deviated laterally within the left ventricle so that they are positioned beneath the zones of apposition between the mural leaflet and the left ventricular components of the two bridging leaflets (Fig. 32).

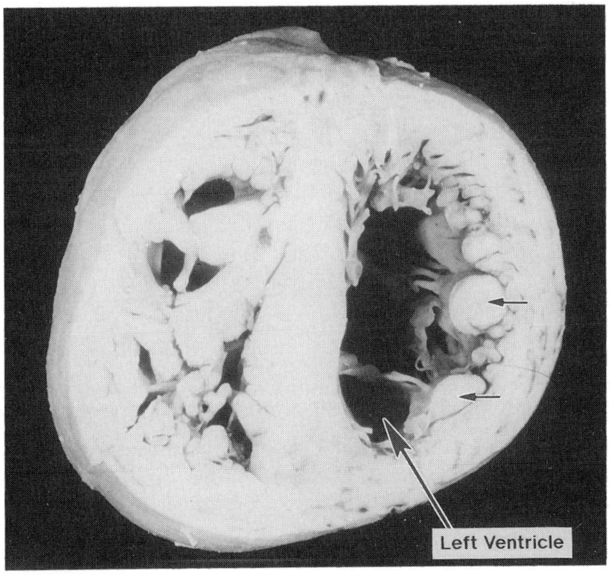

Fig. 32 The left ventricle of a heart with deficient atrioventricular septation and common atrioventricular junction has been sectioned in short axis and is viewed from beneath. Note how the papillary muscles (arrowed) are positioned laterally within the ventricle, lying beneath the end of the zones of apposition between the two bridging leaflets and the mural leaflet.

Further characteristic features are then found in the dimensions of the left ventricle, and in the location of its outflow tract. In the normal heart, the inlet and outlet dimensions of the left ventricle are comparable (Fig. 33 upper). In hearts with atrioventricular septal defect and common atrioventricular junction, the outlet dimension is significantly longer than the inlet (Fig. 33 lower). This difference is comparable be there an ostium primum defect or a common atrioventricular valvar orifice (Fig. 34). This is another reason why the "ostium primum" defect is no more "partial" than is the variant with common orifice. There is, however, a difference found in the group of defects with separate right and left atrioventricular valvar orifices within the common junction. The degree of "scooping" of the ventricular septum is significantly deeper in the presence of a common valvar orifice,[7] although it is not possible to predict in any individual heart, once the valvar leaflets have been removed, whether there had initially been separate valvar orifices or a common orifice guarding the common junction (Fig. 35).

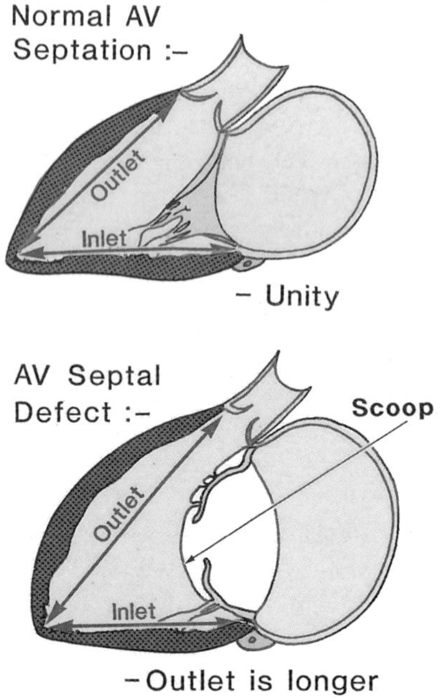

Fig. 33 The inlet and outlet dimensions of the left ventricular septal surface are equal in hearts with normal atrioventricular (AV) septation (upper panel), whereas the outlet dimension is significantly longer in all hearts with deficient atrioventricular septation and a common atrioventricular junction (see Fig. 34). The depth of the scoop is greater in hearts with a common atrioventricular valve as opposed to those with separate valves for the right and left ventricles.

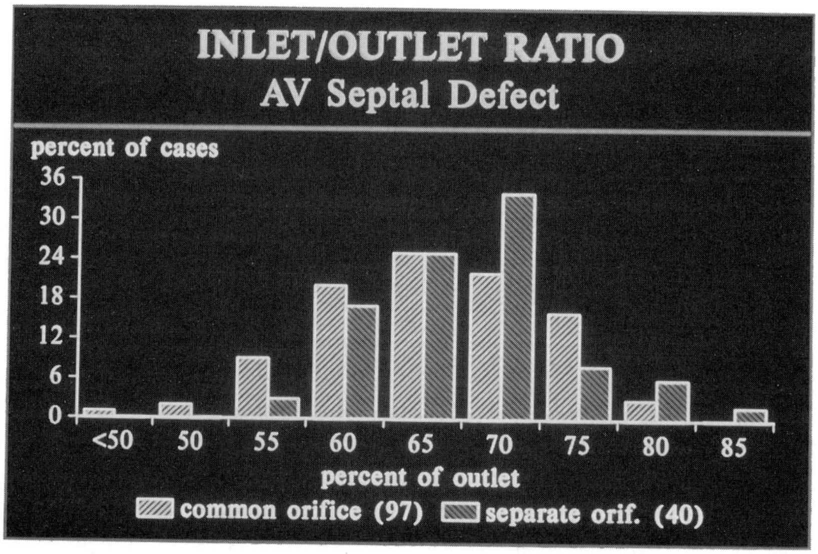

Fig. 34 These measurements, from the study of Penkoske and colleagues,[6] show how the inlet/outlet disproportion is comparable for all hearts with deficient atrioventricular septation and common atrioventricular junction.

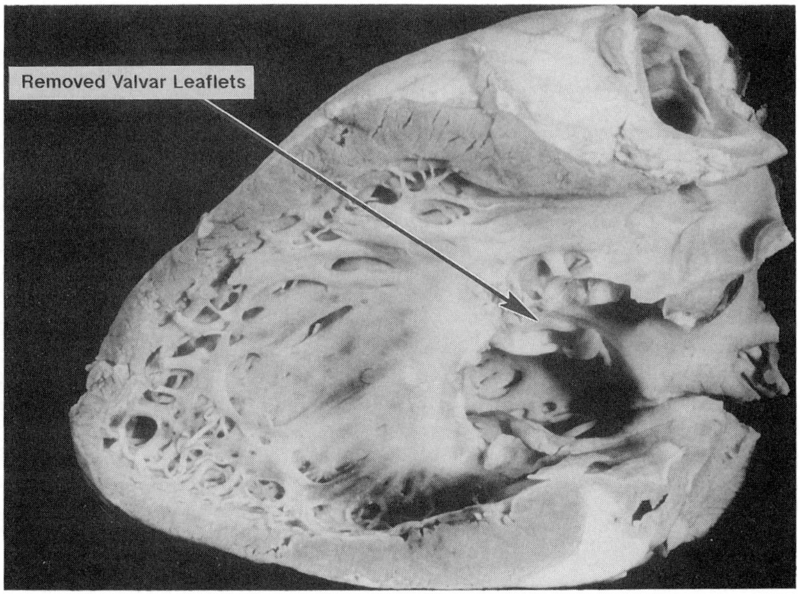

Fig. 35 Once the bridging leaflets are removed from the ventricular mass, it is not possible in any individual heart to know whether, initially, there had been a common atrioventricular valve or separate valvar orifices within the right and left ventricles.

The location of the subaortic outflow tract, as already discussed, is another distinguishing feature of hearts with deficient atrioventricular septation and common atrioventricular junction. Because of the common junction, the outflow tract, of necessity, is wedged between the superior bridging leaflet and the anterosuperior wall of the left ventricle. The capacity of the outflow tract thus formed itself varies according to the extent to which the superior leaflet is bound down to the septal crest. This feature is important with regard to the potential for subaortic obstruction. In the hearts with common valvar orifice, the superior bridging leaflet is hinged only from the anterosuperior margin of the common atrioventricular junction. Although the leaflet is often tethered to the right ventricular aspect of the septum by tendinous cords, a space exists between the septal crest and the undersurface of the bridging leaflet (Fig. 36). The space is greater when the leaflet is free-floating than when it is tethered. In the hearts with separate right and left atrioventricular valvar orifices, in contrast, the superior bridging leaflet is additionally hinged from the crest of the ventricular septum. This not only removes the space seen in the hearts with common valvar orifice, but additionally lengthens the dimensions of the subaortic outlet (Fig. 37). Clinical experience shows that the elongated outflow tract is not intrinsically stenotic. Any additional lesion, however, be it naturally occurring or iatrogenic, rapidly produces stenosis.[8,9] One option for surgical relief is to detach the superior leaflet from the septum and insert an enlarging patch.[10]

Almost all hearts having deficient atrioventricular septation and common atrioventricular junction also have a hole at the anticipated site of the septal deficiency. It is possible, nonetheless, to encounter hearts in which the

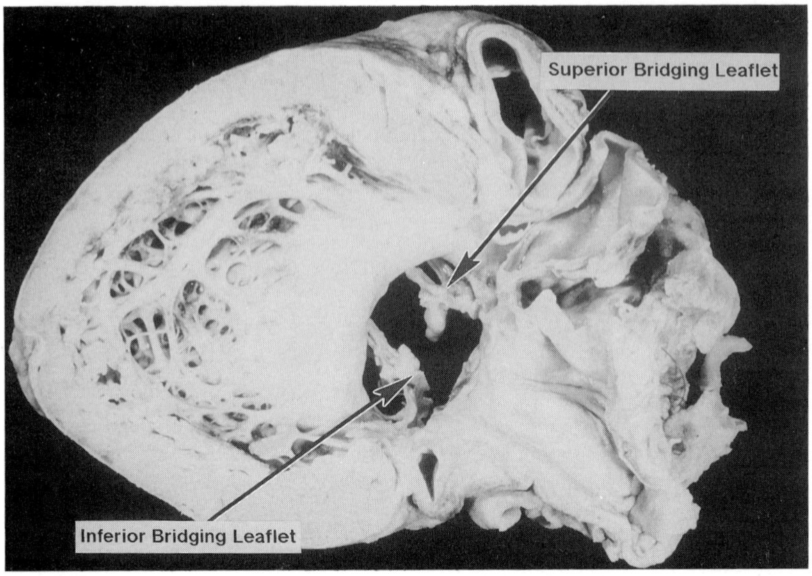

Fig. 36 This heart with a common atrioventricular orifice has been dissected to show the left ventricular aspect of the septum. Note that the two leaflets which bridge the septum float freely within the atrioventricular septal defect. The subaortic outlet is relatively short.

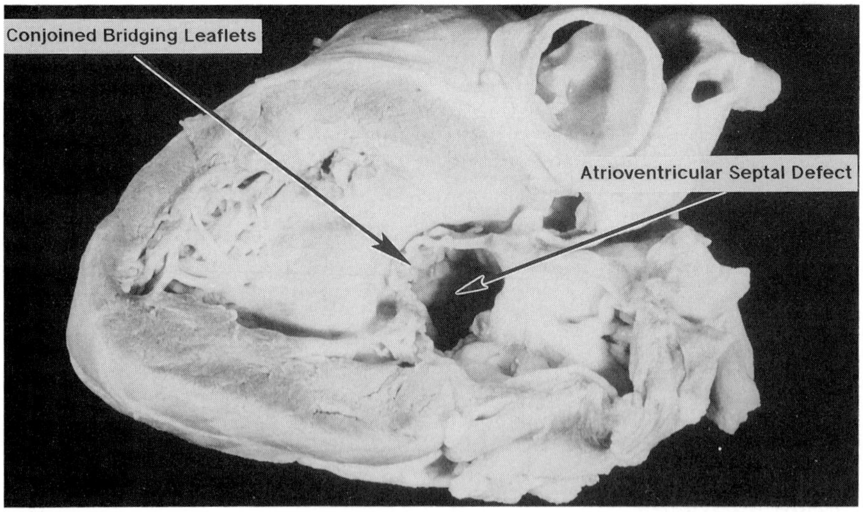

Fig. 37 In this heart, there are separate atrioventricular valvar orifices for the right and left ventricles. The fusion of the superior leaflet to the ventricular septal crest elongates markedly the subaortic outlet (compare with Fig. 36).

initially deficient septal structures have closed together, thus obliterating the communication between the right and left sides of the heart. These hearts have all the anticipated features of deficient atrioventricular septation with a common junction, namely a trifoliate left atrioventricular valve, inlet/outlet septal disproportion, and a narrowed, anterosuperiorly located, and unwedged subaortic outflow tract. The atrioventricular junctions, therefore, still form two parts of an effectively common structure, albeit divided in these cases by the fused septal components. The finding of such hearts with intact septal structures emphasizes once more that the true anatomical hallmark of the group of malformations is the common atrioventricular junction.

ANATOMIC VARIANTS

We have already discussed the most significant variants within the group of hearts unified by the presence of an atrioventricular septal defect in the setting of a common atrioventricular junction. These are the subsets of hearts with common atrioventricular valvar orifice as opposed to the set with separate right and left atrioventricular valvar orifices within the common atrioventricular junction (Fig. 38). We have also discussed the lack of any evidence to support the notion that the two variants can be considered "partial" as opposed to "complete" forms of the anomaly. The difference between the two forms is no more than the presence or absence of a tongue of valvar leaflet tissue joining together the two leaflets of the common

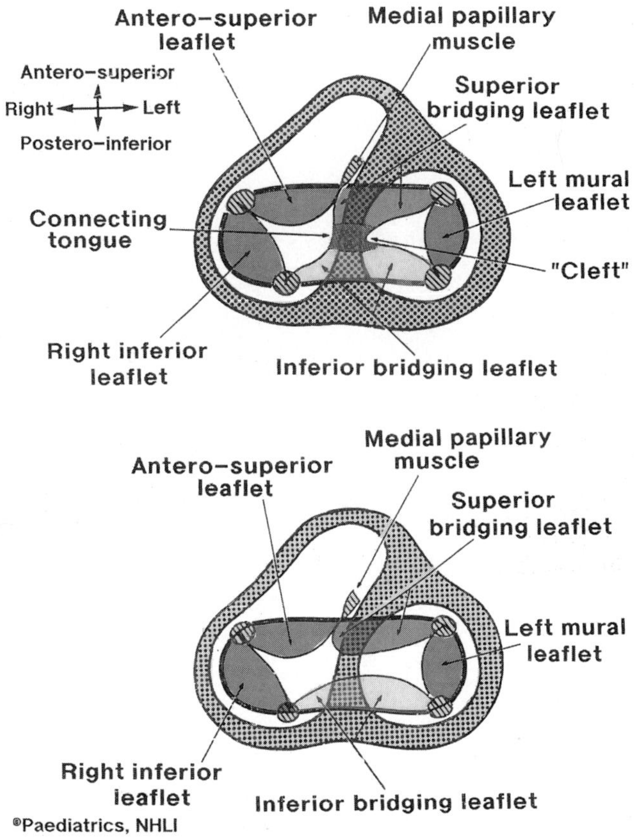

Fig. 38 These diagrams illustrate the valvar structure as seen from beneath in hearts with deficient atrioventricular septation and common atrioventricular junction. The major variation is produced by fusion (upper panel – tongue shown in red) versus non-fusion (lower panel) of the leaflets which bridge the ventricular septum.

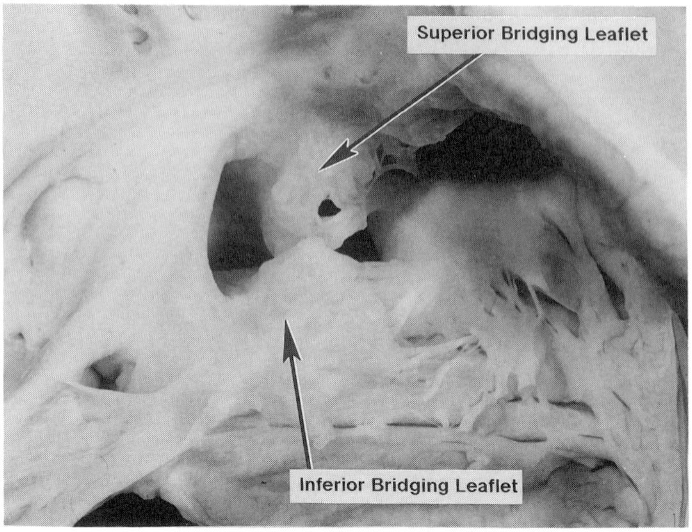

Fig. 39 This heart with deficient atrioventricular septation and a common atrioventricular junction guarded by a common valve is viewed from the right side, and shows the separate nature of the bridging leaflets.

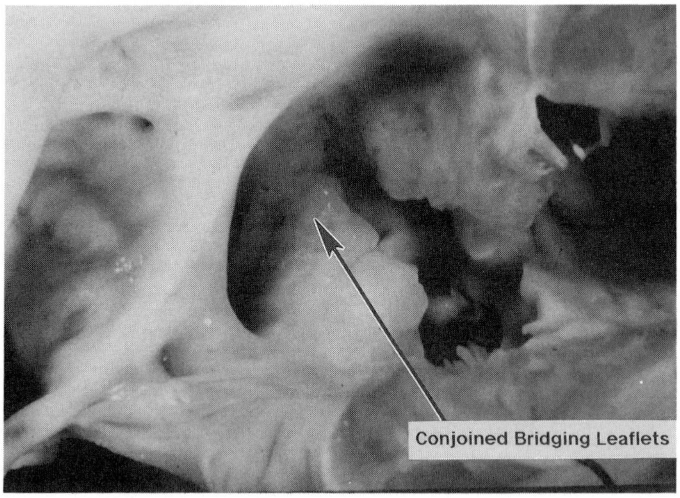

Fig. 40 In this heart, viewed in comparable fashion to Fig. 39, the bridging leaflets are fused to each other to produce separate valvar orifices within the common atrioventricular junction.

atrioventricular valve which bridge the septum (compare Figs. 39, 40). The anatomy also calls into question the convention of describing the variant with separate valvar orifices as an "ostium primum atrial septal defect". The septal deficiency certainly functions as an interatrial communication, and is bounded superiorly by the leading edge of the primary atrial septum and inferiorly by the crest of the muscular ventricular septum. The atrial septum itself, however, can be virtually normal apart from the concavity at its leading edge, and it often extends down to the level of the atrioventricular junction (Fig. 19). The hole between the chambers is an atrioventricular septal defect which permits shunting at atrial level because the bridging leaflets of the atrioventricular valve are depressed into the ventricle so as to become fused to the scooped-out septal crest (Fig. 27). It is the variations in the extent of fusion of the bridging leaflets to the septal components which underscore the second major series of anatomic variations within the overall group.

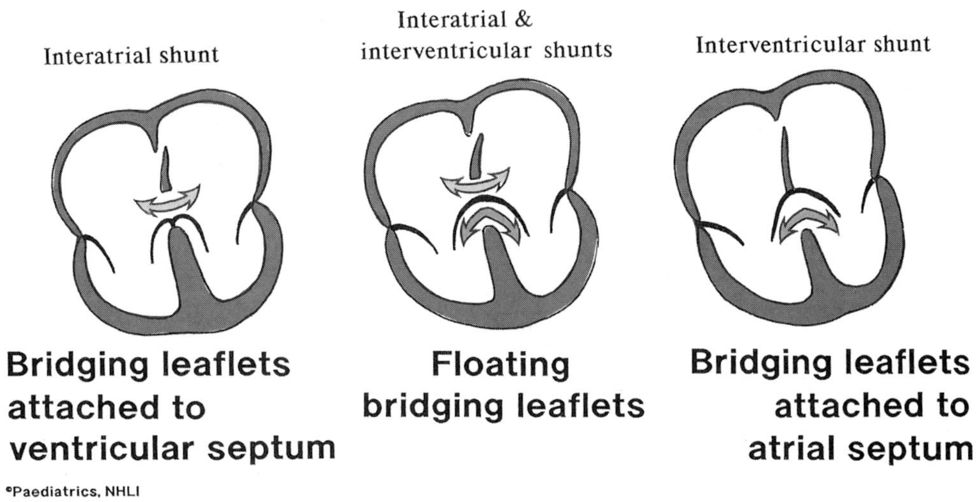

Fig. 41 Shunting across the atrioventricular septal defect when there is deficient atrioventricular septation depends on the relationship of the bridging leaflets to the atrial and ventricular septal structures.

Thus, as discussed above, shunting through the atrioventricular septal defect exists at atrial level when the bridging leaflets, and the tongue of valvar leaflet tissue which connects them, are attached to the crest of the ventricular septum (Fig. 41, *left*). Should the bridging leaflets be unattached to either the atrial or ventricular septal components, then shunting through the septal deficiency will be feasible, depending upon the prevailing haemodynamic conditions, at both atrial and ventricular levels (Fig. 41, *centre*). Presuming the presence of comparable haemodynamics, the extent of ventricular shunting will then depend on the degree of tethering of the bridging leaflets relative to the ventricular septum. This, in turn, will vary for the superior and the inferior leaflet. There is then one further possibility for containment of shunting. That is seen when the bridging leaflets are fused, not to the crest of the ventricular septum, but to the leading edge of the atrial septum. This arrangement confines the anatomic potential for shunting at ventricular level (Fig. 41 *right*). The heart thus produced, with a ventricular septal defect (Fig. 42), will have all the stigmas of a common atrioventricular junction, including a trifoliate left atrioventricular valve, inlet/outlet septal disproportion, and unwedging of the subaortic outflow tract.

In most instances, those hearts which have separate valvar orifices for the right and left ventricles have the potential either for atrial shunting alone, or else for exclusively ventricular shunting. Those with a common valvar orifice, in most instances, have the potential for atrial and ventricular shunting. Unfortunately, these combinations are not absolute. Thus, it is frequent to find hearts with separate valvar orifices for right and left ventricles in which intercordal spaces beneath the bridging leaflets produce limited interventricular communications (Fig. 43). In rare circumstances, the fused bridging leaflets can float freely within the atrioventricular septal defect (Fig. 44). In comparable fashion, although it is usual for there to be atrial and ventricular shunting when there is a common valvar orifice, the separate superior and inferior bridging leaflets can sometimes be fused firmly to the ventricular septum so that shunting occurs only at atrial level. It was attempts to categorize these anomalies as intermediate between the "partial" and "complete" forms which led to description of "transitional" forms,[11] or else the construction of formidable alphanumeric systems to cope with the supposedly intermediate variants.[12] As we have already emphasized, the basic junctional anatomy of all the anomalies is the same. It is only the specific morphology of the bridging leaflets which varies. The two specific features of the bridging leaflets, whether they are fused to each other, or alternatively fused to the

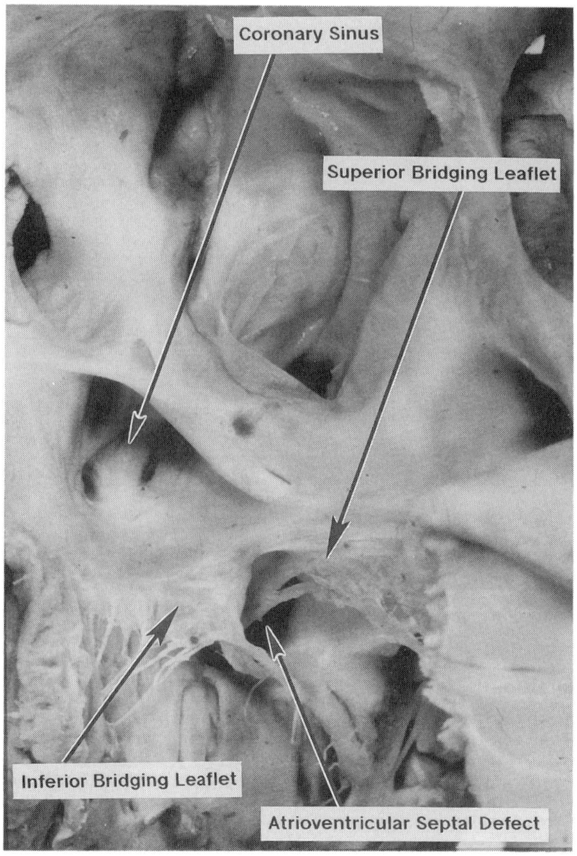

Fig. 42 This heart is viewed from the right side. The leaflets which bridge the ventricular septum are fused to the underside of the atrial septum so that shunting can occur only at ventricular level.

septal components, are mutually exclusive. If, therefore, the two features are described as separate facets of the hearts with deficient atrioventricular septation in the setting of a common atrioventricular junction, there is no need to bother with problems of completeness.

There are, of course, other features which produce variation within the overall group of hearts. These include the degree of sharing of the common atrioventricular junction between the atriums and the ventricles (Fig. 45). This feature accounts for the features of ventricular dominance, and for so-called "double outlet atrium".[13,14] Variation is also produced by associated lesions which can be many and varied, and by the Rastelli classification, which we will discuss below. The major variation, nonetheless, and that which is most important in clinical diagnosis, is provided by the relationship of the bridging leaflets to each other (common valvar orifice versus separate right and left valvar orifices within the common atrioventricular junction: Fig. 38), and by the relationship of the bridging leaflets to the septal structures (attached to atrial septum, to ventricular septum, or free-floating: Fig. 41).

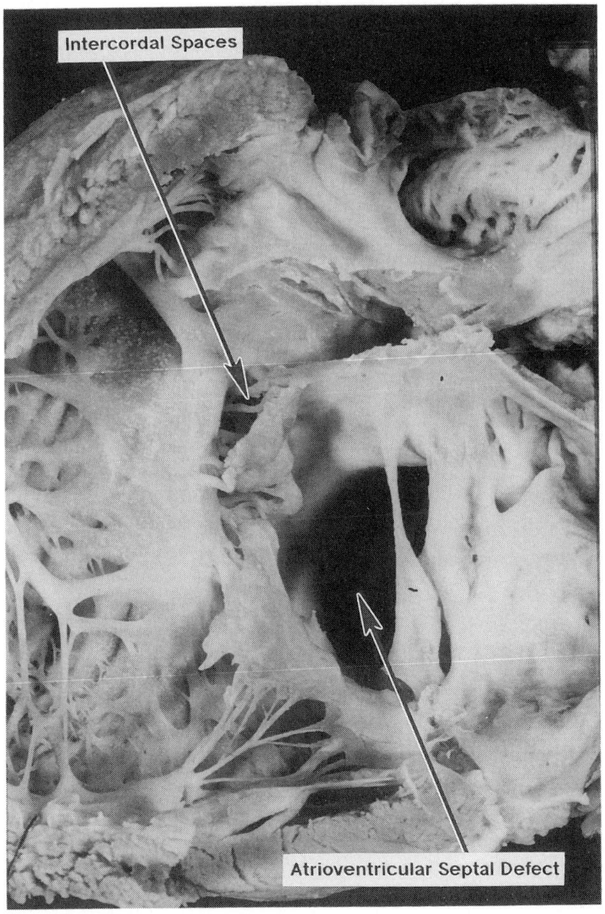

Fig. 43 This heart is viewed from the left ventricular aspect. The intercordal spaces beneath the superior bridging leaflet permit interventricular shunting even though there are separate valvar orifices for the right and left ventricles.

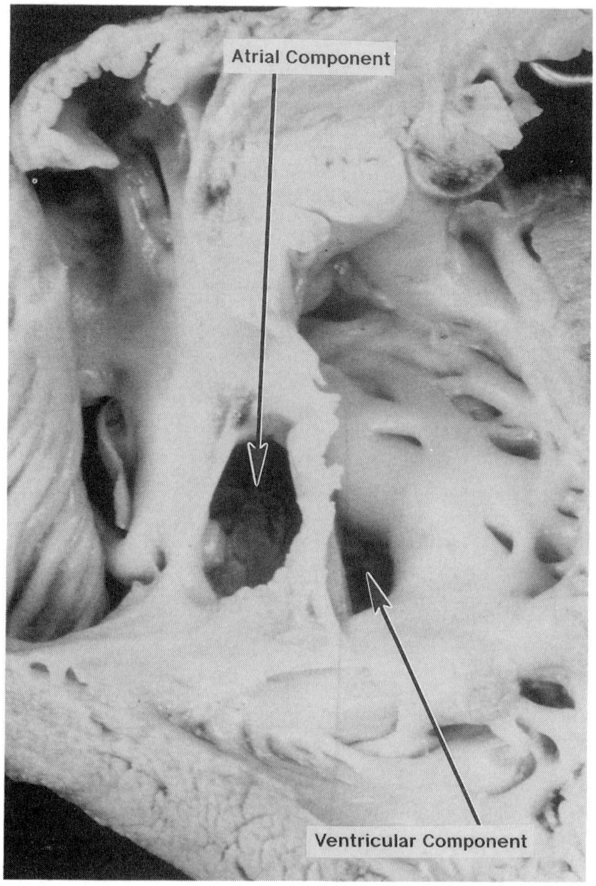

Fig. 44 In this heart, viewed from the right side, the bridging leaflets are fused to each other, but float freely within the atrioventricular septal defect.

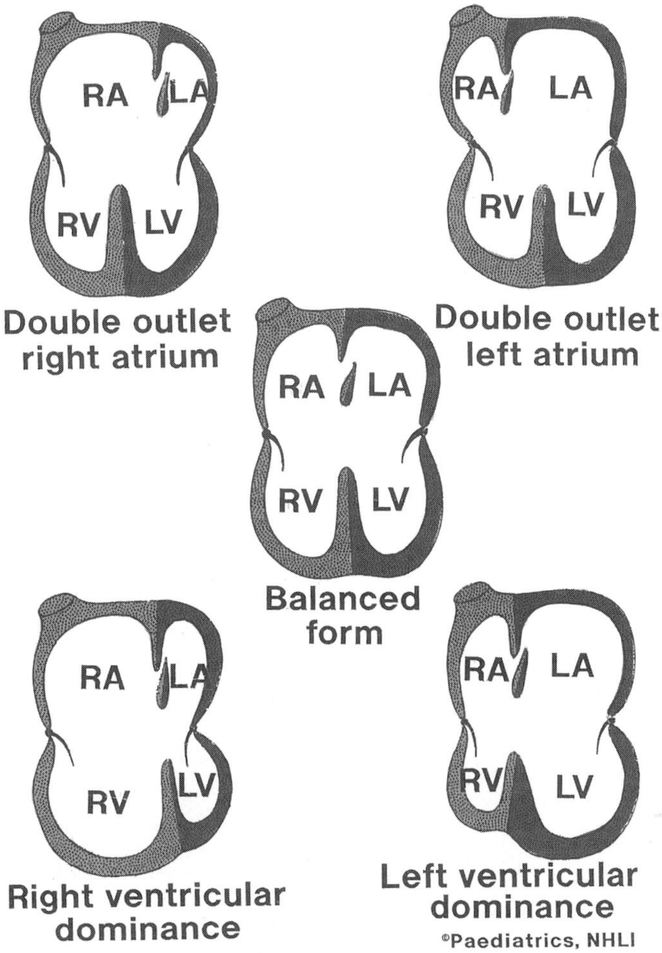

Fig. 45 The sharing of the common atrioventricular junction between the atrial and ventricular chambers produces the variants in morphology known as double outlet atrium (upper panels) or ventricular dominance (lower panels).

THE RASTELLI CLASSIFICATION

One of the earliest works which influenced the surgical repair of atrioventricular septal defect with common atrioventricular junction was the analysis of the morphology of the superior bridging leaflet conducted by Rastelli and his colleagues from the Mayo Clinic.[15] Of late, however, the differences observed by these investigators have lost much of their surgical significance, while the observations themselves have been the subject of debate.[16] Thus, Rastelli and his colleagues highlighted these arrangements within a spectrum of morphology of the superior leaflet, which they labelled Types A through C. In the first pattern, Type A, they argued that the superior bridging leaflet (which they called the anterior leaflet) was divided into two parts, with tethering of the bridging component to the crest of the ventricular septum (Fig. 46). The other two patterns, Types B and C, were held to represent free-floating of the bridging leaflet, with attachment further into the right ventricle in Type C (Fig. 47) than in Type B (Fig. 48). It was Ugarte and his colleagues[16] who first questioned this interpretation, while supporting the concept of the spectrum of morphology. These Spanish investigators argued that the bridging leaflet was no more divided in Type A than in the other variants. They proposed that Type A represented minimal bridging to the right ventricle combined with cordal tethering. As the leaflet bridged further into the right ventricle in the Types B and C varieties, so it became further detached from the crest of the ventricular septum. Our findings support their observations.[17] Thus, we interpret the space between the bridging leaflet and the anterosuperior leaflet of the right ventricle in all of these variants as a zone of apposition in the setting of a five-leaflet common valve. Indeed, our observations suggest that the spectrum of malformation can be extended to include the so-called "ostium primum" defect. This variant, as we have explained, is characterized by the presence of separate right and left valvar orifices. In such hearts, the right atrioventricular valve sometimes has a free-standing septal component (Fig. 49). More usually, the superior bridging leaflet is turned in and attached directly to the ventricular crest (Fig. 50), often with a pouch contained by its left ventricular aspect.[18] In some instances,

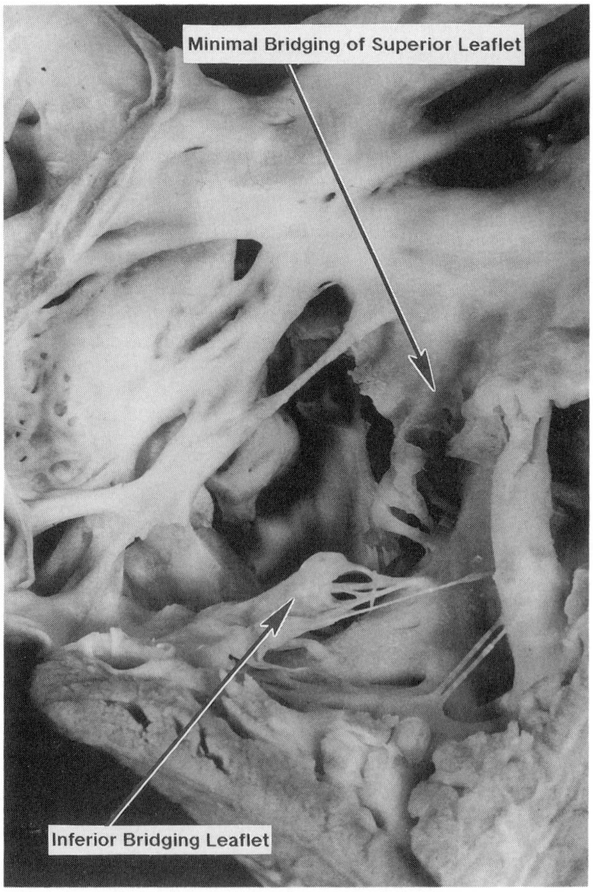

Fig. 46 This heart is viewed from the right side, to show the minimal bridging of the superior leaflet which produces the so-called "Rastelli Type A" morphology.

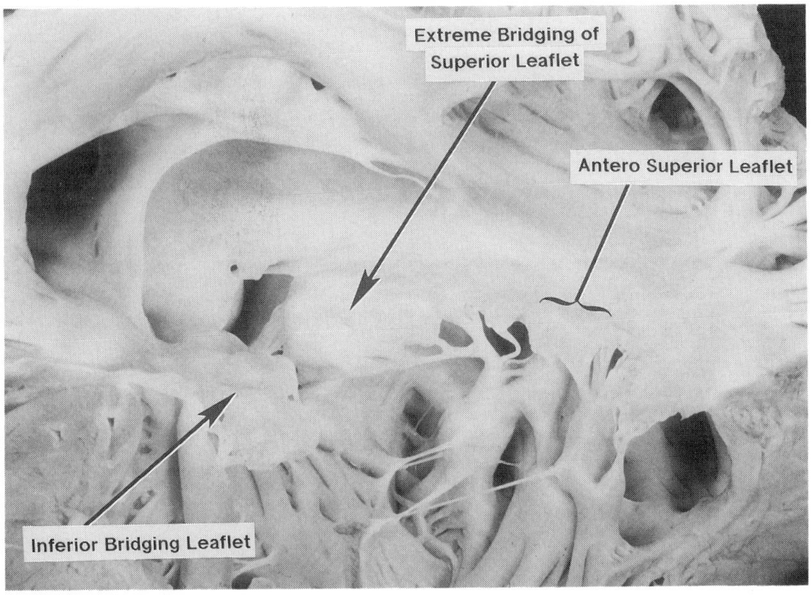

Fig. 47 This heart is viewed in comparable fashion to the one shown in Fig. 46. There is extreme bridging of the superior leaflet, with concomitant diminution in size of the antero-superior leaflet of the right ventricle. This is the so-called "Rastelli Type C" arrangement.

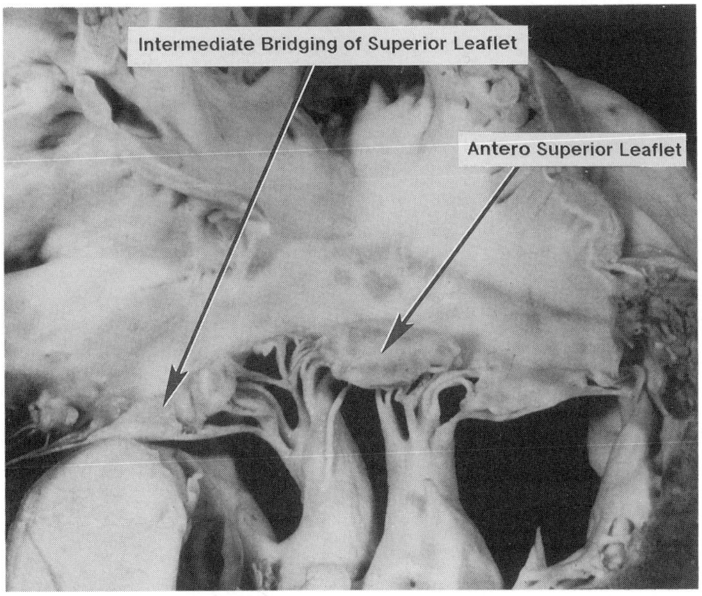

Fig. 48 This heart has been sectioned in its coronal plane, and the anterior segment is viewed from the back. It shows the intermediate bridging of the superior leaflet which gives the so-called "Rastelli Type B" pattern.

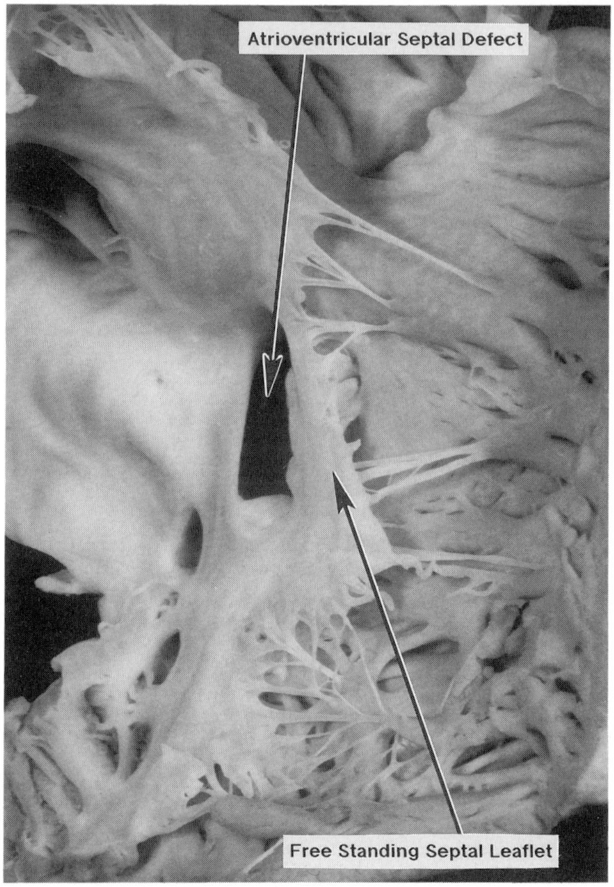

Fig. 49 This heart with deficient atrioventricular septation and common atrioventricular junction has a separate valvar orifice for the right ventricle with a free-standing septal leaflet.

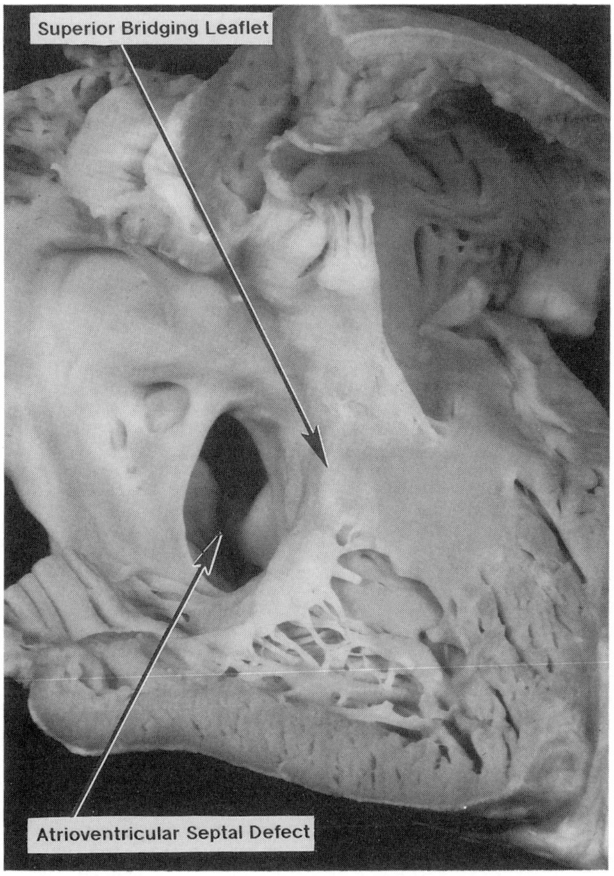

Fig. 50 In this heart with separate valvar orifices (compare with Fig. 49), the superior bridging leaflet is turned in and attached directly to the crest of the ventricular septum so that there is no free-standing septal leaflet for the right atrioventricular valve.

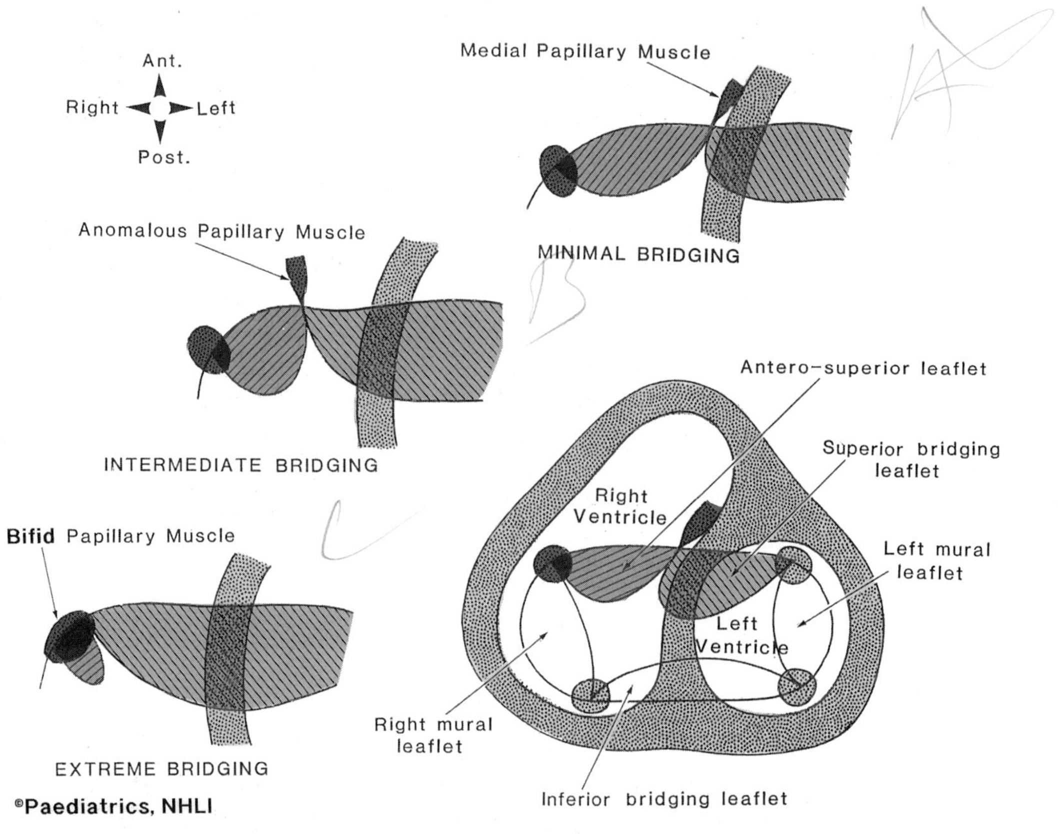

Fig. 51 It is the extent of bridging of the superior leaflet within the right ventricle, coupled with variation in the position of the papillary muscle which supports its zone of apposition with the antero-superior leaflet of the right ventricle, which determines the variation seen in the Rastelli classification. Note the diminution in size of the antero-superior leaflet as the spectrum progresses from Type A to Type C.

however, the attachment to the septum is incomplete, and small intercordal communications provide the capacity for interventricular shunting beneath the superior bridging leaflet (Fig. 43). It is then an easy matter to chart the progression from these hearts with separate valvar orifices and intercordal shunting to those with common valvar orifice and minimal bridging of the superior leaflet: the so-called Rastelli Type A variant (Fig. 46). The remainder of the spectrum through Types B and C then reflects increasing commitment of the superior leaflet to the right ventricle, with concomitant diminution in size of the anterosuperior leaflet of the right atrioventricular valve (Fig. 51).

It should also be noted that the Rastelli classification focused only on the superior bridging leaflet of the common atrioventricular valve. The arrangement of the inferior bridging leaflet is also of importance in determining the most appropriate option for surgical repair, albeit that the anatomic variation is less marked in the inferior bridging leaflet than in the superior leaflet.[19] Thus, the commitment of the inferior leaflet is almost always comparable in the right and left ventricles, be there a common orifice or separate right and left valvar orifices. The variability reflects the degree of tethering to the ventricular septal crest. Sometimes a discrete raphe is seen between divided right and left ventricular components of the leaflet, and the raphe then marks the location of the extensive non-branching component of the atrioventricular conduction axis. More usually, the inferior bridging leaflet is inserted directly on the septal crest, but with no potential beneath it for interventricular shunting, or else shunting is possible only through tight intercordal spaces. Less frequently, the leaflet floats freely relative to the ventricular septum. The degree of tethering of the inferior bridging leaflet is unrelated to the arrangement of the superior leaflet.[6]

THE LEFT ATRIOVENTRICULAR VALVE

The key to diagnosis of hearts with atrioventricular septal defect and common atrioventricular junction, and the key to appropriate surgical treatment, lies in the structure of the left atrioventricular valve (Figs. 25, 52). It is significant in this regard that, although arguments continue to rage as to whether or not this valve can be interpreted, as suggested by Rokitansky,[4] in terms of a mitral valve with a cleft in the aortic leaflet, all illustrations of which we are aware demonstrate clearly the trifoliate pattern of closure of the valve (Fig. 52). Examination of all these illustrations, amongst which we can cite those of Rastelli and colleagues[15] Van Mierop,[20] Carpentier,[21] and Castaneda and co-workers,[2] shows that, when the left atrioventricular component of the common junction is considered in isolation, the mural leaflet of this trifoliate valve guards less than one-third of the orificial circumference. This observation is then supported by the extensive measurements made by Penkoske *et al.*[6] and by Ebels and his co-workers,[22] both in autopsied hearts and in the operating room. Taken together, the findings show that, even if the surgeon were to suture together completely this zone of apposition between the left ventricular components of the two leaflets which bridge the ventricular septum, the manoeuvre would in no way restore the morphology to that of a

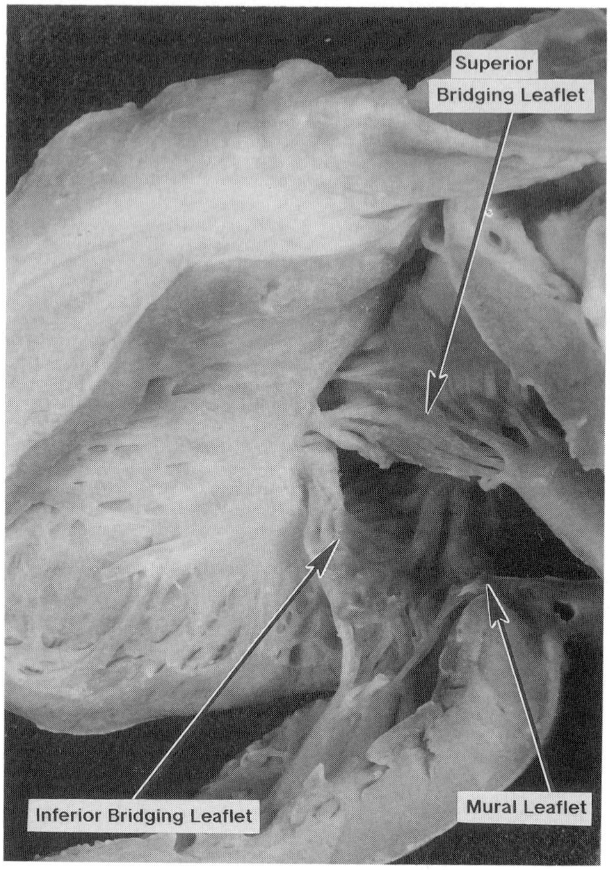

Fig. 52 This "ostium primum" defect is opened through the left ventricle so as to display the structure of the left atrioventricular valve. It has three leaflets, and the so-called cleft is the zone of apposition between the left ventricular components of the two bridging leaflets.

normal mitral valve. In the morphologically mitral valve, the mural leaflet guards two-thirds of the overall valvar circumference.

The fact that suturing of the zone of apposition between the bridging leaflets does not restore a mitral valve cannot be taken as evidence that the surgeon does not need to close this zone of apposition during repair. Arguments concerning the advisability of closing surgically this zone have unduly coloured the debate concerning valvar anatomy, as have disagreements concerning whether or not the zone of apposition should be considered as a cleft or a commissure. The latter point is readily resolved when it is appreciated that, irrespective of its label, the zone of apposition is the meeting point between the left ventricular components of the leaflets which bridge the ventricular septum. It is then important to note, as was drawn to our attention by Ebels (personal communication), that the angle of this meeting point relative to the ventricular septum varies considerably between hearts with common valvar orifice and free-floating leaflets and in those with separate valvar orifices. It is only in the hearts with free-floating superior and inferior leaflets that the zone of apposition subtends a right angle to the septum (Fig. 24). In hearts with separate right and left atrioventricular valvar orifices, the zone of apposition, which now extends between the superior bridging leaflet and the tongue of valvar leaflet tissue which joins together the two bridging leaflets, can subtend a markedly acute angle to the septum (Fig. 53). The nature of this feature, along with the arrangement of other aspects of the valve, including the extent of the mural leaflet,[22] need to be taken into account by the surgeon wishing to establish the most effective means of providing a competent left atrioventricular valve after repair. Such competence will most readily be achieved when it is appreciated that the basic format of the left valve is a mechanism with three leaflets closing together over three zones of apposition.

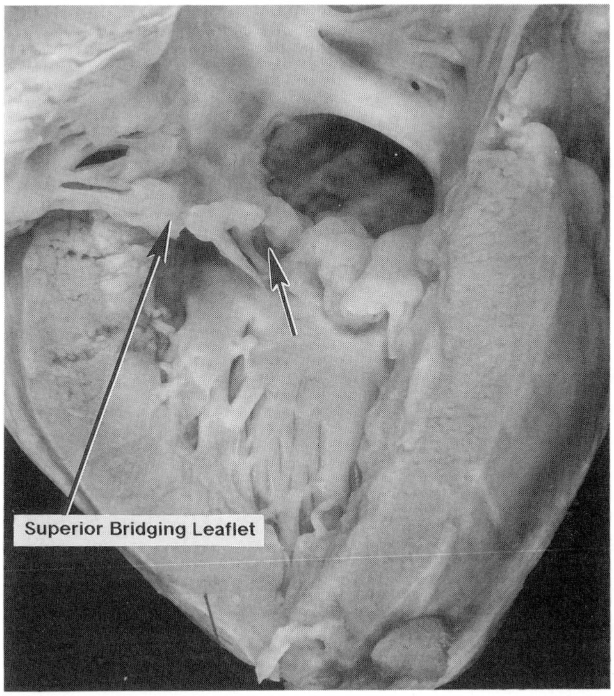

Fig. 53 When there are separate valvar orifices for the right and left ventricles, the zone of apposition between the bridging leaflets in the left ventricle extends onto the tongue which unites the two leaflets, thus producing a markedly acute angle of the so-called cleft relative to the septum (arrow) compare this with the angle seen in the presence of common valvar orifice (Fig. 24).

This trifoliate arrangement can be distorted in some cases when the left valve itself is abnormal, and this also has major surgical significance. The classical distortion is seen in the so-called "Parachute" malformation. In this lesion, all the tendinous cords of the left valve focus together on one papillary muscle, usually because the mural leaflet is either grossly hypoplastic or lacking.[22] The valvar orifice is then represented only by the zone of apposition between the bridging leaflets. Ebels has commented[5] that a parachute thus formed, with an open canopy, would be a lethal instrument, but for better or worse the anatomy is described in this fashion. The key point of surgical significance is that the valve has only two leaflets, and it is not possible in this setting to suture the "cleft".

THE ATRIOVENTRICULAR CONDUCTION AXIS

As may be expected, the disposition of the atrioventricular conduction axis reflects both the deficient atrioventricular septation and the common atrioventricular junction, and deviates from the arrangement seen in the normal heart.[23–25] In the normal heart, the atrioventricular axis contained at the apex of the triangle of Koch has only to penetrate the central fibrous body to reach the crest of the ventricular septum in the subaortic outflow tract (Fig. 6). As we have already emphasized, the presence of the common atrioventricular junction in the hearts with deficient atrioventricular septation splits up the central fibrous body. The conduction tissue still sits on the crest of the ventricular septum, but is now no longer related to the unwedged subaortic outflow tract. Instead, an extensive non-branching atrioventricular bundle runs to the posterior margin of the atrioventricular junction, the atrioventricular node being formed at the point of union of the ventricular septum with the junction. Usually this is in line with the atrial septum, and the node is then contained in a triangle delimited by the leading edge of the atrial septum, the atrioventricular junction, and the mouth of the coronary sinus (Fig. 54). The only exception to this rule occurs when there is malalignment between the atrial and ventricular septums, usually associated with left ventricular dominance. The atrioventricular node is then positioned along the right posterior atrioventricular junction at the point of attachment of the malaligned ventricular septum (Fig. 55). The long non-branching bundle is buried beneath the inferior bridging leaflet. The branching bundle occupies the free margin of the ventricular septum when there is a common valvar orifice, but is covered over by the connecting tongue of valvar tissue in the presence of separate right and left atrioventricular valvar orifices (Fig. 56).

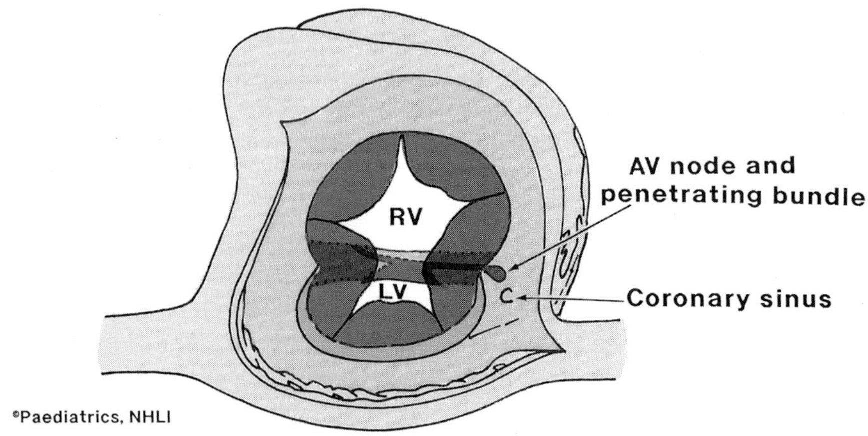

Fig. 54 The disposition of the atrioventricular conduction axis is dictated by the deficient atrioventricular septation combined with the common atrioventricular junction. The arrangement is shown here as seen with common valvar orifice, and as viewed by the surgeon in the operating room.

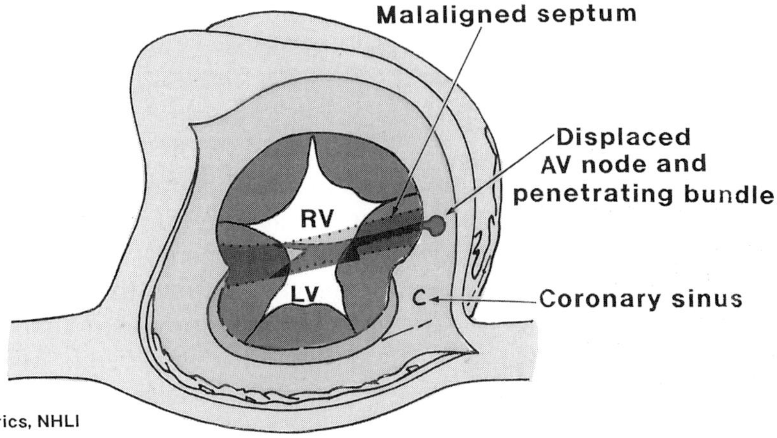

Fig. 55 The major exception to the rule that the atrioventricular node is found with the postero-inferior nodal triangle is when there is malalignment of the ventricular septum. The node is then formed at the point where the ventricular septum meets the common atrioventricular junction, shown here in surgical orientation.

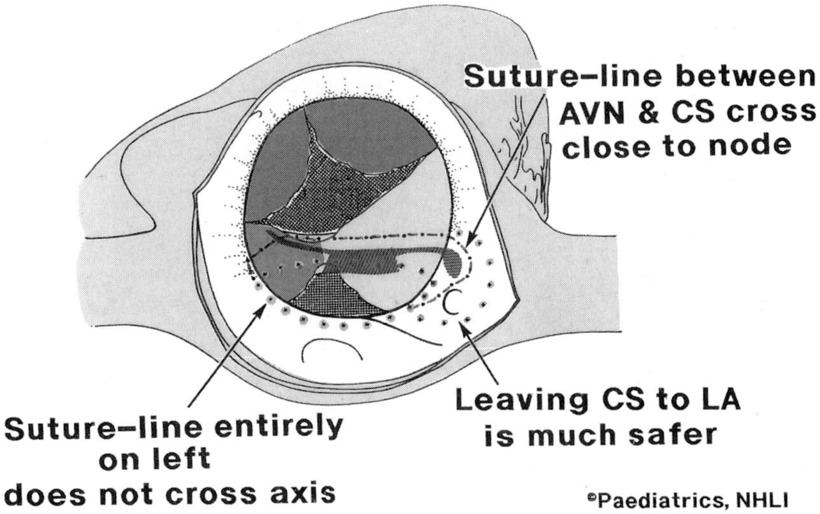

Fig. 56 The presence of separate valvar orifices for the right and left ventricles means that the bridging leaflets cover over the entirety of the atrioventricular conduction axis as it runs down the ventricular septal crest. The dotted lines show the options available to the surgeon to avoid the axis during repair of the atrioventricular septal defect, with the heart displayed as it would be seen in the operating room.

HEARTS WHICH ARE NOT ATRIOVENTRICULAR SEPTAL DEFECT WITH COMMON JUNCTION

Further disagreement in the categorization of "atrioventricular canal malformation" has centered on those hearts which might be considered "formes frustes" of the anomaly. Included in this group are those with straddling of the tricuspid valve,[26] deficiency of the atrioventricular component of the membranous septum (see Ref. 27, Fig. 20), large perimembranous defects opening to the inlet of the right ventricle,[28] and isolated clefts of the otherwise normally structured mitral valve (see Ref. 29, Fig. 26). Some of these malformed hearts, such as the so-called Gerbode defect,[27] do represent atrioventricular septal defects (Fig. 20). Others show some of the anatomic features of the group of hearts described in this chapter, such as bridging of the ventricular septum by valvar leaflets as in straddling tricuspid valve, or scooping of the ventricular septum as in the perimembranous inlet ventricular septal defect. In none of the hearts, however, is there the cardinal feature of the group presently described, namely a common atrioventricular junction. All these other purported variants of "atrioventricular canal malformation", including those with an isolated cleft of an otherwise normal mitral valve, have completely separate right and left atrioventricular junctions (Fig. 57). Their left atrioventricular valves are all furnished with a mural leaflet guarding about two-thirds of the circumference of the left atrioventricular junction. Disagreements are avoided, therefore, when hearts are entered into

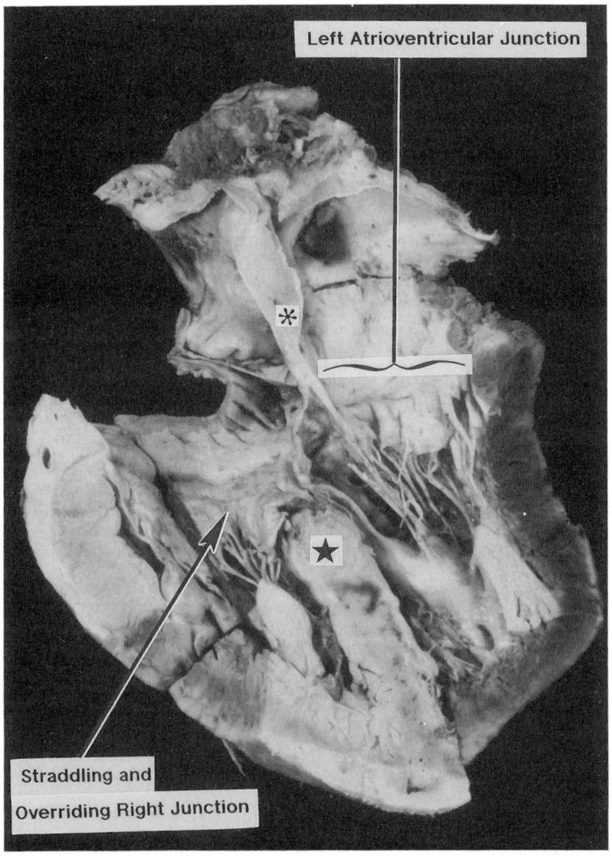

Fig. 57 The malalignment of the septum (asterisk) versus the ventricular septum (star) illustrated in Fig. 55 is comparable to that seen with straddling and overriding of the tricuspid valve. As shown in this four-chamber section, however, the major difference is that straddling tricuspid valve co-exists with a separate left atrioventricular junction guarded by a normally structured mitral valve.

the category discussed in this chapter only when they show evidence of deficient atrioventricular septation existing in the setting of a common atrioventricular junction.

DEVELOPMENTAL CONSIDERATIONS

We have discussed at length how the major difficulties which still exist concerning the morphology of hearts with deficient atrioventricular septation reflect the failure to distinguish between a mitral valve as opposed to a common atrioventricular valve. Exactly the same problem besets the comprehension of mechanisms of development. Conventional wisdom holds that the malformation reflects failure of fusion of the atrioventricular endocardial cushions, and that the lack of fusion produces clefts in the leaflets of the mitral and tricuspid valves.[30] If we divorce these two premises, however, and concentrate only on the role of the endocardial cushions, it is then possible to construct an entirely plausible sequence of events which account for the underlying anatomy, albeit that this sequence does not involve clefts developing in the mitral and tricuspid valves. So as properly to appreciate the events involved, it is also necessary to consider separately the formation of the atrioventricular valvar leaflets as opposed to the atrioventricular junctions. It is also necessary to consider precisely what is derived from the atrioventricular endocardial cushions.

The accepted view in the late 1960s, as displayed by the diagrams drawn by Netter in the Ciba Atlas,[31] for long dictated that the endocardial cushions gave rise to the "septal" leaflets of both atrioventricular valves, as well as the crest of the ventricular septum and the base of the atrial septum. Absence of these contributions from the cushions was presumed to produce not only the atrioventricular valvar malformations, but also the septal deficiencies which are so characteristic of atrioventricular septal defect with common atrioventricular junction. We are unaware of any evidence, however, which shows that the tissues of the atrioventricular endocardial cushions become muscularized to form the muscular atrioventricular septal components. For several recent years, it was also argued that the cushions did not contribute in any marked extent to the formation of the atrioventricular valvar leaflets, these structures instead being formed largely by ingrowth of the tissues of the atrioventricular grooves. We do now have good evidence that the cushions form a significant component of the leaflets, with part being derived by undermining of the surface layer of the ventricular myocardium.[32] It has also long been argued that fusion of the two atrioventricular endocardial cushions themselves is a key process in the formation of the membranous septum and the central fibrous body.[33] It is concentration on this latter structure which provides the key to understanding of the morphogenesis of deficient atrioventricular septation in the setting of a common atrioventricular junction.

It was Van Mierop who first, to our knowledge, emphasized the significance of failure of formation of the central fibrous body in the genesis of atrioventricular septal defect. Speaking at the Henry Ford Symposium in Detroit in 1977,[34] he argued that it was the anchorage provided by a properly-constituted fibrous body which then permitted expansion of the mitral and tricuspid orifices and incorporation of the aorta into the left ventricle between the newly-expanded mitral valve and the septum (Fig. 58). This explanation remains entirely credible, and fits in well with the time-honoured account of closure of the embryonic interventricular communication provided by investigators such as Odgers.[33] This sequence of events, however, placed the anticipated line of fusion between the endocardial cushions at right angles to the axis of the muscular ventricular septum, but also at right angles to the axis of the aortic leaflet of the normal mitral valve. Thus, it is an easy matter to understand how failure of fusion of the cushions would prevent formation of the central fibrous body (Fig. 59), and would permit development of a common rather than separate atrioventricular junctions as proposed by Van Mierop.[34] It is also easy to see that the location of these unfused superior and inferior cushions within the common junction accounts readily for the location of the bridging leaflets of the common atrioventricular valve (Fig. 60). It is very difficult, in contrast, to appreciate how the failure of fusion of two structures aligned at right angles to the developing subaortic outflow tract could also produce a cleft in the aortic leaflet of an otherwise normally-structured mitral valve. This postulate is the more difficult to accept when we recognize that the central fibrous body itself can normally be formed in the presence of "isolated" cleft of the mitral valve. Once more, therefore, we find that it is the aspects concerning the mitral valve which produce the impediment in the understanding of atrioventricular septal defect with common atrioventricular junction. The inferences to be drawn from the developmental events support, instead, the anatomic evidence we have already shown, namely that atrioventricular septal defect with common atrioventricular junction is a fundamentally different malformation than those lesions held previously to be closely related, such as straddling tricuspid valve, defects of the atrioventricular membranous septum, and perimembranous inlet ventricular septal defect. In all of these latter anomalies, the formation of separate atrioventricular junctions points to appropriate initial formation of the

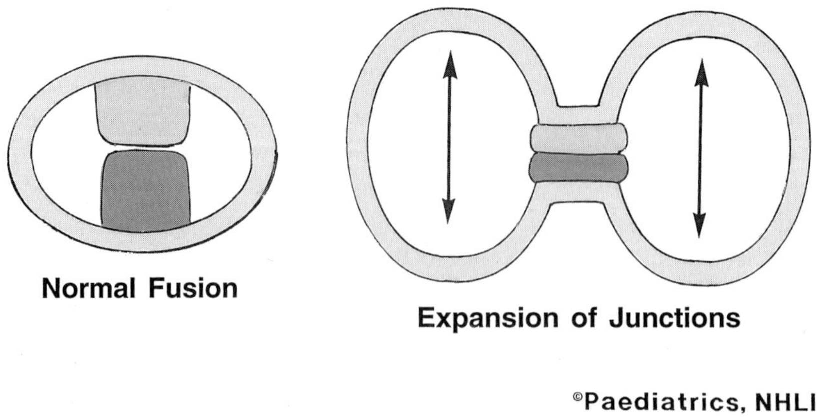

Fig. 58 Normal fusion of the atrioventricular endocardial cushions permits the developing right and left junctions to grow out from the middle, and provides room for the aorta to become connected to the left ventricle.

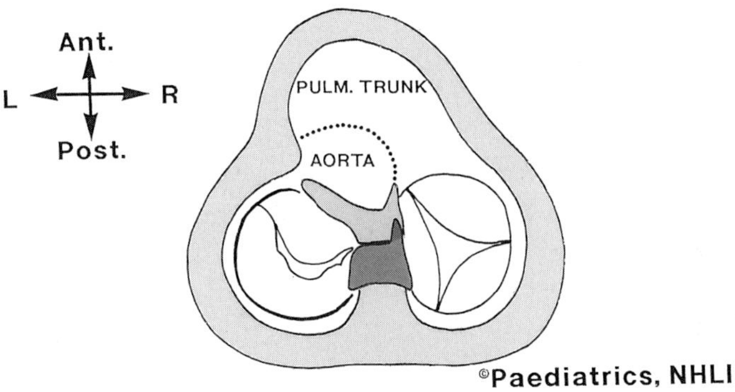

Fig. 59 The normal cushions fuse so as to cement together the centre of the heart at the central fibrous body. If the cushions fuse in this fashion, however, it is difficult to imagine how failure of fusion could give a "cleft" in the aortic leaflet of the mitral valve, since this leaflet is derived exclusively from the superior cushion.

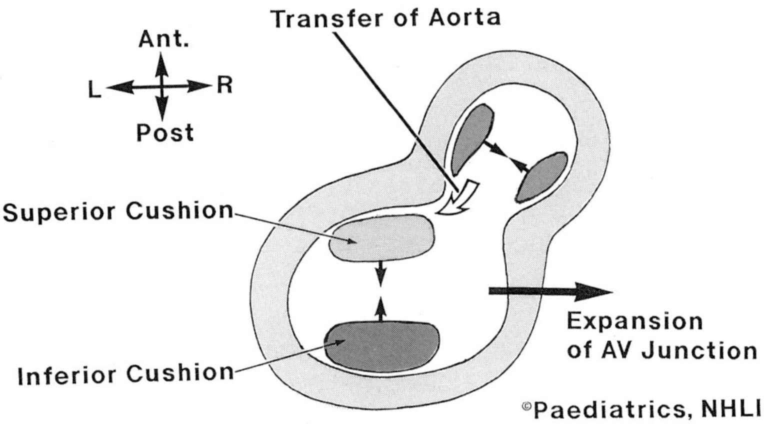

Fig. 60 Although it is difficult to account for a cleft in the aortic leaflet of the mitral valve on the postulated basis of failure of fusion of the atrioventricular endocardial cushions (See Fig. 59), it is easy to see how, after expansion of the developing atrioventricular junctions, these cushions would provide the basis for formation of the bridging leaflets in atrioventricular septal defect with common atrioventricular junction, and how the position of the superior leaflet would produce difficulties in transfer of the aorta.

endocardial cushions, a mechanism which is almost certainly at fault in those hearts which develop subsequently with a common atrioventricular junction.

Other inferences to be drawn from the study of hearts within the group of atrioventricular septal defect with common atrioventricular junction, however, suggest that the situation is not quite as straightforward as may be imagined. It has usually been suggested that the variant of atrioventricular septal defect with a common atrioventricular orifice is a "complete" defect, whereas the so-called "ostium primum" variant, with separate right and left atrioventricular valvar orifices and the potential only for interatrial shunting, is a "partial" defect. Yet the structure of the atrioventricular junction is, as we have seen, identical in the two variants (Fig. 22), as is the degree of disproportion between the inlet and outlet dimensions of the ventricular mass (Fig. 34). The only morphologic feature which discriminates between the variants, other than the arrangement of the bridging leaflets themselves, is the degree of scooping of the septal component of the ventricular mass.[7] Thus, in terms of developmental events, it is difficult to offer a plausible explanation which depends upon variation in development of the junctions.

When we compare the morphology of hearts with atrioventricular septal defect having common atrioventricular orifice with those having separate right and left valves within the common atrioventricular junction (Fig. 22), then the similarities observed also raise questions concerning developmental mechanisms which are presently widely accepted. As we have discussed, recent evidence has supported the long-held notion that the endocardial cushions contribute to the substance of the leaflets of the atrioventricular valves.[32] But, when we study the variant with separate right and left atrioventricular junctions (the "ostium primum" variant), we note that the two leaflets which bridge the ventricular septum, and which we presume are derived from the superior and inferior cushions, are also fused to each other! And such fusion of the leaflets is also to be seen when they float freely relative to the septal components (Fig. 44). Here, therefore, we have a major paradox. We can explain the formation of the common atrioventricular junction on the basis of the lack of any central fibrous body due to failure of fusion of the endocardial cushions (Fig. 59). Yet, if the cushions also produce the leaflets, then it would seem that they need to fuse so as to provide the linking tissue which produces separate right and left atrioventricular valvar orifices within the common atrioventricular junction. Could it be that different events are responsible for formation of the common junction as opposed to the arrangement of the valvar leaflets? And has too much emphasis been placed previously on the role of the cushions themselves? Future investigations may well show that the problem resides in the atrioventricular junctional musculature as well as the endocardial cushions.

CONCLUSIONS

The essence of the group of congenital cardiac malformations which we have described in this chapter is deficient atrioventricular septation occurring in the setting of a common atrioventricular junction. The common junction itself typically has right and left components committed to their respective ventricles. The left component, with its contained valvar apparatus, bears no morphologic resemblance to the mitral valve and the left atrioventricular junction as seen in the normal left ventricle. If considerations of the mitral valve, and notions of clefts in its anterior or aortic leaflet, are removed from the equation, then little fault can be found in the concept of the malformation representing an atrioventricular canal defect. Indeed, the development of the anomaly is readily understood on the basis of an abnormality occurring in the atrioventricular junction, almost certainly involving the atrioventricular endocardial cushions in some way or other. We can now extend the apposite aphorism of Joseph Hyrtl, therefore, to comment that the mitral valve came not only into the normal heart, but also into atrioventricular septal defect with common atrioventricular junction, like the devil into the baptismal font.[5] It is exclusion of considerations of the mitral valve from these abnormal hearts which will clarify their understanding.

REFERENCES

1. Becker AE, Anderson RH. Atrioventricular septal defects. What's in a name? *J Thorac Cardiovasc Surg* 1982;**83**:461–469.
2. Castaneda AR, Jonas RA, Mayer JE, Jr., Hanley FL. *Cardiac Surgery of the Neonate and Infant.* Philadelphia: W.B. Saunders Company. 1994: pp 167–186.
3. Peacock TB. Malformation of the heart consisting in an imperfection of the auricular and ventricular septa. *Trans Pathol Soc (London)* 1846;**1**:61–62.
4. Rokitansky CF. *Die Defecte der Scheidewande des Herzens.* Vienna: Pathologisch-Anatomisch Wilhelm Braumuller 1875: pp 27–36.
5. Ebels T. New surgical aspects of atrioventricular septal defect. Thesis. Groningen: Drukkerij Van Denderen B.V. 1989.
6. Penkoske PA, Neches WH, Anderson RH, Zuberbuhler JR. Further observations on the morphology of atrioventricular septal defects. *J Thorac Cardiovasc Surg* 1985;**90**:611–622.
7. Anderson RH, Neches WH, Zuberbuhler JR, Penkoske PA. Scooping of the ventricular septum in atrioventricular septal defect. (Letter). *J Thorac Cardiovasc Surg* 1988;**95**:146–147.
8. Lappen RS, Muster AJ, Idriss FS, Riggs TW, Ilbawi M, Paul MH, Bharati S, Lev M. Masked subaortic stenosis in ostium primum atrial septal defect: recognition and treatment. *Am J Cardiol* 1983;**52**:336–340.
9. Piccoli GP, Ho SY, Wilkinson JL, Macartney FJ, Gerlis LM, Anderson RH. Left sided obstructive lesions in atrioventricular septal defects. *J Thorac Cardiovasc Surg* 1982;**83**:453–460.
10. Chang CI, Becker AE. Surgical anatomy of left ventricular outflow tract obstruction in complete atrioventricular septal defect. A concept for operative repair. *J Thorac Cardiovasc Surg* 1987;**94**:897–903.
11. Wakai CS, Edwards JE. Developmental and pathologic considerations in persistent common atrioventricular canal. *Proc Staff Meet Mayo Clin* 1956;**31**:487–500.
12. Bharati S, Lev M, McAllister HAJ, Kirklin JW. Surgical anatomy of the atrioventricular valve in the intermediate type of common atrioventricular orifice. *J Thorac Cardiovasc Surg* 1980;**79**:884–889.
13. Corwin RD, Singh AK, Karlson KE. Double-outlet right atrium: A rare endocardial cushion defect. *Am Heart J* 1983;**105**:1156–1157.
14. Horiuchi T, Saji K, Osuka Y, Sato K, Okada Y. Successful correction of double outlet left atrium associated with complete atrioventricular canal and l-loop double outlet right ventricle with stenosis of the pulmonary artery. *J Cardiovasc Surg* 1976;**17**:157–161.
15. Rastelli GC, Kirklin JW, Titus JL. Anatomic observations on complete form of persistent common atrioventricular canal with special reference to atrioventricular valves. *Proc Staff Meet Mayo Clin* 1966;**41**:296–308.
16. Ugarte M, Enriquez de Salamanca F, Quero M. Endocardial cushion defects: an anatomical study of 54 specimens. *BHJ* 1976;**38**:674–682.
17. Piccoli GP, Wilkinson JL, Macartney FJ, Gerlis LM, Anderson RH. Morphology and classification of complete atrioventricular defects. *Br Heart J* 1979;**42**:633–639.

18. Kudo T, Tokoyama M, Imai Y, Konno S, Sakakibara S. The tricuspid pouch in endocardial cushion defect. *Am Heart J* 1974;**87**:544–549.
19. Akiba T, Becker AE, Neirotti R, Tatsuno K. Valve morphology in complete atrioventricular septal defect: variability relevant to operation. *Ann Thorac Surg* 1993;**56**:295–299.
20. Van Mierop LHS, Alley RD. The management of the cleft mitral valve in endocardial cushion defects. *Ann Thorac Surg* 1966;**2**:416–423.
21. Carpentier A. Surgical anatomy and management of the mitral component of atrioventricular canal defects. In: Anderson RH, Shinebourne EA (eds). *Paediatric Cardiology 1977.* Edinburgh: Churchill Livingstone 1978: pp 477–490.
22. Ebels T, Ho SY, Anderson RH, Meijboom EJ, Eijgelaar A. The surgical anatomy of the left ventricular outflow tract in atrioventricular septal defect. *Ann Thorac Surg* 1986;**41**:483–488.
23. Lev M. The architecture of the conduction system in congenital heart disease. I. Common atrioventricular orifice. *Arch Pathol* 1958;**65**:174–191.
24. Feldt RH, DuShane JW, Titus JL. The atrioventricular conduction system in persistent common atrioventricular canal defect: correlations with electrocardiogram. *Circulation* 1970;**42**:437–444.
25. Thiene G, Wenink ACG, Frescura C, Wilkinson JL, Gallucci V, Ho SY, Mazzucco A, Anderson RH. The surgical anatomy of the conduction tissues in atrioventricular defects. *J Thorac Cardiovasc Surg* 1981;**82**:928–937.
26. LaCorte MA, Fellows KE, Williams RG. Overriding tricuspid valve. Echocardiographic and angiocardiographic features. 8 cases of ventricular septal defect of atrioventricular canal type. *Am J Cardiol* 1976;**37**:911–919.
27. Gerbode F, Hultgren H, Melrose D, Osborn J. Syndrome of left ventricular-right atrial shunt, successful surgical repair of defect in five cases with observation of bradycardia on closure. *Ann Surg* 1958;**148**:433–446.
28. Van Praagh R, Geva T, Kreutzer J. Ventricular septal defects: how shall we describe, name and classify them? *J Am Coll Cardiol* 1989;**14**:1298–1299.
29. Di Segni E, Edwards JE. Cleft anterior leaflet of the mitral valve with intact septa. A study of 20 cases. *Am J Cardiol* 1983;**51**:919–926.
30. McGoon DC, Puga FJ, Danielson GK. Atrioventricular canal. In: Sabiston DC, Spencer FC (eds). *Gibbon's Surgery of the Heart.* Philadelphia: WB Saunders Co. 1983: pp 1051–1066.
31. Netter FH. The Heart. The Ciba Collection of Medical Illustrations Volume 5 1969:13.
32. Odgers PNB. The development of the pars membranacea septi in the human heart. *J Anat* 1938;**72**:247–259.
33. Van Mierop LHS. Pathology and pathogenesis of endocardial cushion defects. Surgical implications. In: Davila JC (ed) *Second Henry Ford Hospital International Symposium on Cardiac Surgery.* New York: Appleton-Century-Crofts 1977: pp 201–207.

Chapter 3
Isomerism of the Atrial Appendages

INTRODUCTION

The association between characteristic constellations of congenital cardiac malformations and an abnormal arrangement of the organs elsewhere within the body has long been recognized. The classical association of the most complex lesions within the heart is with absence of the spleen. Patients lacking a spleen had been reported at autopsy for centuries, but most of the early reports are held to reflect acquired absence subsequent to tuberuculous infection. The report by Martin from Paris, published in 1826,[1] is generally acknowledged to be the first account of congenital absence of the spleen occurring as part of the complex which includes congenital cardiac anomalies. It is with the name of Ivemark, however, that congenital asplenia is most associated, since Ivemark charted closely the developmental history of the spleen, linking this to that of the cardiac lesions.[2] But, as Devine has considered,[3] what would have been the consequences had Ivemark focused the primary attention upon the heart? This is the more pertinent since, over the same period, Putschar and Mannion[4] had made the critical observation that the essence of the malformation of the organs which accompanied the cardiac anomalies, far from representing some degree of mirror imagery as was generally thought, reflected the presence of a symmetric as opposed to a lateralized arrangement of the paired organs of the body. Had more note been taken of these early crucial observations, following the review of Van Mierop[5] which stressed the presence of bilateral right- or left-sidedness, many of the subsequent polemics could well have been avoided. Yet even Van Mierop, who illustrated exquisitely the symmetry of the lungs, bronchial tree and atrial appendages in the variants of the syndrome of visceral heterotaxy associated with absent and multiple spleens, respectively, chose to describe the overall arrangement in terms of ambiguity ("situs ambiguus"). The subset of the syndrome generally found with multiple spleens, and associated with bilateral left-sidedness, had been recognized as a harbinger of cardiac malformations even earlier than the variant associated with absence of the spleen, Abernethy having documented the conjunction of multiple spleens in a patient with double outlet right ventricle at the end of the eighteenth century.[6] The cardiac malformations typically associated with symmetrical left-sidedness had then been clearly charted by Moller and his colleagues.[7] Despite all these careful observations, it remained a fact that the presence of symmetrical features within the heart had not been agreed upon by the end of the 1970s, and that the combinations of lesions within the heart were described in the ambiguous fashion favoured by Van Mierop,[5] or else in terms of subsets labelled as "asplenia" and "polysplenia".[8] Evidence already existed, however, that the status of the spleen was a relatively poor guide to the malformations found within the heart,[9–11] and discovery of patients with bilateral right-sidedness who possessed a spleen[12] led to the rather comical description of splenic tissue existing in the patient with "asplenia". It had also been well demonstrated by this time[13] that the obvious syndromes of symmetry displayed by the bronchial tree provided a much better marker to happenings within the heart than did the status of the spleen. The question that faces us now, therefore, is whether there is truly evidence for symmetry within the atrial segment of the heart, as suggested by our own studies conducted during the 1980s and 1990s,[14–16] or whether the apparent morphologic evidence of atrial symmetry serves as no more than a general guide,[17] with all patients having visceral heterotaxy fitting into the groups of usual or mirror imaged arrangements according to the patterns of venous drainage.[18] These are the problems on which we will focus in this chapter, centering our attention on the critical morphology of the atrial appendages.[19]

SYMMETRY VERSUS LATERALIZATION

Before we get to grips with the problem of whether there is evidence of symmetry in the atrial chambers of the hearts from patients with visceral heterotaxy, we will start by reviewing the concepts of symmetry versus lateralization within the overall structure of the body. In the normal person, the two sides of the body, in terms of their skeletal and muscular structure, are mirror images of each other, or in other words the basic plan of the somatic structure is one of symmetry, making allowance for the changes superimposed on the basic plan by features such as exercise or disease. Thus, the right hand has as its mirror image the left hand, the position of the component parts in space, or their topology, serving always to distinguish between the individual right-sided or left-sided components of these symmetrical structures. Another way of describing the relationships between the hands, and the related symmetrical structures of the body, is to label them as being isomeric. Within this basic isomeric structure of the musculo-skeletal components of the body, however, and the neurovascular structures which supply them, the normal organs of the body, even those which are paired, show a distinctly lateralized arrangement. The evidence of lateralization is most obvious in the unpaired organs, which are rarely centrally located within the body. Thus, the liver in the normal person is predominantly to the right, while the stomach and spleen occupy exclusively left-sided positions. The gut has a characteristic pattern for the attachment of its mesentery to the body wall. The heart is normally positioned within the mediastinum so that two-thirds of its bulk are to the left, and its long axis points downwards and to the left. The aorta is left-sided, while the inferior caval vein is to the right of the spine. The paired organs then show further evidence of this characteristic lateralization. The right lung has three lobes, compared to the two lobes found in the left lung. The pattern of lateralization is even more obvious within the bronchial tree, with the bronchus supplying the right lung being short, and being crossed by the artery to the middle and lower lobes only after it has given off its first branch, making this an eparterial bronchus (Fig. 1). In contrast, the long left bronchus is crossed by the artery supplying the lower lobe before it gives rise to its first branch, which is, in consequence, hyparterial (Fig. 2). Similar anatomic differences are to be found in the position and structure of the other paired organs, such as the kidneys, testes, and even the cerebral hemispheres. The overall pattern of this lateralization, which includes the location of the major vessels of the body, is described as "situs solitus" which, when translated into english, simply means a usual arrangement (Fig. 3).

It has always been recognized that the usual arrangement of the body can, in some individuals, occur in a totally mirror imaged arrangement. The mirror imaged variant can, exceedingly rarely, be the standard pattern for those who, apart from the mirror imagery, are perfectly normal. In these individuals, therefore, the lung with three lobes supplied by the short, eparterial, bronchus is to the left, while the bilobed lung with its hyparterial bronchus is right-sided. (Fig. 4). The liver is a left-sided structure, but the stomach and spleen are found in the right upper quadrant of the abdomen (Fig. 5). This pattern has, traditionally, been described as showing "situs inversus". The inversion, however, is one of mirror imagery rather than "upside-downness". Our preference, therefore, is simply to describe the pattern as a mirror image arrangement. Patients with this type of mirror imagery can, as described, be found with otherwise normal hearts. When patients with mirror imagery

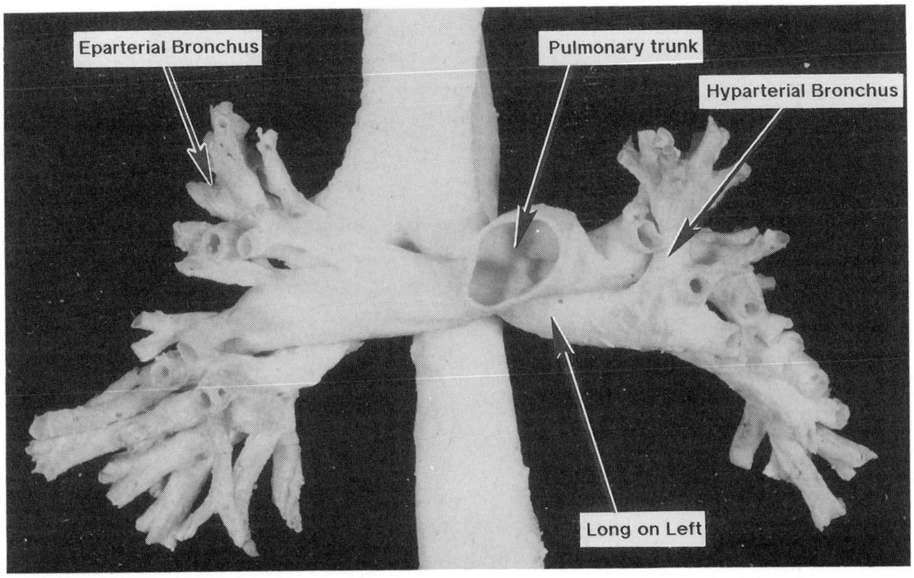

Fig. 1 The normal bronchial tree has been dissected to show its relationship to the pulmonary arteries, and is viewed from the front. The bronchus to the right lung branches before it is crossed by the pulmonary artery to the middle and lower lobes, making it eparterial. In contrast, the left bronchus is crossed by the pulmonary artery before it branches, making it long and hyparterial.

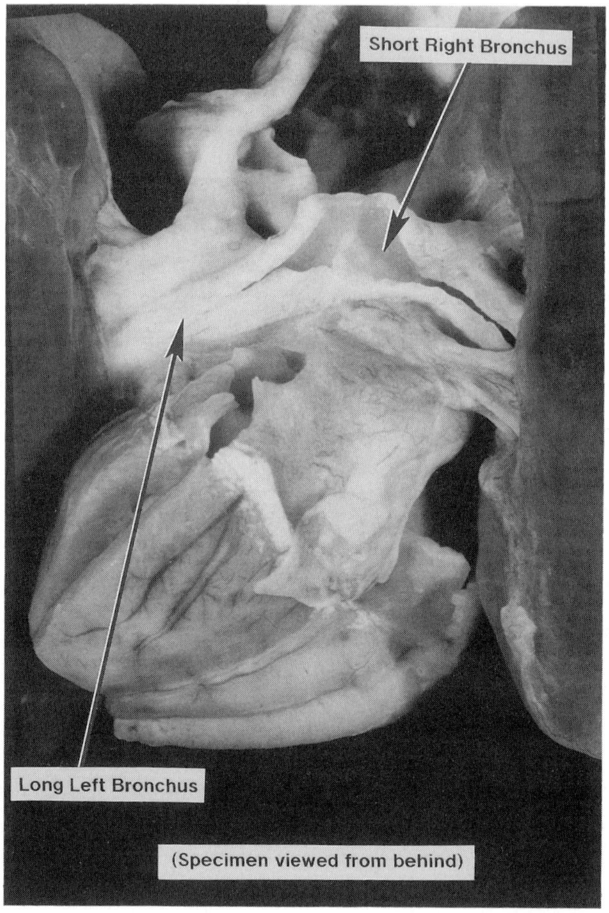

Fig. 2 This normal bronchial tree is viewed from behind, showing the discrepancy in length between the short morphologically right and the long morphologically left bronchuses.

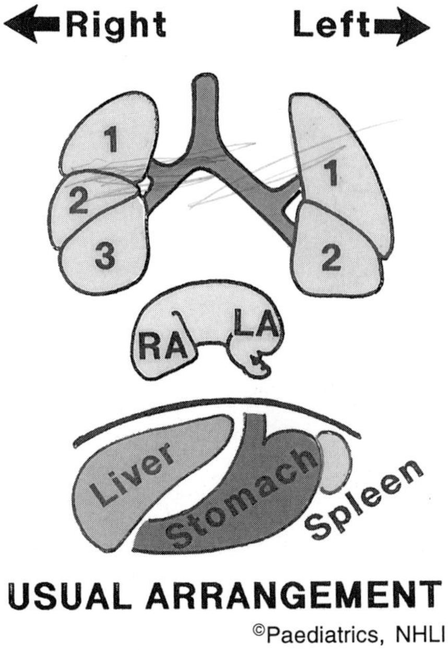

Fig. 3 The diagram shows the usual (solitus) arrangement of the lateralized organs of the body. RA – morphologically right atrial appendage; LA – morphologically left atrial appendage. 1–3 – lobes of the lungs.

are referred to the paediatric cardiologist, nonetheless, it is usually because they have intracardiac malformations such as complete or corrected transposition. All the features of these abnormal hearts are then mirror imaged when compared to the more typical malformations found in those individuals with usual arrangement.

In the middle part of this century, when pathologists and cardiologists started to take more interest in congenitally malformed hearts, it soon became clear that a group of complex combinations of intracardiac lesions was found in patients who showed some of the features of mirror imagery. Thus, the hearts of such patients were frequently in the right rather than the left half of the chest. The cardiac apex often pointed to the right, or directly downward. The aortic arch was frequently right-sided. Initially, these hearts tended to become lumped together as "situs inversus",[20] although as we have already discussed, prescient observers such as Putschar and Mannion[4] had observed the symmetry which is the essence of these malformations. Conventional wisdom, nonetheless, dictated that, when these syndromes, which were generally lumped together as showing visceral heterotaxy, were distinguished from the usual and mirror imaged arrangements, they were described in terms of "situs ambiguus".[5,8] The two subsets of the heterotaxic group were identified in terms of asplenia and polysplenia, and attention tended to be focused on the jumbled-up arrangement of the abdominal organs, this being the feature which justified the terms such as heterotaxy and "ambiguus".

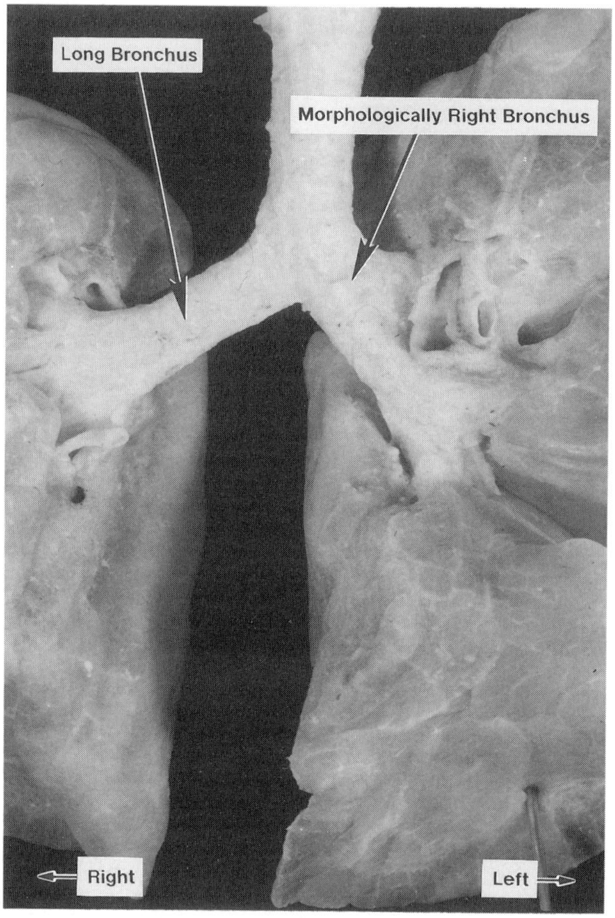

Fig. 4 This bronchial tree, viewed from the front, is from an individual with mirror imaged bodily arrangement. The long bronchus is right-sided.

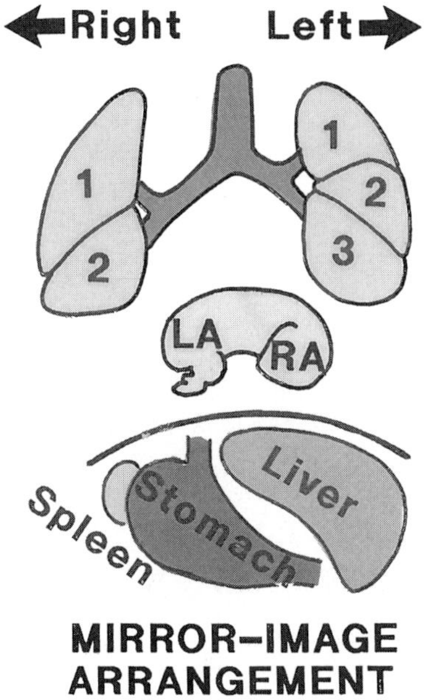

Fig. 5 This diagram shows the mirror imaged arrangement of the lateralized organs of the body. Abbreviations as for Figure 3.

It had already been shown that there was nothing ambiguous about the arrangement of the lungs and bronchial trees of these patients.[13] Thus, attention to the arrangement of these lungs revealed just as much symmetry, or isomerism, as in the skeleto-muscular systems of normal or mirror imaged individuals. In the greater majority, but not all, of the patients lacking a spleen, both lungs were trilobed, and both bronchuses were short and eparterial (Fig. 6). Similarly, in most, but not quite all, of the patients who possessed multiple spleens, it was shown that the right-sided and left-sided lungs each had two lobes, and were supplied by bronchuses both of which were long and hyparterial (Fig. 7). Interestingly, over the same period, it was also recognized that a subset of the patients with multiple spleens had the anticipated left pulmonary and bronchial isomerism, but that their hearts were normal, albeit with the venous return from the abdomen reaching the heart through the azygos system, the inferior caval vein being interrupted. The patients also had congenital biliary atresia.[21] When attention is directed to the lungs and bronchuses in patients with visceral heterotaxy, therefore, it is clear that the morphology is seen in the arrangements of right and left isomerism (Fig. 8). Significantly, no one has ever proposed, as far as we are aware, that these characteristic patterns of bronchopulmonary morphology should be distinguished in terms of "asplenia" and "polysplenia". Why, then, should this convention be proposed for the heart if it can be shown that the atrial segment of the heart in patients with visceral heterotaxy shows just as much evidence of isomerism as do the lungs and bronchuses? In the next section we will demonstrate the anatomy which supports this contention, but first we will review the criterions used to recognize atrial morphology.

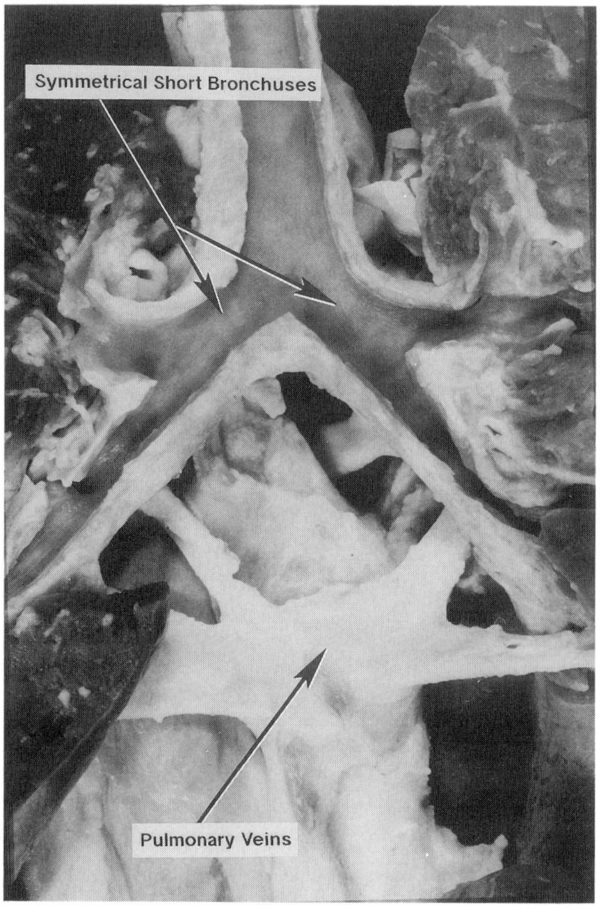

Fig. 6 This bronchial tree, viewed from behind, shows a symmetrical arrangement, with both bronchuses being short. Note the anomalous connection of the pulmonary veins to the heart.

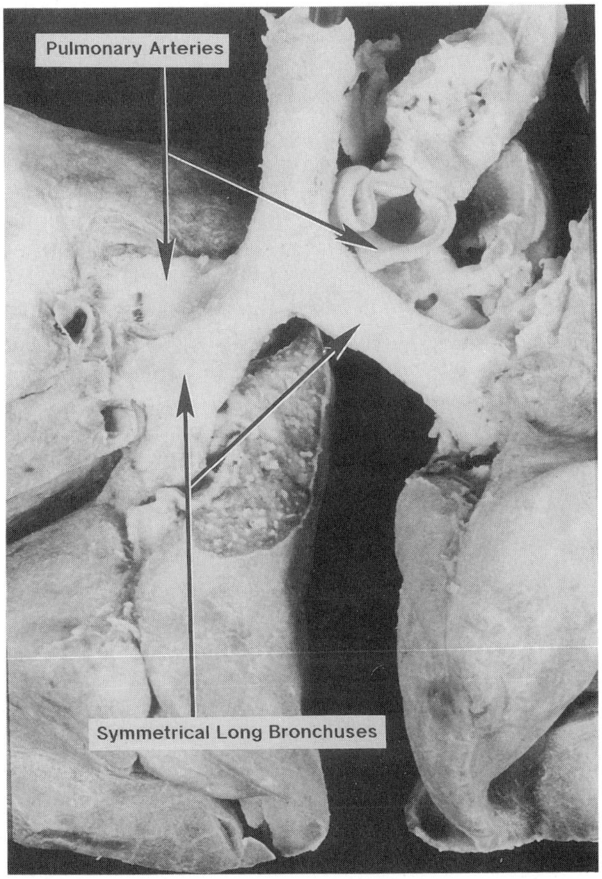

Fig. 7 This bronchial tree, viewed from the front, is again symmetrical, but both the bronchuses are long and hyparterial. Compare with Fig. 6.

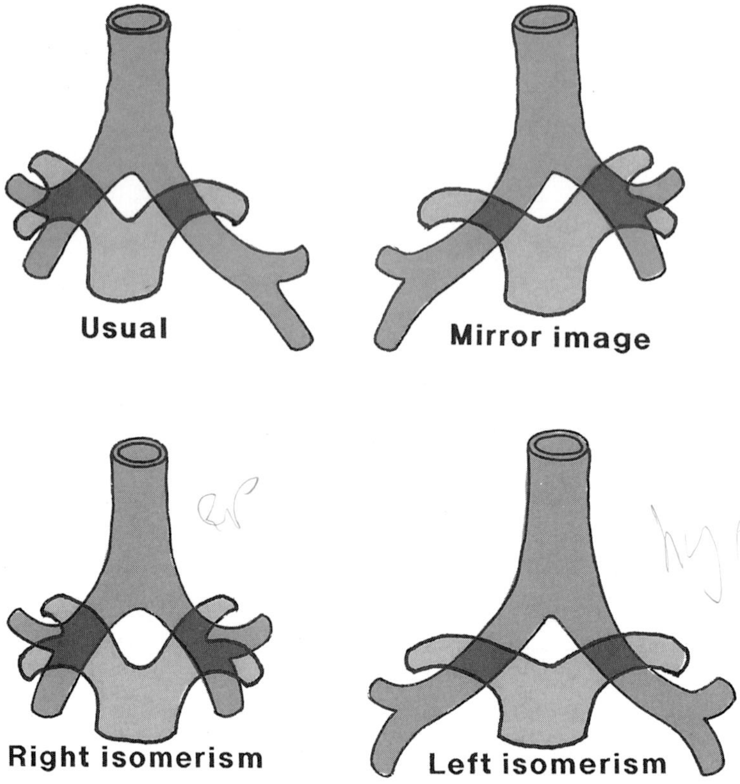

Fig. 8 This diagram shows the four patterns of bronchial arrangement.

MORPHOLOGY OF THE ATRIUMS RELEVANT TO ISOMERISM

In our introductory chapter (see p. 1), we emphasized the significance of the morphological method[22,23] in recognizing structures within the heart. In essence, the method states that structures which are themselves variable should not, in the ideal world, be used as determining features of other cardiac structures. In the context of the atrial chambers, the venous components, the vestibules, and the septum, all of which can be markedly abnormal or lacking in congenitally malformed hearts, are ruled out by this principle as arbitrating features for distinguishing morphologically rightness or leftness. Fortunately, one component of the atriums remains for use in distinction of morphology, namely the appendage. It is also the case that the structure of the normal morphologically right appendage (Fig. 9) is markedly different from that of the left appendage (Fig. 10). In a series of studies through the 1980s and 1990s, we showed that the morphology of the appendages could also be distinguished in patients with visceral heterotaxy, even when the atrial chambers were viewed in isolation.[14] We also showed that, when the appendages were examined in isolation in a very large series of congenitally malformed hearts,[15] their characteristic morphology permitted us to select from the overall series those hearts which came from patients with visceral heterotaxy. This was done without us having any knowledge of the arrangement of the abdominal organs. In diagnosing the existence of morphologically right as opposed to left appendages, however, we had relied upon their characteristic shape as the defining criterion, along with the size of the junction of the appendage with the body of the atrium. Thus, when Van Praagh and Van Praagh argued that these features may simply be a consequence of abnormal haemodynamics,[17] and that there was no such thing as isomerism of the atrial appendages, our extensive experience suggested that this was not the case, but we could not prove our beliefs on the basis of morphologic evidence. Working together with Uemura, therefore, we extended our investigations to establish whether the atrial appendages had morphological features independent of the shape and size of their junctions with the bodies of the atriums. Examination of a large number of normal hearts revealed that there was an additional feature of which we had not taken account in our previous studies. This was the extent of the pectinate muscles relative to the vestibule of the atrioventricular junctions. In the normal morphologically right atrium (Fig. 11), these pectinate muscles are extensive, running all round the vestibule to abut the septum at the crux in the region of the post-Eustachian sinus. In the normal morphologically left atrium, in contrast, the pectinate muscles are almost completely confined within the tubular appendage, and the smooth muscular vestibule of the mitral valve is directly continuous with the smooth-walled pulmonary venous component (Fig. 12). This difference in the extent of the pectinate muscles,

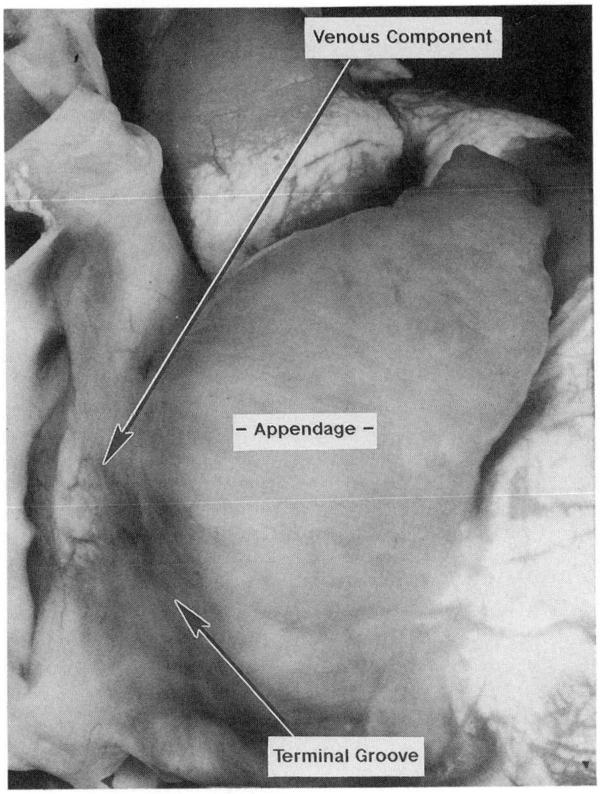

Fig. 9 The morphologically right atrial appendage seen from its right side. It has a characteristic triangular shape, and a broad junction with the systemic venous component across the terminal groove.

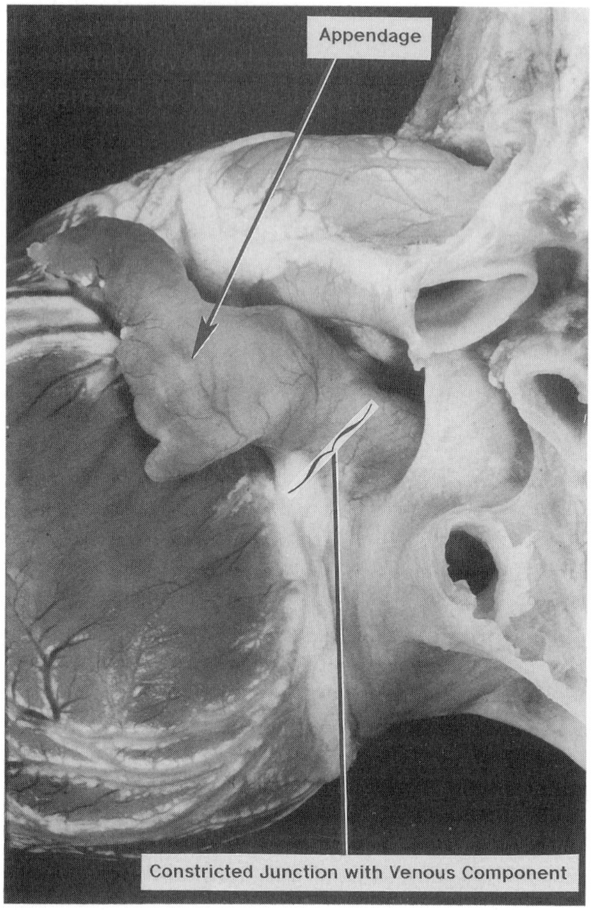

Fig. 10 In comparison to the normal morphologically right atrial appendage (see Fig. 9), the morphologically left appendage is long and tubular, with a constricted junction with the pulmonary venous component.

found in all normal hearts we examined, is an obvious feature in the drawings made by Van Praagh to illustrate atrial morphology in one of his authoritative reviews.[24] A further feature of note is that the smooth-walled posterior vestibule of the morphologically left atrium contains a prominent transverse venous structure, the coronary sinus (Fig. 13). Such a prominent venous structure is absent from the pectinated morphologically right atrioventricular vestibule (Fig. 16). When Uemura examined a large number of hearts from patients with visceral heterotaxy,[19] this feature of the extent of the pectinate muscles enabled all the appendages examined to be designated as morphologically right or morphologically left. All the hearts, indeed, had either morphologically right or morphologically left appendages bilaterally. Thus, on the basis of the structure of the pectinate muscles, all the hearts could be diagnosed as having either isomeric left or right atrial appendages (Fig. 14). It should be noted that, in this same series of hearts, it had been possible to diagnose isomerism of the appendages in virtually all the cases using our previously favoured criterions. Only the extent of the pectinate muscles, however, proved to be an absolute distinguishing feature.

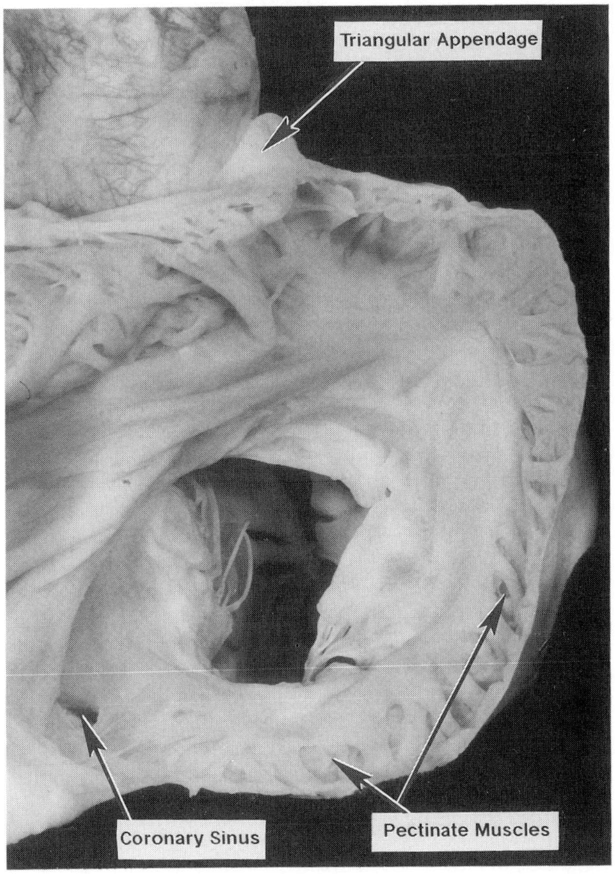

Fig. 11 The morphologically right atrium has been opened through the appendage so as to show the vestibule. Note how the pectinate muscles extend all round the vestibule to the mouth of the coronary sinus.

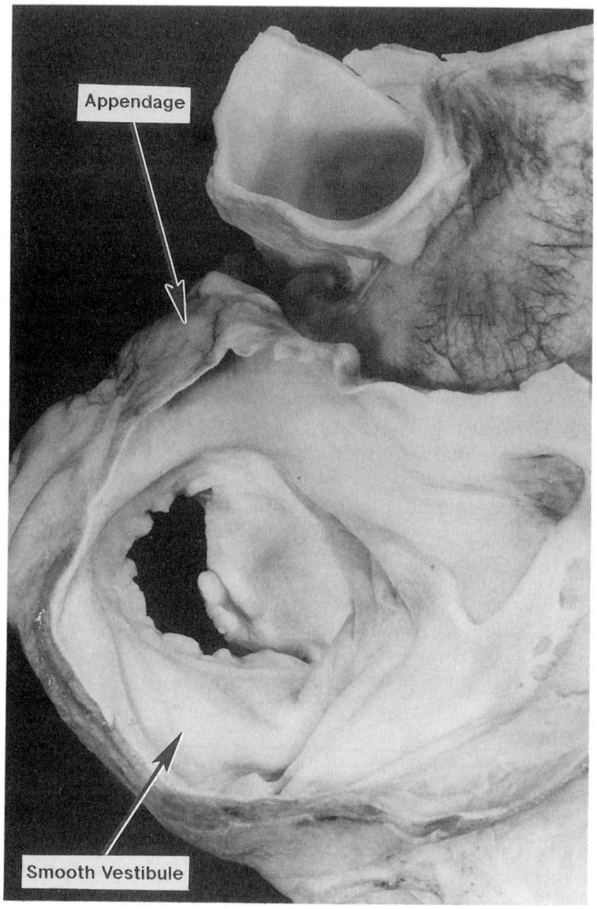

Fig. 12 The morphologically left atrium is viewed through the pulmonary venous component. Note that the appendage has minimal relation to the vestibule, which is smooth continuous with the smooth venous component. Compare with Fig. 11.

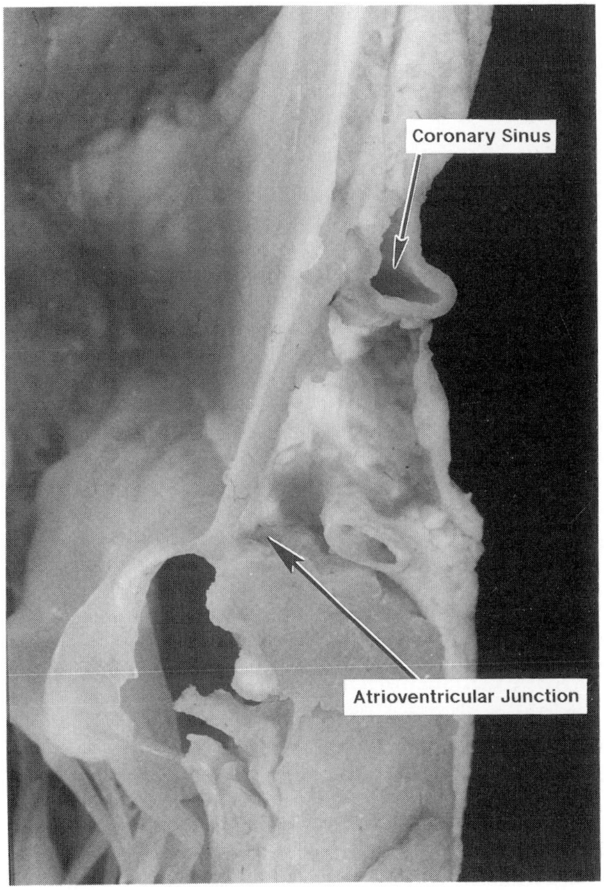

Fig. 13 This section across the morphologically left atrioventricular junction shows the characteristic coronary sinus.

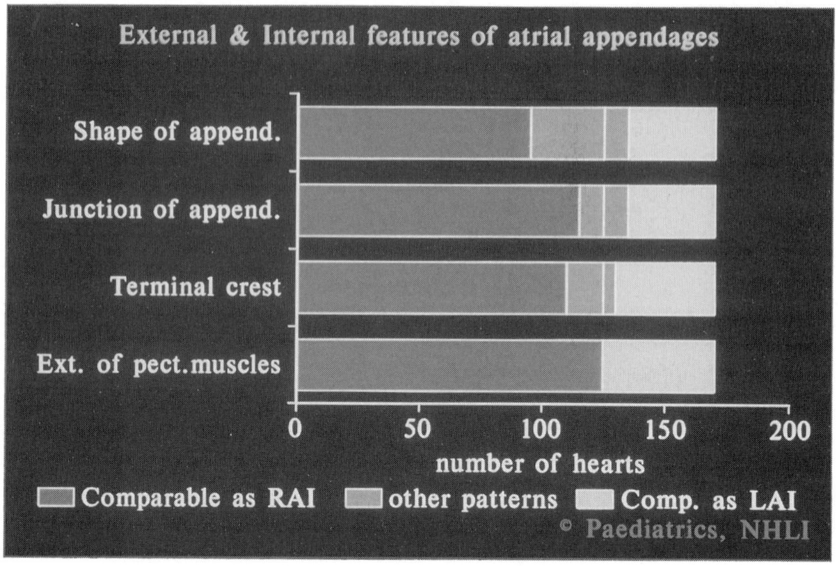

Fig. 14 Examination of 182 hearts from patients with visceral heterotaxy by Uemura *et al.*[19] showed that, when judged on the shape, the nature of the junction or the presence of a terminal crest, it was not always possible to recognize isomerism of the atrial appendages (append.). When examined on the basis of the extent (ext.) of the pectinate (pect.) muscles, however, it proved possible to segregate all hearts as having either isomeric right (RAI) or isomeric left (LAI) atrial appendages.

When Uemura then studied the concordance between the morphology of the appendages and that of the bronchial tree, there was harmony in the greater majority of the cases.[19] Comparisons with splenic status, however, showed major discrepancies. Of the patients who had isomerism of the appendages, and the constellation of cardiac anomalies anticipated for "asplenia", 17% proved to have either multiple spleens or else a solitary spleen on either the right or left side (Fig. 15). In similar fashion (Fig. 16), 10% of those with isomeric left appendages, who would be anticipated to possess multiple spleens, had absence of the spleen, or else solitary spleens on one or other side.[19] These data are not cited in an attempt to suggest that splenic status is unimportant. Rather that, in patients with visceral heterotaxy, the status of the spleen is of less value as a guide to the findings within the heart than is the morphology of the atrial appendages, with significant variation emerging when large series are analyzed on the basis of these two features.[25] One further important aspect then emerges when analysis is based upon the structure of the atrial appendages. The sinus node is an integral part of the junction between the morphologically right appendage and the body of the right atrium. In all the cases with isomeric right atrial appendages of which we are aware in which histological studies have been conducted,[26–28] with the exception of one case,[29] the sinus nodes have also been bilaterally symmetrical structures, a fact first emphasized by Van Mierop and Wiglesworth.[26] In the greater majority of cases studied with isomeric left appendages, in contrast, it is either impossible to find a sinus node, or else a rudimentary nodal structure is found adjacent to the atrioventricular junctions.[27,19] Combining together the

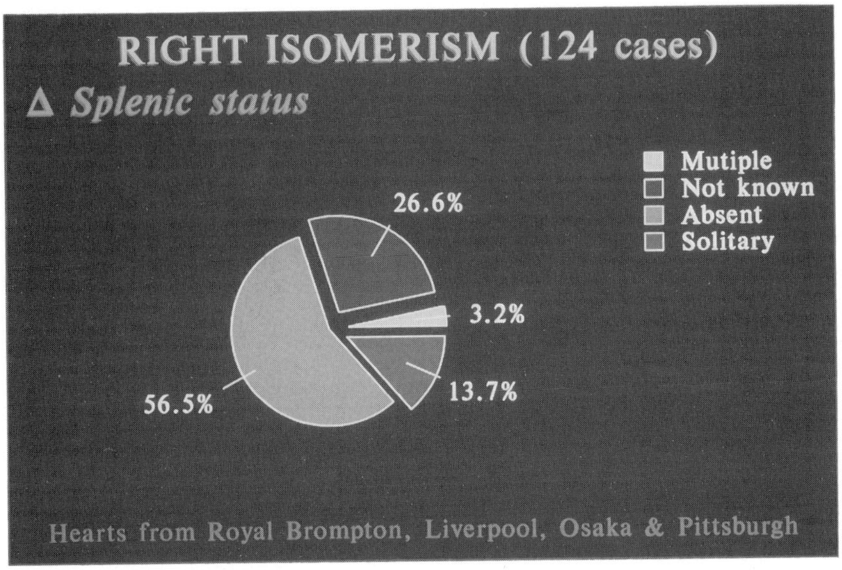

Fig. 15 Analysis of splenic state in the 124 patients shown to have isomeric atrial appendages according to the extent of the pectinate muscles by Uemura *et al.*[19] — see Fig. 14 — revealed that only 56.5% had the anticipated absence of splenic tissue.

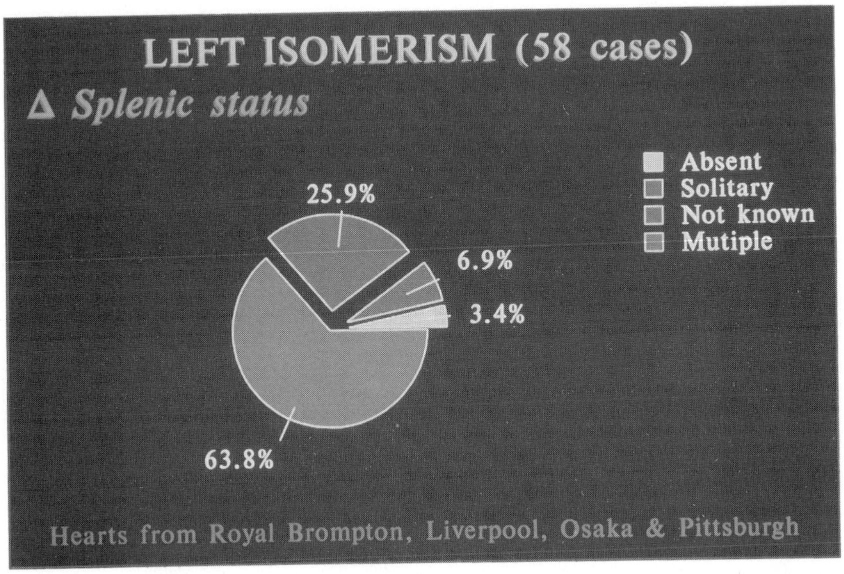

Fig. 16 Analysis of the patients with isomeric left appendages in the study of Uemura *et al.*[19] showed that only 63.8% had the anticipated multiple spleens.

evidence from the location of the sinus node with that related to the extent of the pectinate muscles, it is evident that hearts from patients with visceral heterotaxy can readily be segregated into subsets with isomerism of either the morphologically right or the morphologically left atrial appendages (Fig. 17). Indeed, when this concept is then extended to analysis of the overall spectrum of congenitally malformed hearts, it is clear that all patients can be

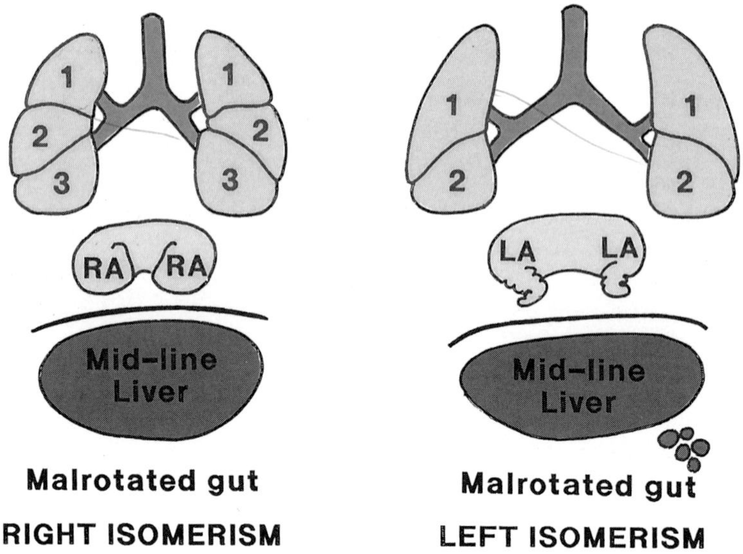

Fig. 17 Analysis of the overall arrangement of the organs in patients with visceral heterotaxy shows that the structure of the thoracic organs is basically one of isomerism when the atrial chambers are judged on the morphology of the appendages based on the extent of the pectinate muscles (see Figs. 11 and 12). In any individual case, nonetheless, it may be necessary to describe each system of organs separately, since the arrangements are not always absolute. The structure of the appendages remains the best guide to the segmental arrangement of the heart.

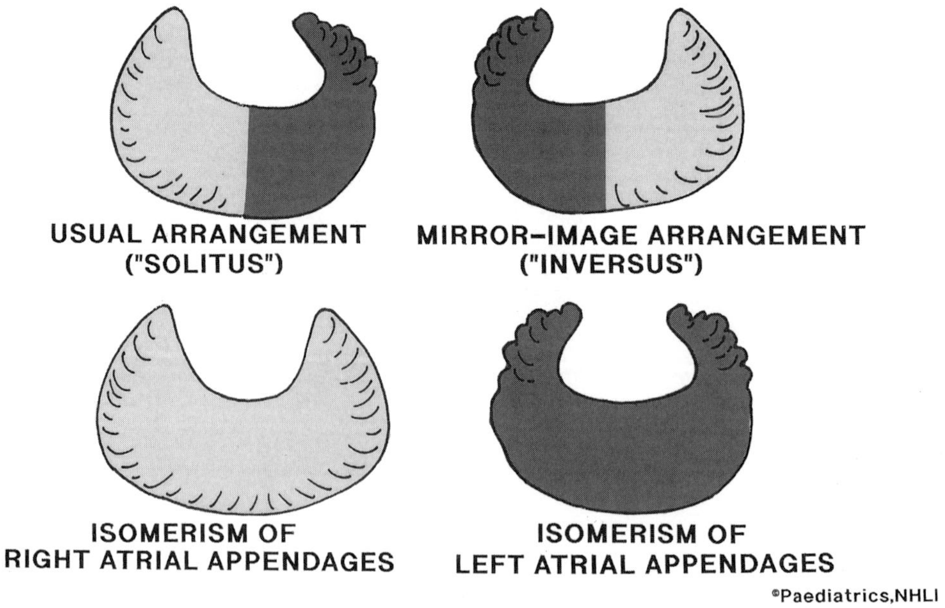

Fig. 18 When the atrial chambers are analysed on the basis of the extent of the pectinate muscles within the appendages, then all hearts fit into one of the four groups shown. The diagram illustrates the short axis of the atrial chambers viewed from the ventricular aspect. Venoatrial connections are variable, and must be described separately.

placed into one of four groups according to the morphology of their atrial appendages. These groups are the usual arrangement, its mirror image, or the variants with isomerism of either the morphologically right or morphologically left appendages (Fig. 18).

MORPHOLOGY OF HEARTS WITH ISOMERIC ATRIAL APPENDAGES

It is well known that the combinations of lesions to be found in hearts from patients with visceral heterotaxy are the most complex in the overall spectrum of congenitally malformed hearts. Not all patients, however, exhibit complex combinations. Of these, notably those with isomeric left appendages, some can have relatively simple combinations of lesions, such as an "ostium primum" atrioventricular septal defect. For the purposes of diagnosis, therefore, it is necessary to treat each patient on an individual basis, following a strict sequential segmental approach which starts with the recognition of the isomeric appendages. In reality, however, it will often be the specific combination of lesions within the heart which points to the likely presence of isomeric atrial appendages. This can then be confirmed by direct echocardiographic recognition,[30] by examination of the penetrated chest

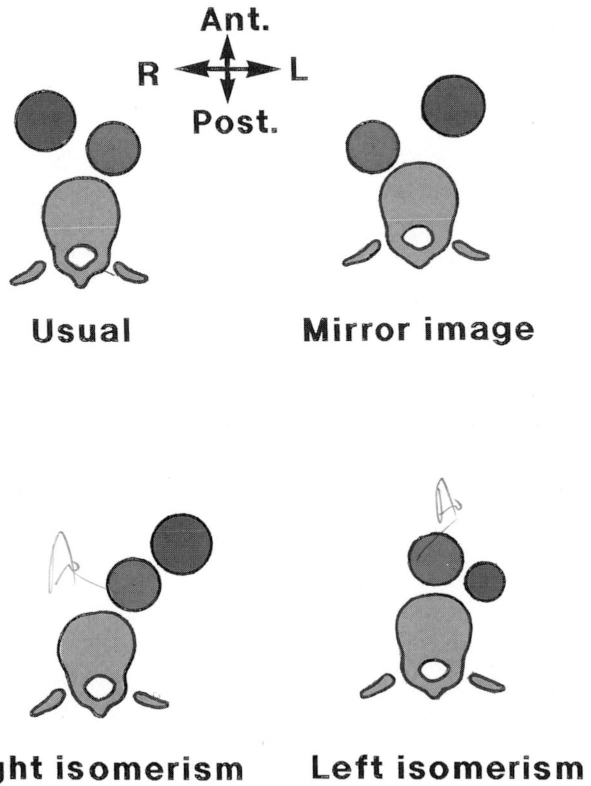

Fig. 19 In most cases, but not all, the presence of isomerism can be inferred from the arrangement of the abdominal great vessels relative to the spine. In the final analysis, nonetheless, it may be necessary to describe each system in its own right.

radiograph to determine bronchial morphology[31] (Fig. 8), or by ultrasonic examination of the relationship of the abdominal great vessels to each other and to the spine[32] (Fig. 19). The latter two methods, of course, are inferential. It is much preferable, if possible, to make the diagnosis directly, but this may not always be feasible prior to surgery. It is also important to be aware, therefore, of the particular combination of lesions which presage the likely presence of right or left isomerism.

The atrial anatomy is dominated by the presence of the isomeric appendages (Figs. 20, 21) coupled with grossly abnormal venoatrial connections. In patients with right isomerism, the cardinal feature is the pectinate muscles extending symmetrically round both atrioventricular junctions to meet at the crux (Fig. 22). Most frequently, the atrial septum is also grossly deficient, often represented merely by a muscular strand spanning the common atrial cavity. There is a common atrioventricular valve in the majority of cases (Fig. 22). Bilateral superior caval veins are also found in most cases and, when present, each drains directly to the atrial roof, almost always being separated from the morphologically right appendage by bilateral terminal crests (Figs. 23, 24). Terminal crests can be absent on one side or

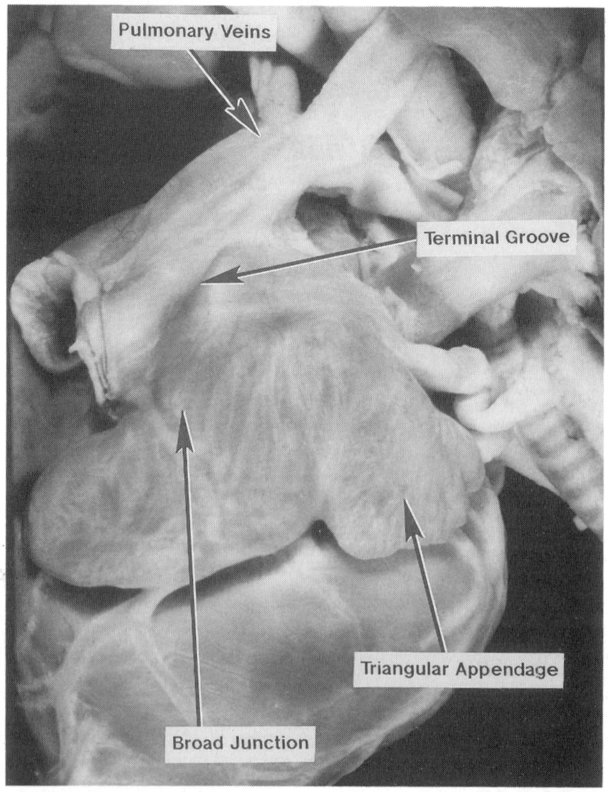

Fig. 20 The typical triangular right-sided appendage of right morphology from a patient with right isomerism. Note the terminal groove, the broad junction with the venous component, and the anomalous connection of the pulmonary veins. These features are present in the greater majority of cases.

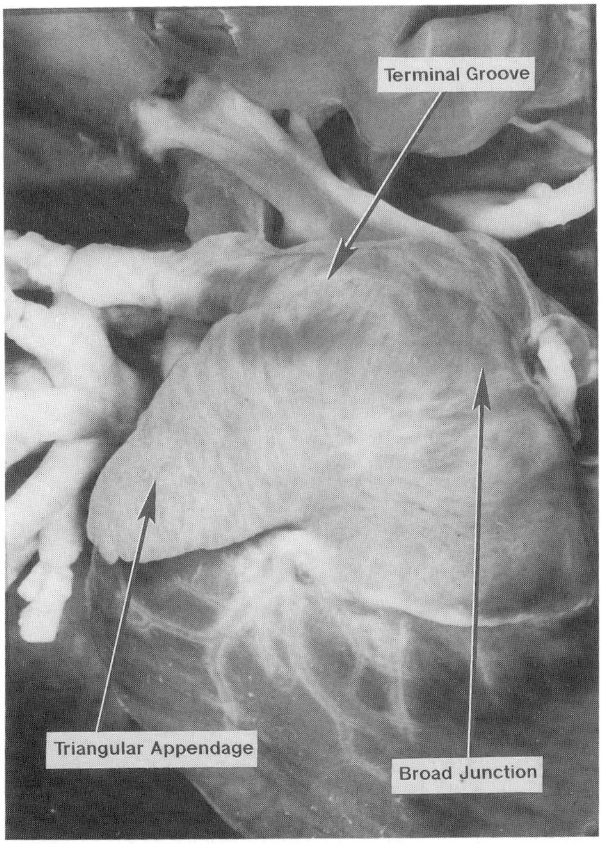

Fig. 21 The left-sided appendage of the heart illustrated in Fig. 20. It is also triangular, with a broad junction across a terminal groove with the systemic venous component. As with the right-sided appendage, it is of right morphology.

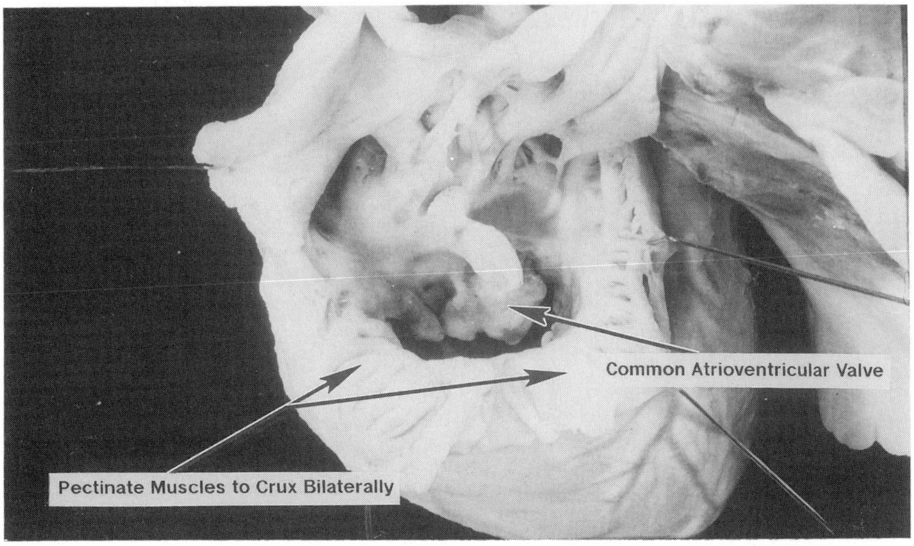

Fig. 22 Although the shape of the appendages is characteristic (see Figs. 20 and 21), it is the extent of the pectinate muscles, as illustrated in this heart by reflecting the atrial dome, which always serves to identify the presence of right isomerism within the atrial segment of the heart.

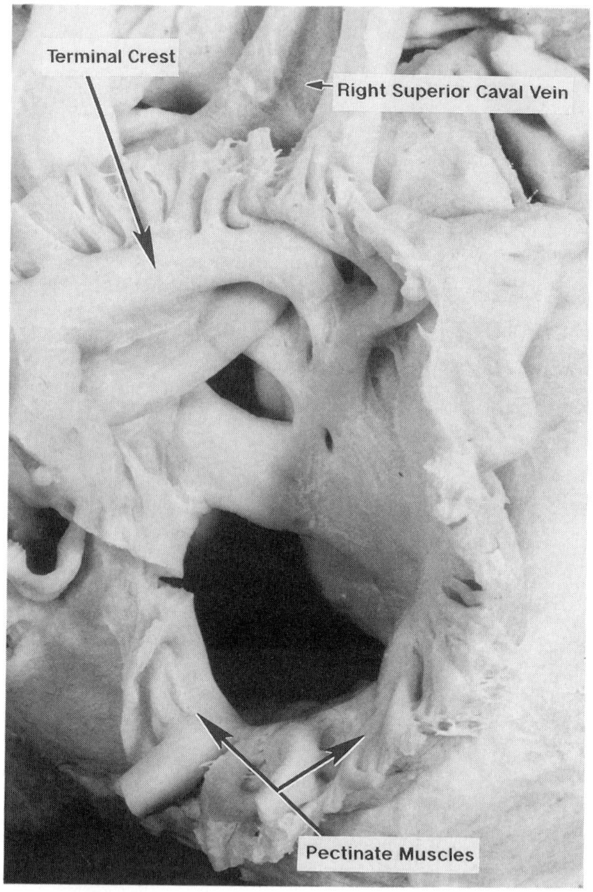

Fig. 23 The right-sided atrium from a heart with isomeric right appendages is opened to show the extent of the pectinate muscles and the opening of the right superior caval vein relative to the terminal crest. Note the absence of the coronary sinus.

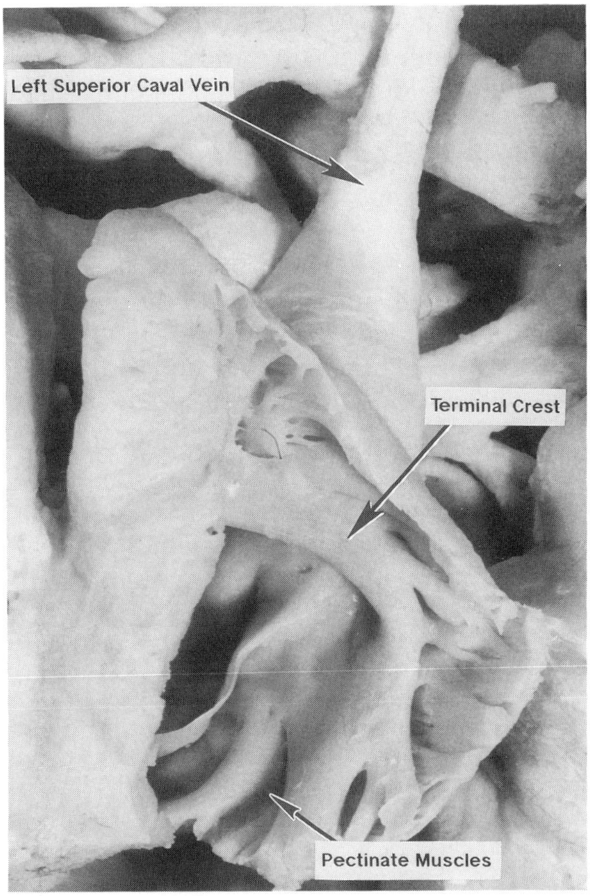

Fig. 24 The left-sided atrium from the heart shown in Fig. 23. Note the extent of the pectinate muscles, the terminal crest, and the opening of the left superior caval vein. This atrium also has an appendage of unequivocal right morphology.

other in a small proportion of cases (Fig. 14). In some instances, one of the bilateral superior caval veins may be atretic, or a unilateral superior caval vein may be present, either on the right or on the left (Fig. 25). Irrespective of the number of superior caval veins present, the most characteristic feature of atrial anatomy in the presence of isomeric right atrial appendages is complete absence of the coronary sinus. In keeping with the absence of any transverse channel in the atrioventricular junctions, the drainage of the coronary veins is grossly abnormal. Uemura identified three specific patterns,[33] which he designated as direct, crooked, and distant return (Fig. 26). The coronary veins with distant return are particularly significant, since they can extend for appreciable distances through the atrial myocardium, entering the atrial chamber well away from the atrioventricular junctions (Fig. 27). They are at major risk during surgical procedures for correction of the abnormal venoatrial connections.[33] In contrast to the absence of the coronary sinus, the inferior caval vein almost always drains directly to the atriums in patients with isomeric right appendages, sometimes bilaterally but more usually unilaterally, with connection to either the right- or left-sided atrium (Fig. 28). We are aware of only two cases reported with interruption of the inferior caval vein in the setting of right isomerism, and no cases were encountered in the extensive series studied by Uemura *et al.*[19] (Fig. 29), nor in the subset of the large series of patients with visceral heterotaxy stratified in terms of "asplenia" by Rubino and his colleagues.[18] The pulmonary veins, in contrast, are always connected in anomalous fashion in patients with isomeric right appendages, even when they drain directly to the atriums (Figs. 6, 30, 31). Cardiac connection occurred in 43% of the cases examined by Uemura *et al.*[19] Rubino and his colleagues[18] argued that drainage to the atriums could occur in normal fashion

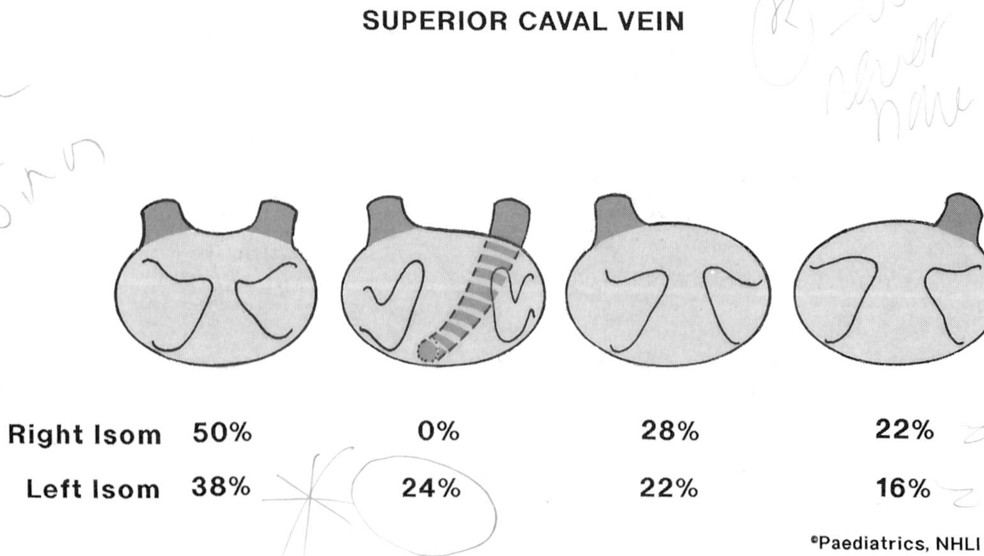

Fig. 25 The connections of the superior caval veins in the overall series of hearts studied by Uemura *et al.*[19] and shown to have isomerism on the basis of the structure of the atrial appendages. Note that drainage via the coronary sinus is found only in the setting of left isomerism.

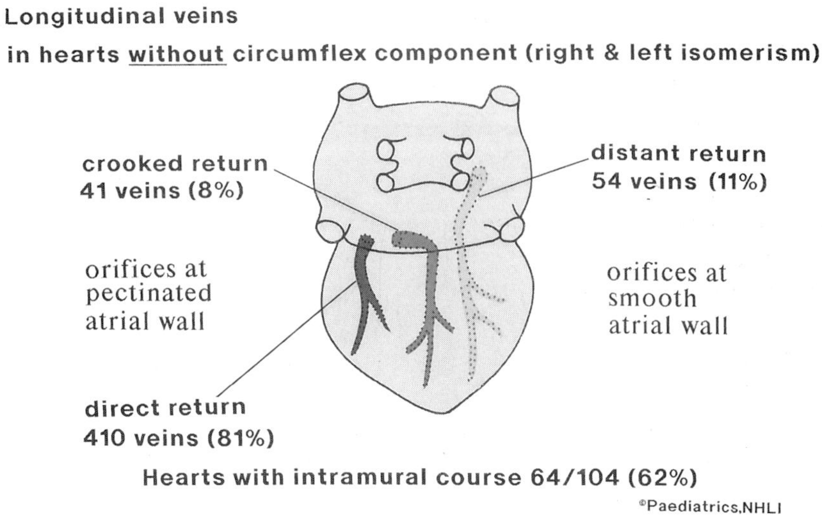

Fig. 26 In the absence of the coronary sinus, the venous return from the heart itself is abnormal. This diagram shows the arrangement of the ventricular veins in the hearts studied by Uemura *et al.*,[19] and includes cases with right and left isomerism.

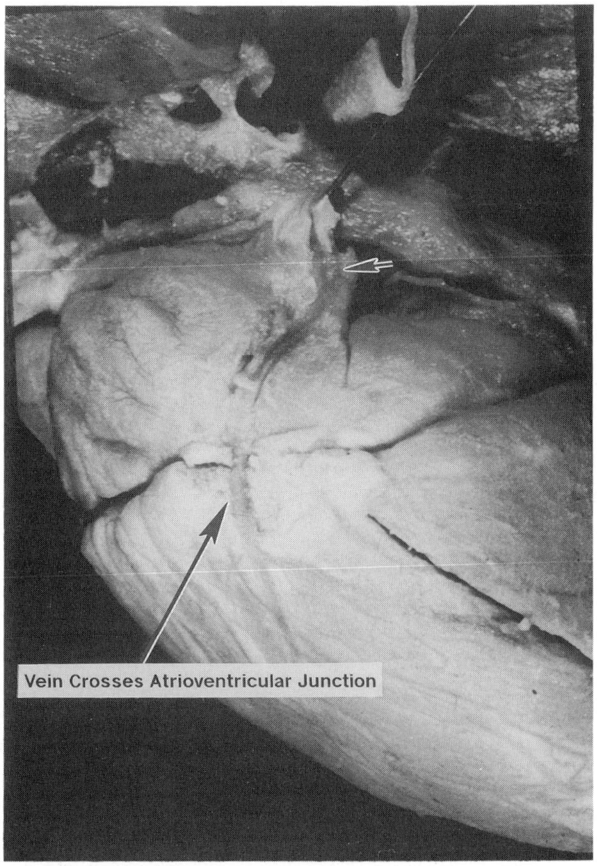

Fig. 27 A typical example of distant return of a coronary vein in a case with isomeric right atrial appendages. Note the termination close to the orifice of a pulmonary vein (arrowed).

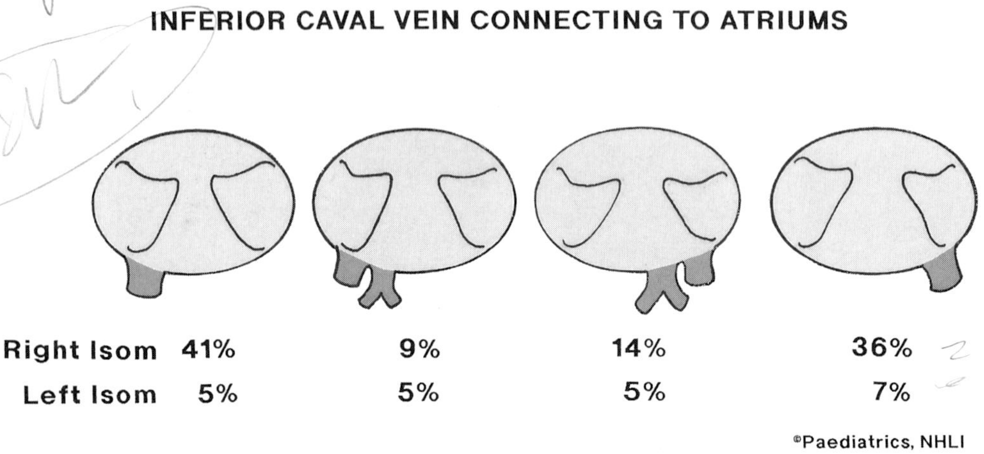

Fig. 28 The drainage of the inferior caval vein in the overall series of the hearts with isomeric appendages studied by Uemura *et al.*[19] Of the hearts with isomeric left atrial appendages, 78% had interruption of the inferior caval vein, with return through the azygos venous system. The bifurcating venous channels represent separate drainage of the hepatic veins.

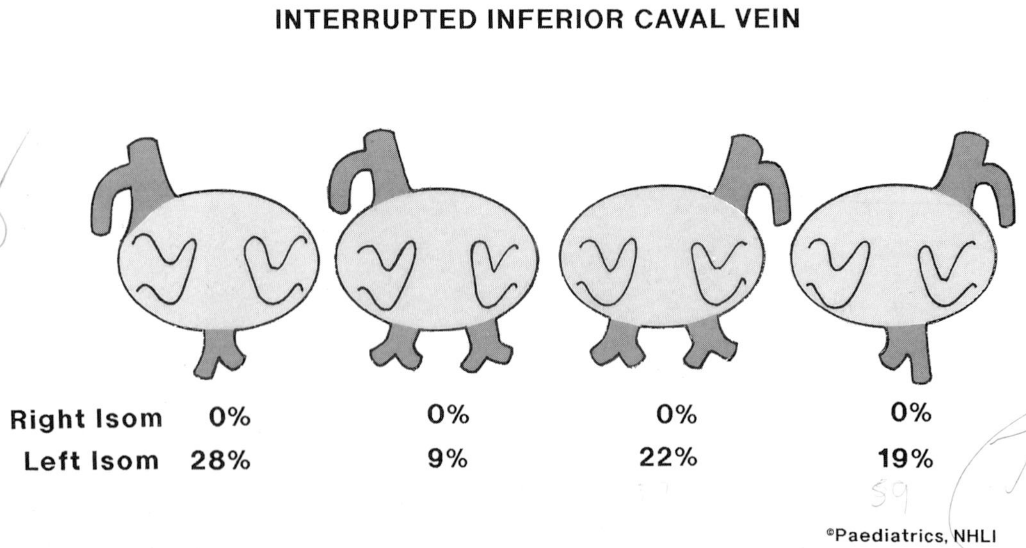

Fig. 29 Details of the arrangement of the venous connections in the hearts with interruption of the inferior caval vein in the series studied by Uemura *et al.*[19] Note that no patients with right isomerism had interruption of the inferior caval vein.

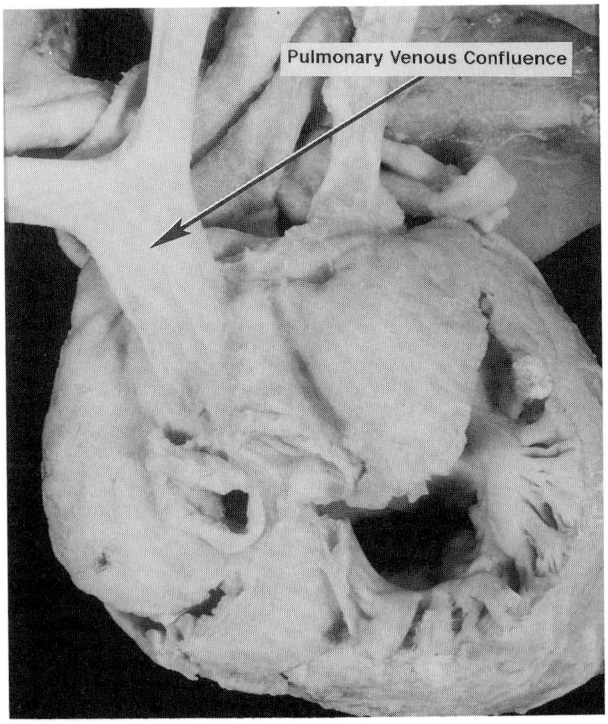

Fig. 30 The typical arrangement of anomalous connection of the pulmonary veins to the atrial roof in a heart with isomeric right atrial appendages. Note the absence of muscle in the pulmonary venous confluence.

in their patients with asplenia, and be explained on the basis of malposition of the atrial septum. Even taking note of the fact that some of the patients described by Rubino *et al.*[18] may have shown absence of the spleen in association with usual atrial arrangement, we have major problems with their concept of malposition of the primary septum. If we examine the normal drainage of the pulmonary veins in hearts with usual atrial arrangement, we see that one vein is attached at each corner of the extensive pulmonary venous component of the morphologically left atrium (Fig. 32). Furthermore, the dome of the left atrium between the pulmonary veins is made up of muscle, with a characteristic array of internal fibres surrounding each of the venous orifices. We have never seen such an arrangement in a heart from a patient with isomeric right atrial appendages. When the pulmonary veins drain to the atriums in right isomerism, they usually connect to the midpoint of an effectively common atrial chamber, draining through a fibrous pulmonary venous sinus (Fig. 30) which lacks the normal musculature found in the dome of a morphologically left atrium. We have encountered two hearts in which all four pulmonary veins drained to the right-sided atrium, and all the systemic veins to the left-sided atrium, and in which the atrial septum was virtually intact. Even in these hearts, the presence of the pectinate muscles and terminal crest in the right-sided atrium meant that the pulmonary venous connection was anatomically abnormal (Figs. 31–33), while the left-sided atrium, although possessing a morphologically right appendage, received the

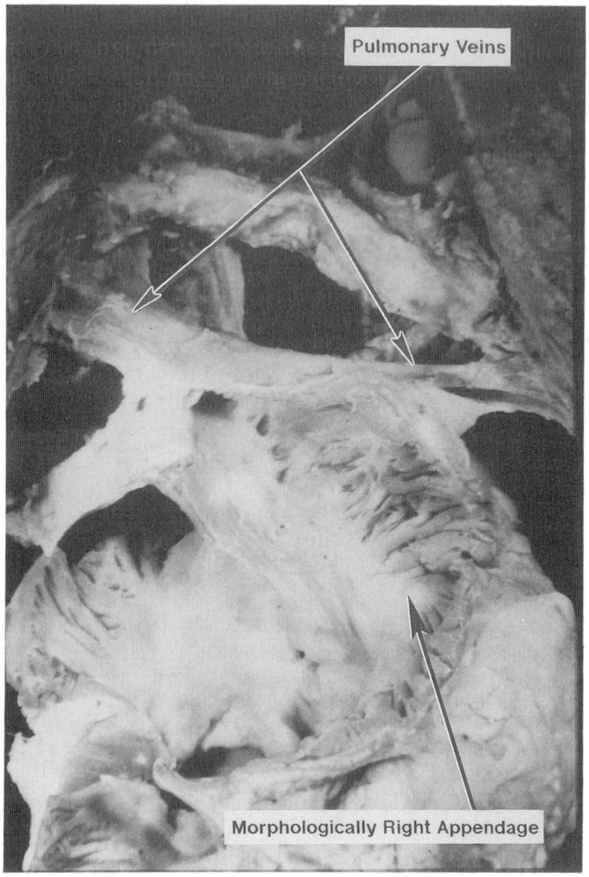

Fig. 31 In this heart, the pulmonary veins are abnormally attached to an atrium with a morphologically right appendage.

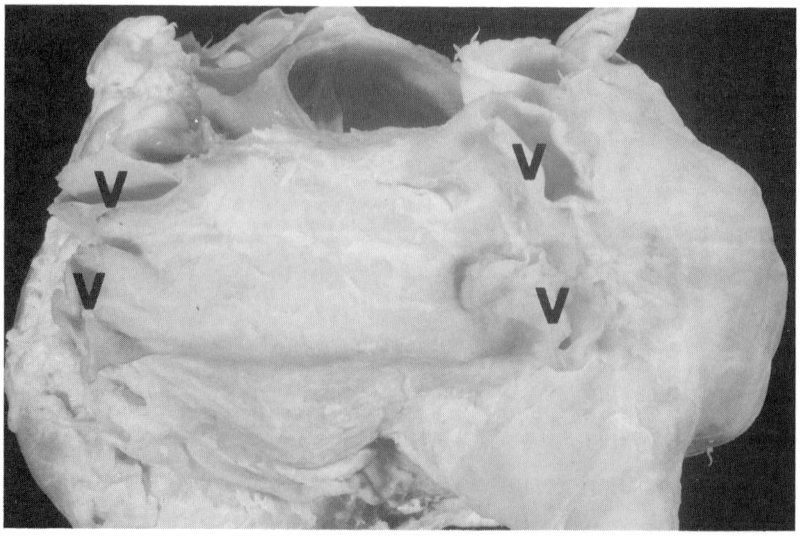

Fig. 32 The usual arrangement of connection of the pulmonary veins (V) to the morphologically left atrium, with one vein at each corner of the chamber, and with a muscular dome between the venous orifices.

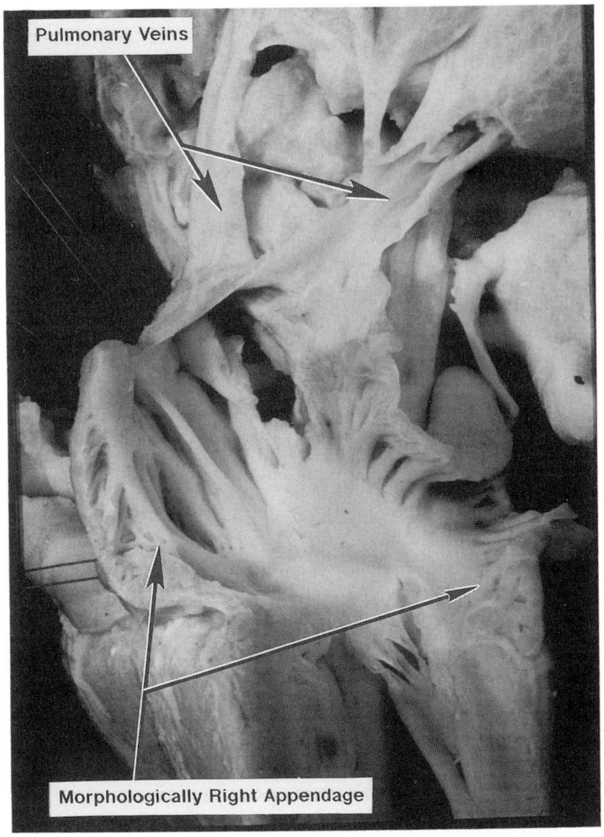

Fig. 33 Another heart with anomalous connection of the pulmonary veins to a right-sided atrium with a morphologically right appendage. The atrial septum was initially intact.

superior and inferior caval veins (Fig. 34). Furthermore, had the surgeon designated mirror imaged arrangement in these cases on the basis of the venoatrial connections, inappropriately placed incisions could well have damaged the sinus nodes, which are anticipated bilaterally because of the presence of the isomeric right appendages. In the majority of cases, however, there is no question about the abnormality of the pulmonary venous drainage because it is to an extracardiac sump. This can be supracardiac (Fig. 35) or infracardiac, or can be mixed. Drainage cannot occur through a coronary sinus, since this structure is always absent in patients with isomeric right atrial appendages.

The atrial septum is usually much better formed in patients with isomeric left atrial appendages although, on occasion, there can be a common chamber, characterized then by the bilateral smooth vestibules posteriorly (Fig. 36), and the connection bilaterally of two pulmonary veins to the left-sided and right-sided extremities of the common atrial chamber (Fig. 37). More usually, the atrial septum is intact, or else there is an atrioventricular septal defect present (Fig. 38). Bilateral superior caval veins are found in left isomerism just as frequently as in right (Fig. 25). Their connections to the atrial chambers, in contrast, are markedly different. Terminal crests are lacking in atriums with

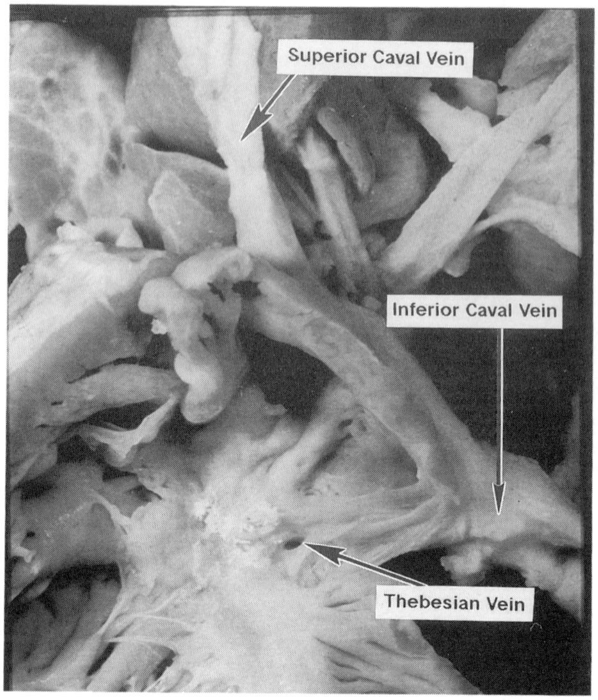

Fig. 34 The left-sided atrium from the heart shown in Fig. 33 is seen to receive all the systemic venous return, but also to have an appendage of morphologically right type. Thus, although the venoatrial connections are mirror imaged, the heart has isomeric right atrial appendages. Note the absence of the coronary sinus, with a Thebesian vein at its anticipated site of drainage.

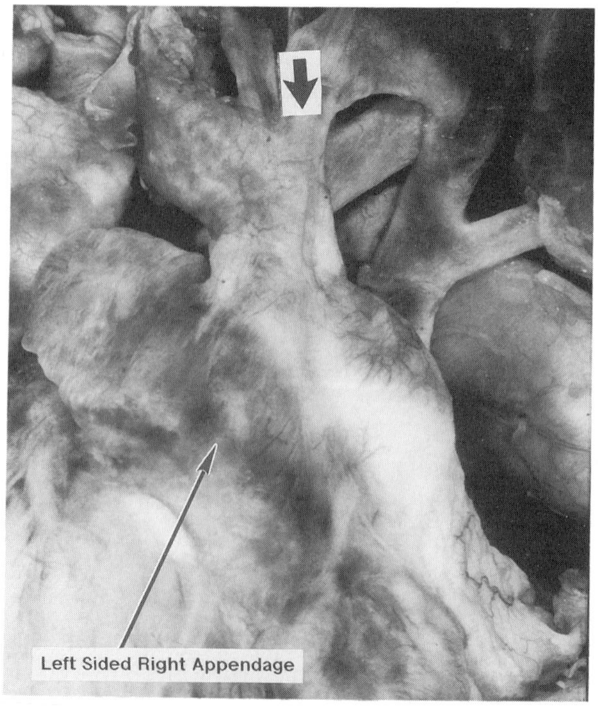

Fig. 35 Anomalous connection of the pulmonary veins to the left superior caval vein (arrowed) in a heart with isomeric right atrial appendages.

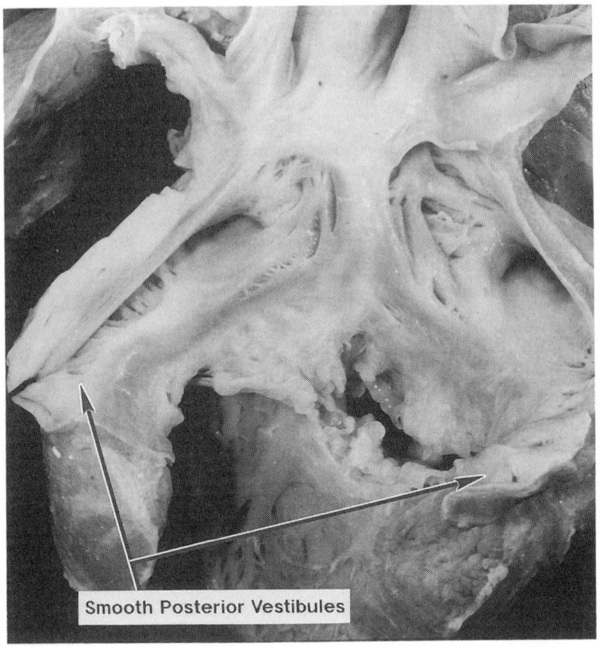

Fig. 36 The characteristic smooth posterior vestibules, confluent with the venous components, in a heart with isomeric left atrial appendages.

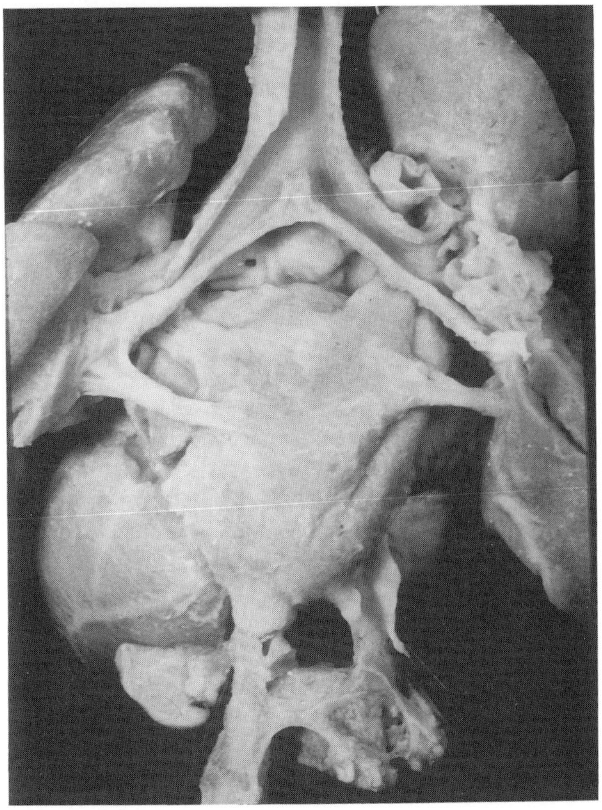

Fig. 37 Symmetrical pulmonary veins, hepatic veins and bronchial tree in a heart with isomeric left atrial appendages viewed from behind.

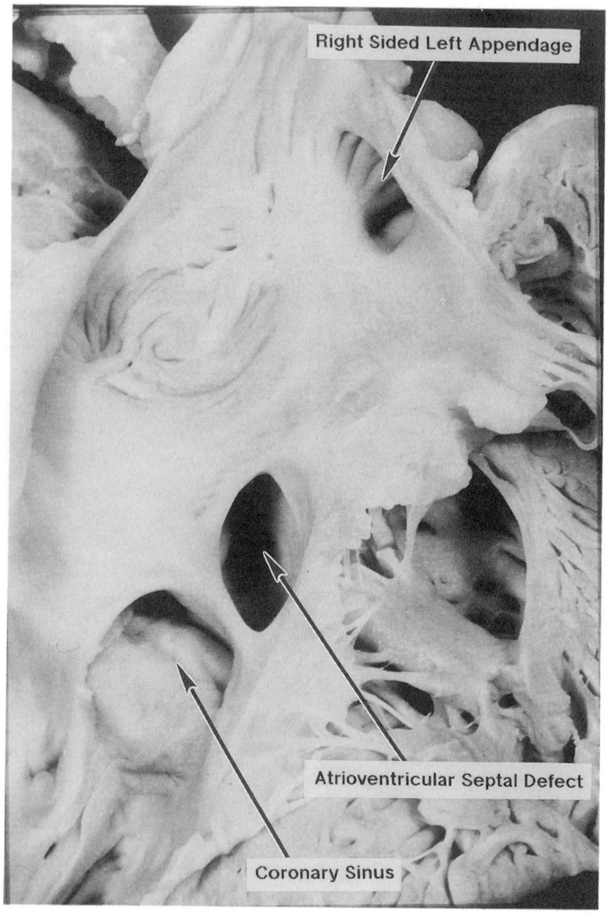

Fig. 38 This heart with isomeric left atrial appendages (note the narrow opening of the right-sided appendage) has an atrioventricular septal defect with separate right and left atrioventricular orifices, and the left superior caval vein draining through the coronary sinus to the right-sided atrium.

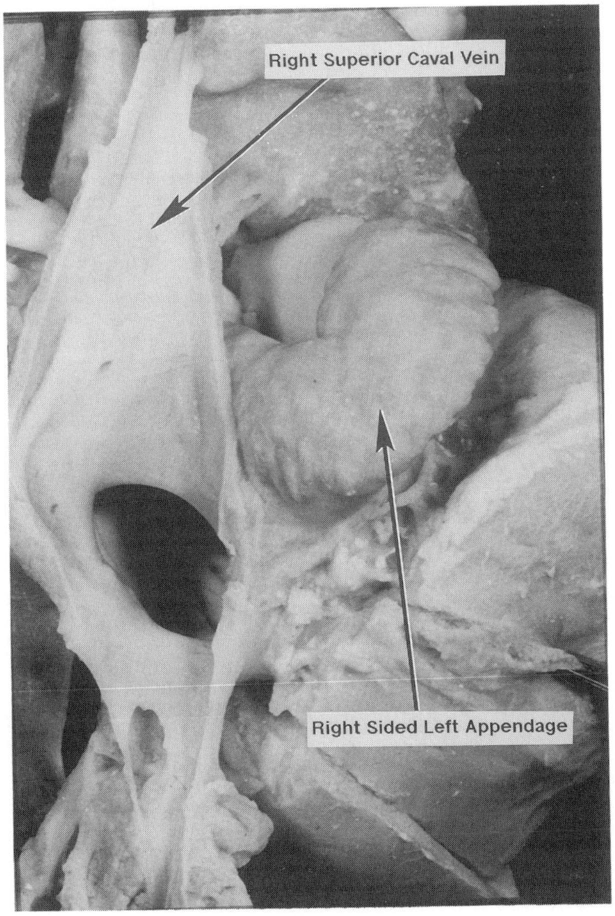

Fig. 39 The typical drainage of the right superior caval vein relative to a morphologically left atrial appendage in a heart with isomeric left appendages. Note the absence of the terminal crest.

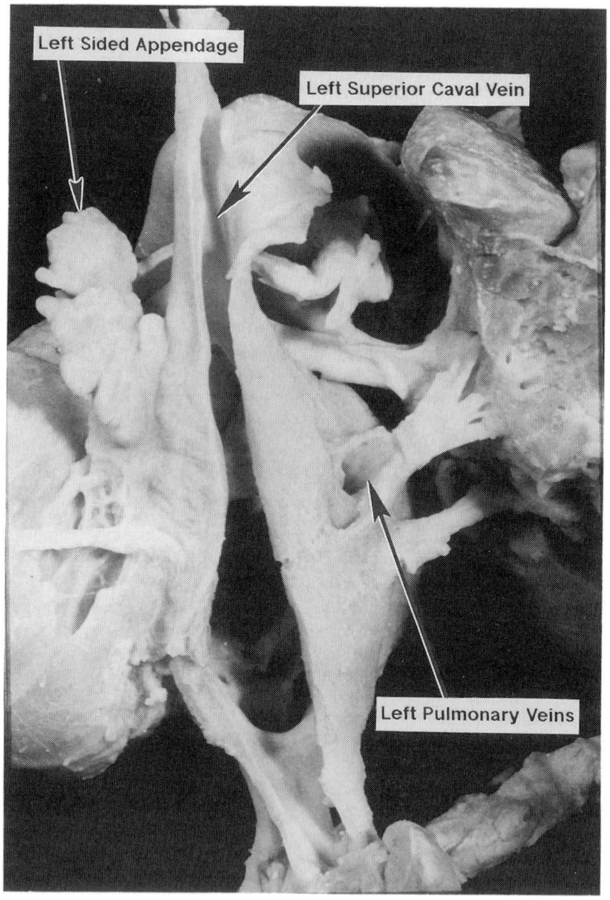

Fig. 40 The typical drainage of the left superior caval vein between the appendage and the pulmonary veins in a heart with left isomerism.

morphologically left appendages (Fig. 39), and the caval venous opening is usually sandwiched between the orifice of the appendage and the pulmonary venous connections (Fig. 40), often marked by extensive folds. In patients with isomeric left appendages, the coronary sinus can be present (Fig. 38) and, when found, can drain one of the superior caval veins as well as the venous return from the heart itself (Fig. 41). The coronary sinus, nonetheless, is not universally present. In its absence, the termination of the coronary veins can be as abnormal as in right isomerism[33] (Figs. 26, 41). The major venous anomaly found in hearts with isomeric left appendages, nonetheless, is interruption of the abdominal inferior caval vein, with continuation and drainage through the azygos system of veins (Fig. 42). Strictly speaking, since patients with left isomerism have symmetry of morphologically left structures, the veins should be considered to be hemiazygos. But they can be found to the left or the right, so it is simpler to describe them as left or right azygos systems. Such azygos return, on either side, was found in 77% of the cases with left isomerism studied by Uemura *et al.*[19] (Fig. 29). It had been thought that, in patients with interruption of the inferior caval vein, the presence of a confluent venous channel draining the hepatic veins to one or other atrium distinguished those with lateralized atrial arrangement from those with left isomerism, bilateral hepatic venous drainage being considered the rule in the latter setting[32] (Fig. 37). Unfortunately, observation of hearts with isomeric left appendages does not bear out this supposition. A confluent suprahepatic venous channel (Fig. 42) was found by Uemura *et al.*[19] in 43% of those cases with interrupted abdominal inferior caval veins (Fig. 29). Direct return of the abdominal systemic veins through an inferior caval vein was also found in

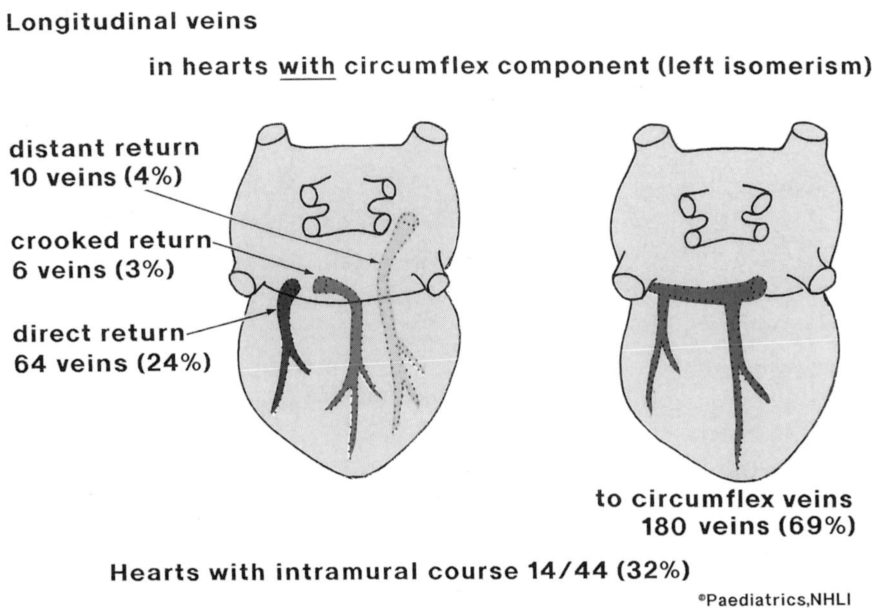

Fig. 41 The arrangement of drainage of venous return from the heart itself in those patients with left isomerism studied by Uemura *et al.*[19] in which a circumflex component of the coronary venous system was present in the atrioventricular grooves.

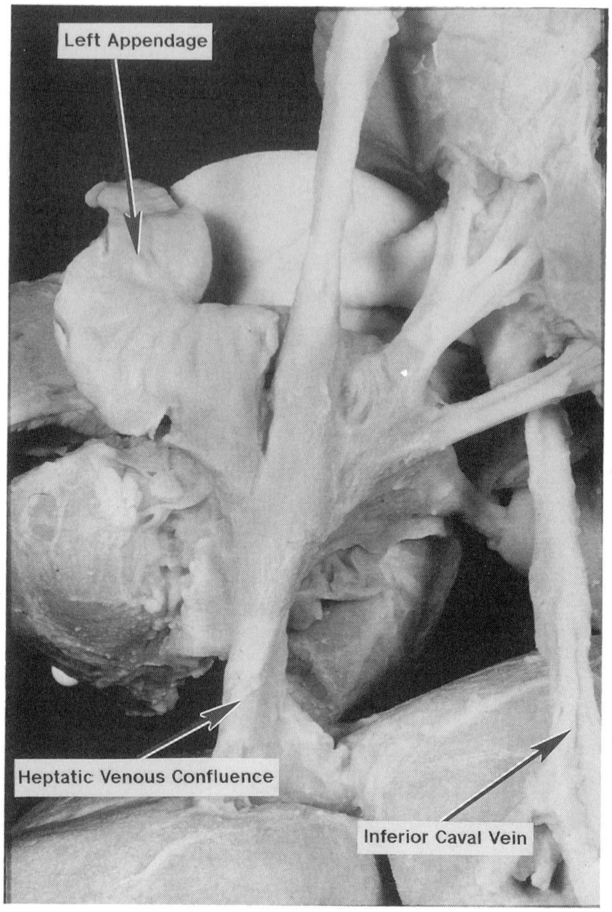

Fig. 42 An example of the interrupted inferior caval vein, with return through the azygos venous system, which is so typical of left isomerism. Note the hepatic venous confluence connecting directly to the atrium.

20% of cases, and bilateral inferior caval veins, each draining to a separate atrial chamber with a morphologically left appendage, were present in a small number (Fig. 28). It is difficult to reconcile the finding of an inferior caval vein draining bilaterally to atrial chambers each possessing a morphologically left appendage with the hypothesis that the morphologically right atrium can always be identified on the basis of the connection of the inferior caval vein.[17] Using this hypothesis, we would have major problems in categorizing some of the hearts studied by Uemura *et al.*[19] The patients had multiple spleens, so would have been labelled "polysplenia". Yet the presence of bilateral inferior caval veins, each draining to an atrium, would have pointed to bilateral right atriums, a condition held not to exist by those who use venoatrial connections to predict atrial morphology.[17] In reality, such patients have two atriums, each with a morphologically left atrial appendage and each receiving an inferior caval vein. It is findings of this kind which emphasize the need to describe atrial arrangement according to the morphology of the appendages in addition to specifying the venoatrial connections.

Whenever the pulmonary veins connect to the atrial chambers in the setting of isomerism of the morphologically left appendages, they do so in anatomically normal fashion, but the veins can be connected so that two veins join to each of the atrial components (Fig. 37). Alternatively, all four veins drain to the same atrium, which can be right-sided or left-sided. Usual or mirror imaged patterns of venous drainage, with all pulmonary veins connected to one atrium with a left appendage and all systemic veins connected to the other atrium, also with a left appendage, were found in 14% of the material studied by Uemura *et al.*[19] Such quasi-usual or quasi-mirror-imaged patterns of drainage were present in only 12.5% of the overall group of hearts obtained from patients with isomeric atrial appendages.[19] These data contradict in no uncertain terms the contention of Rubino *et al.*[18] that patterns of venous drainage in patients with visceral heterotaxy can always be distinguished as "solitus" or "inversus". They emphasize still more strongly the need to describe atrial arrangement, determined according to the morphology of the appendages, as well as venoatrial connections. The overall findings in the setting of visceral heterotaxy show that the venoatrial connections are too variable to provide any realistic inferential guide to atrial "situs" (Figs. 25, 26, 28).

The majority of patients with isomeric atrial appendages possess a common atrioventricular junction. In those with isomeric right appendages, this common junction is most usually part of a double inlet atrioventricular connection, usually to either a dominant left (Fig. 43) or a dominant right ventricle, but not infrequently to a solitary and indeterminate ventricle. Double inlet ventricle can also occur through two separate atrioventricular valves, but is much rarer, as is absence of one of the atrioventricular connections. Right isomerism co-existing with a common atrioventricular junction and biventricular atrioventricular connections,

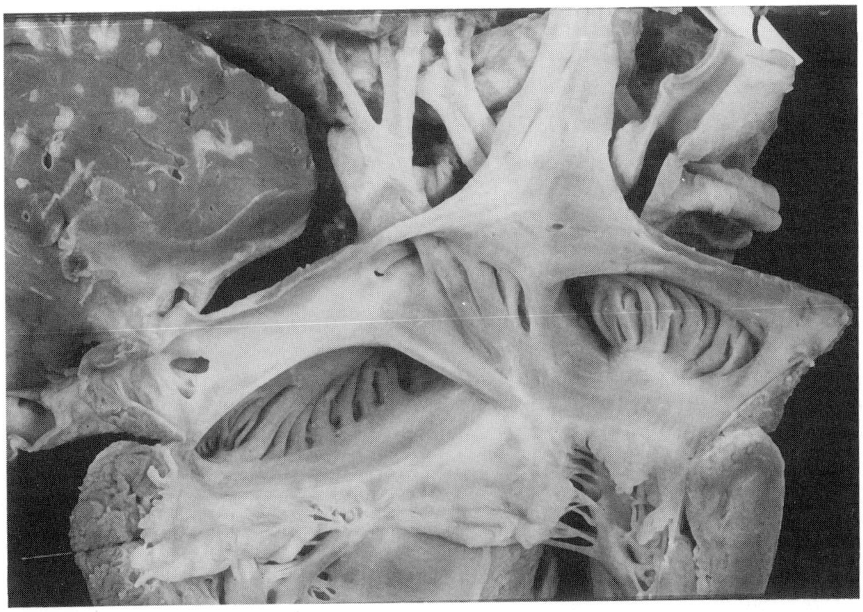

Fig. 43 Double inlet to a dominant left ventricle through a common atrioventricular valve in a heart with isomeric right atrial appendages. Note the bilateral pectinate muscles.

however, is also a frequent finding. In this setting, because of the symmetry of the appendages, the biventricular connection will be ambiguous irrespective of whether the right-sided atrium is connected to a morphologically right ventricle (right-hand topology) or to a morphologically left ventricle (left-hand topology). It is because of the truly ambiguous nature of the biventricular atrioventricular connections found in patients with isomeric atrial appendages that, for full description, it is always necessary to specify both the type of isomerism present and the ventricular topology (Fig. 44). This holds equally good for the rarer examples of right isomerism which exist with a common atrioventricular junction but separate right and left atrioventricular valves, and for those with separate right and left atrioventricular junctions with mitral and tricuspid valves. The same goes for left isomerism, which much more frequently is found with a common atrioventricular junction and separate right and left atrioventricular valves ("ostium primum" defect), or with separate right and left atrioventricular junctions guarded by tricuspid and mitral valves.

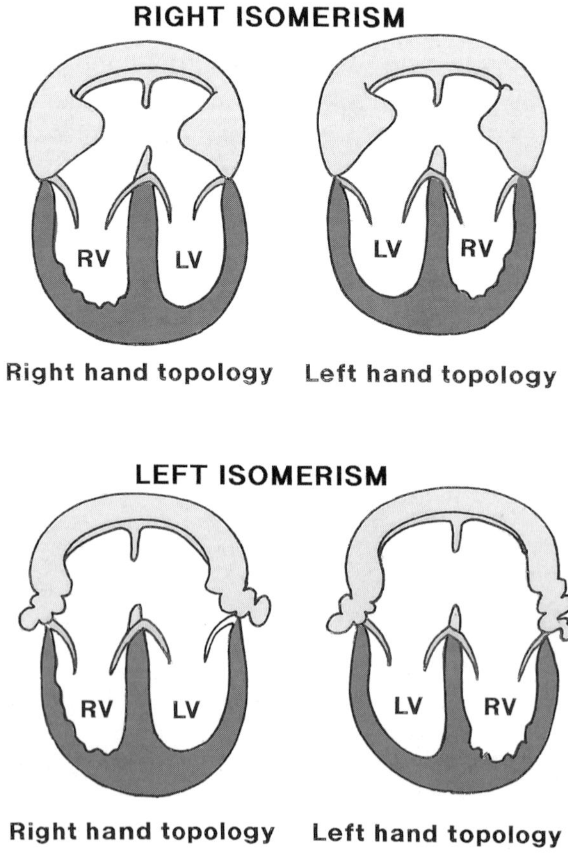

Fig. 44 When each atrium connects to its own ventricle in hearts with isomeric atrial appendages, then the atrioventricular connection, of necessity, is biventricular and ambiguous. It is necessary to account for ventricular topology as well as the nature of the isomerism.

The importance of identifying ventricular topology in patients with isomeric atrial appendages is related to predicting the location of the ventricular conduction tissues. When there is a univentricular atrioventricular connection, most typically double inlet, then the conduction tissues are disposed as for the patient with usual atrial arrangement. Thus, the atrioventricular conduction axis will arise from an anterior node in those with double inlet left ventricle, and in double inlet right ventricle with left-hand ventricular topology. Double inlet right ventricle with right-hand topology has a regular node. Bizarre patterns of the conduction axis are found when hearts with isomeric atrial appendages have a solitary ventricle of indeterminate morphology.[27] With biventricular atrioventricular connections, however, and either right or left isomerism, the conduction axis arises from a posterior node when there is right-hand topology, but from an anterior node or a "sling" in the presence of left-hand topology (Figs. 45, 46). This fact provides still further evidence why it is important to recognize the morphology of the atrial appendages as well as the pattern of venous drainage. Thus, in the heart illustrated in Figs. 33 and 34, there is isomerism of the right atrial appendages and left-hand ventricular topology. This combination indicates that the conduction axis will arise from an anterior atrioventricular node, or else there will be a sling of conduction tissue joining anterior and posterior nodes. The venoatrial connections in this heart, however, are mirror imaged. Following the concept based exclusively on venoatrial connections,[17] this combination of mirror imagery and left-hand topology would be interpreted as indicating concordant atrioventricular alignments, in which, of course, the conduction axis arises from a regularly positioned posterior node.[34] Thus, ignoring the presence of isomeric right atrial appendages in this particular heart (Figs. 33, 34) would lead not only to an erroneous interpretation concerning the site of the sinus node, but also the location of the atrioventricular conduction axis.

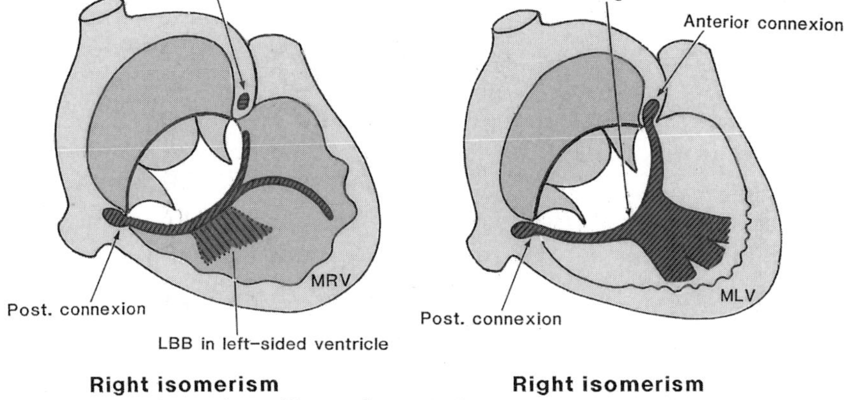

Fig. 45 The variation in the course of the atrioventricular conduction axis in hearts with isomeric right atrial appendages studied histologically.

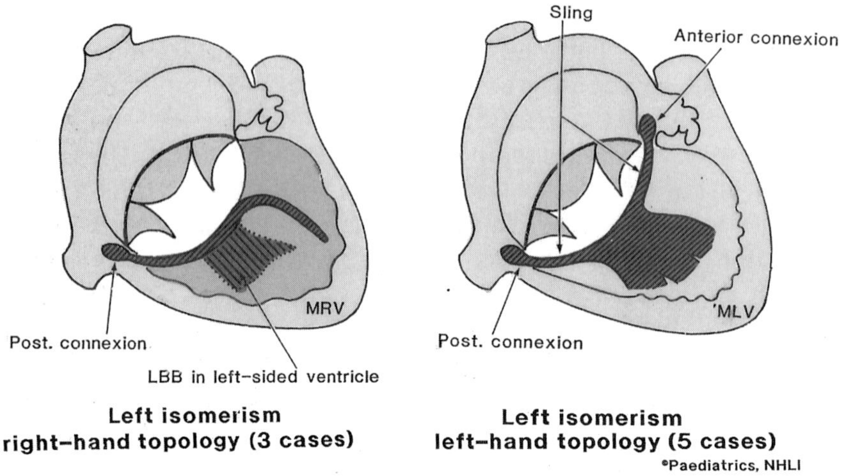

Fig. 46 The course of the atrioventricular conduction axis in patients with isomeric left atrial appendages studied histologically. Note the variation according to the ventricular topology.

Abnormalities of the ventricular outflow tracts are much more frequent in the setting of right isomerism, but can also be found with left isomerism.[35] It is rare to find concordant ventriculo-arterial connections when there are right-sided appendages bilaterally. Most usually, there is a double outlet right ventricle, with bilateral infundibulums in most cases, or else the ventriculo-arterial connections are discordant. These connections themselves are then further complicated by pulmonary stenosis or atresia, but pulmonary atresia can also be found in the setting of tetralogy of Fallot with the aorta connected predominantly in the left ventricle. When there is pulmonary atresia and right isomerism, then almost always the pulmonary arteries are fed through the arterial duct, which may be present bilaterally. Systemic-to-pulmonary collateral arteries can feed the pulmonary circulation in right isomerism, but are rare.

The ventricular outflow tracts are much more frequently normally arranged in the setting of isomeric left atrial appendages, although the concordant connections can be compromised by the presence of aortic stenosis, atresia or coarctation. Other ventriculo-arterial connections and abnormal infundibular morphology, must also be anticipated on occasion.

The cardiac position, and the location of the cardiac apex and the aortic arch, are frequently abnormal in patients with isomerism of either the right or the left atrial appendages. The two subsets of isomerism, nonetheless, cannot be separated statistically on the basis of any of these features.

SYNTHESIS OF FINDINGS

The hearts from patients with visceral heterotaxy unequivocally show symmetry in their atrial segments. The symmetry is seen consistently in the appendages and, while certain of the venoatrial connections can themselves also be symmetrical, it is certainly not the case that the entire atriums are bilaterally symmetrical. Although our initial description can be criticized on the basis that we described "atrial isomerism", it was clear from all our writings[14,15,35] that our arguments concerning symmetry were based on the structure of the atrial appendages. It would be reducing the debate to the absurd to suggest that the heart with left atrial isomerism would be expected to have eight pulmonary veins. Be that as it may, such a criticism can readily be negated by specifying that the isomerism involves the atrial appendages. Recognition of this feature, coupled with full description of venoatrial connections and other intracardiac malformations, then provides a simple account of the pertinent morphology. This must then be rounded out with a description of the arrangement of the remainder of the thoraco-abdominal organs. This is because the different systems of organs are not always arranged in harmonious fashion.[36] While the morphology of the atrial appendages provides the best guide to what is happening within the heart, the state of the spleen is always important in immunologic terms, and should also be specified. Description of all these features, namely atrial appendages, venoatrial connections, and splenic status, then removes all arguments concerning priorities for categorization.[17,18] Attention to the extent of the pectinate muscles within the appendage should then remove the doubts expressed by those who questioned the very existence of isomerism within the atrial segment of the heart.[17]

DEVELOPMENTAL CONSIDERATIONS

Having established that symmetry within the hearts of patients with visceral heterotaxy is found within the atrial appendages, it follows that those who seek clues to the development of symmetry as opposed to lateralization should also focus upon the atrial appendages. This fact is particularly important for those who seek a genetic basis of isomerism and mirror imagery. The patient with so-called "situs inversus" is just as lateralized as is the usually arranged person. Comparison of individuals with these two arrangements, therefore, is crucial if the agents which determine normal versus mirror imaged lateralization are to be discovered. The playing field will become decidedly uneven if such studies include also patients with isomerism. The patients with symmetry of the paired organs, including the appendages, need to be segregated from those with usual or mirror imaged arrangement if the correct answers are to be found. It had been suggested that abnormalities of the gene Connexin 43 may be present in patients with visceral heterotaxy,[37] but subsequent investigators[38,39] could not substantiate the initial claims. It was also thought initially that studies of the iv/iv mutant mouse would shed light on the problem of lateralization, since half of these mutants were held to develop in usual pattern and the other half as mirror imaged variants.[40] Attention to the details of atrial structure with emphasis once more on the extent of the pectinate muscles showed that some of these animals developed symmetry rather than lateralization, and exhibited all the features of both right and left isomerism.[41] Work with the iv/iv mouse, therefore, should take account of these complications.

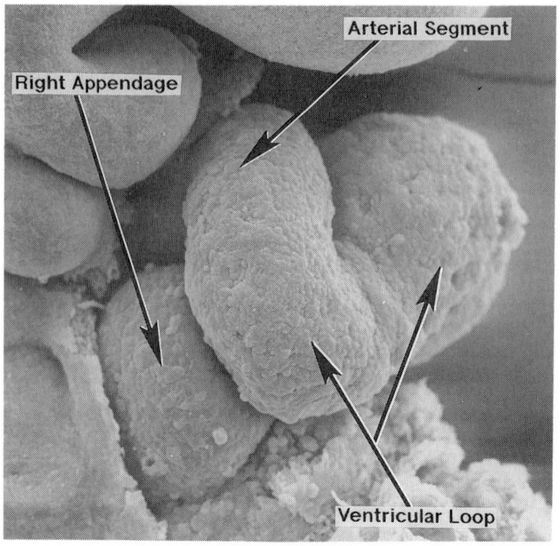

(a)

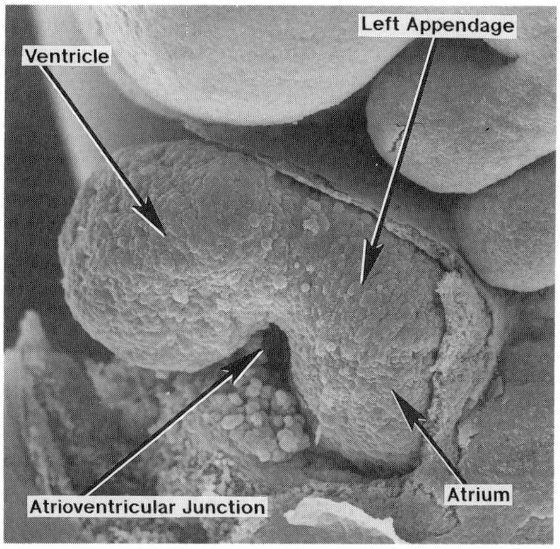

(b)

Fig. 47 The atrial appendages are markedly different in the structure as soon as they are recognizable as such in the mouse heart. These scanning electron micrographs taken at the early stage of ventricular looping in the mouse heart are reproduced by kind permission of Dr Nigel Brown, St George's Hospital, London.

Recognition from the outset, however, of the animals which are isomeric now gives us the opportunity to investigate the steps involved in the production of the isomeric features and the abnormal venoatrial connections. It is certainly the case that, from the time of their earliest growth from the atrial segment of the heart tube, it is possible to distinguish the structure of the morphologically right as opposed to the morphologically left appendage (Fig. 47). This finding, showing that the left appendage buds from the outset as a tubular extension from the anterior component of the atrioventricular junction, whereas the right appendage is always related to the full extent of the expanding right part of the junction, is strong evidence contradicting the suggestion of those who believe that the differences in the structure of the appendages are related to haemodynamic effects.[17] Studies of developing normal mice also show that, initially, the systemic venous sinus is bilaterally symmetrical, and has a particular relationship to the constituents of the musculature of the heart tube with the bodywall which form the portal through which, eventually, the pulmonary veins enter the heart (Fig. 48). Comparison of development of these structures in mice with isomeric appendages is likely to reveal the changes which lead to the intracardiac malformations. It should also be noted that, while the atrial segment of the heart can unequivocally show evidence of symmetry, it is exceedingly rare for the ventricular loop to develop in symmetrical fashion. We have encountered only one heart in which both ventricles were of comparable morphology, both being right ventricles in our specimen. This specimen is, in fact, very difficult to explain in the light of our present knowledge concerning ventricular development. It is generally accepted that, unlike the atriums, the ventricles develop in series. Thus, the atrial appendages grow from either side of a common atrial chamber (Fig. 49) which becomes differentiated into morphologically right and left parts only after the subsequent incorporation of the systemic and pulmonary venous components. It is easy to envisage how the development of this part of the heart could proceed along the lines of symmetry as opposed to lateralization. In the case of the ventricles, in contrast, the left ventricle develops from the proximal, or the inlet, part of the ventricular loop while the right ventricle develops from the distal, or outlet, component. Right-hand or left-hand topological patterns are associated with rightward or leftward looping of the ventricular component. These ventricular arrangements are still lateralized rather than symmetrical. It is of significance, therefore, that genes such as lefty and nodal have been shown to be mirror imaged in animals with left-hand ventricular topology.[42,43] This should not be interpreted in terms of asymmetry, but rather as mirror imaged lateralization. It is also, perhaps, significant that the earliest morphological evidence of incipient ventricular looping is found on the atrial side of the atrioventricular junctions.[44]

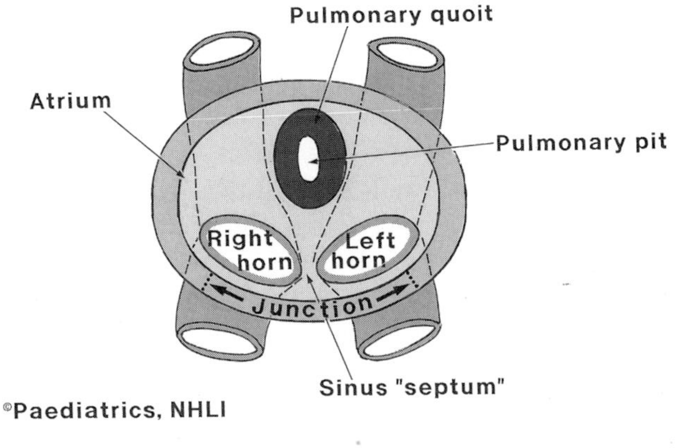

Fig. 48 Diagrammatic representation of the symmetrical arrangement of the horns of the systemic venous sinus relative to the prospective pulmonary portal at the stage of development in which the primary atrial component of the heart tube is undivided.

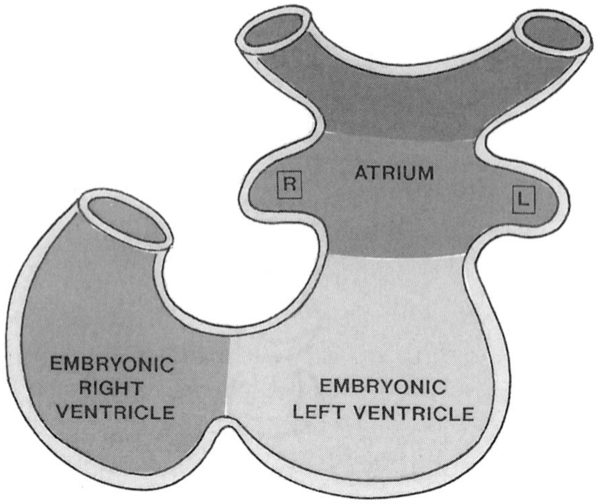

Fig. 49 The atrial appendages bud out in parallel from the atrial component of the primary heart tube, whereas the ventricles develop in series. There is the potential, therefore, for isomerism of the atrial appendages, but not of the ventricles.

REFERENCES

1. Martin G. Observation d'une deviation organique de l'estomac, d'une anomalie dans la situation et dans le configuration du coeur et des vaisseaux qui en partent ou qui s'y rendant. *Bull Soc Anat Paris* 1826;**1**:40–48.
2. Ivemark BI. Implications of agenesis of the spleen on the pathogenesis of conotruncus anomalies in childhood. An analysis of the heart; malformations in the splenic agenesis syndrome, with 14 new cases. *Acta Paediatr Scand* 1955;**44** (Suppl. 104):1–110.
3. Devine WA. Editorial. What if Ivemark had suggested the term "Syndrome of Visceral Symmetry with Asplenia" instead of "Asplenia, a Teratologic Syndrome of Visceral Heterotaxy"? *Cardiol Young* 1992;**2**:108–113.
4. Putschar WGJ, Manion WC. Congenital absence of the spleen and associated anomalies. *Am J Clin Pathol* 1956;**26**:429–470.
5. Van Mierop LHS, Gessner IH, Schiebler GL. Asplenia and polysplenia syndromes. In: Bergsma D (ed). Birth Defects: Original Article Series, Volume VIII, No. 5. The Fourth Conference on the Clinical Delineation of Birth Defects. Part XV The Cardiovascular System. The National Foundation — March of Dimes. Baltimore: Williams and Wilkins Company. 1972: pp 36–44.
6. Abernethy J. Account of two instances of uncommon formations in the viscera of the human body. *Philos Trans* 1793;**83**:59–66.
7. Moller JH, Nakib A, Anderson RC, Edwards JE. Congenital cardiac disease associated with polysplenia: A developmental complex of bilateral "left-sidedness". *Circulation* 1967;**36**:789–799.
8. Van Praagh R. The segmental approach to diagnosis in congenital heart disease. In: Bergsma D (ed). Birth Defects: Original Article Series, Volume VIII, No. 5. The Fourth Conference on the Clinical Delineation of Birth Defects. Part XV The Cardiovascular System. The National Foundation — March of Dimes. Baltimore: Williams and Wilkins Company. 1972: pp 4–23.
9. Lev M, Liberthson RR, Golden JG, Eckner FAO, Arcilla RA. The pathology of mesocardia. *Am J Cardiol* 1971;**28**:428–435.

10. Lev M, Liberthson RR, Eckner FAO, Arcilla RA. Pathologic anatomy of dextrocardia and its clinical implications. *Circulation* 1968;**37**:979–999.
11. Liberthson RR, Hastreiter AR, Sinha SN, Bharati S, Novak GM, Lev M. Levocardia with visceral heterotaxy — isolated levocardia: pathologic anatomy and its clinical implications. *Am Heart J* 1973;**85**:40–54.
12. Layman TE, Levine MA, Amplatz K, Edwards JE. "Asplenic syndrome" in association with rudimentary spleen. *Am J Cardiol* 1967;**20**:136–140.
13. Landing BH, Lawrence TK, Payne VC, Wells TR. Bronchial anatomy in syndromes with abnormal visceral situs, abnormal spleen and congenital heart disease. *Am J Cardiol* 1971;**12**:456–462.
14. Macartney FJ, Zuberbuhler JR, Anderson RH. Morphological considerations pertaining to recognition of atrial isomerism. Consequences for sequential chamber localisation. *Br Heart J* 1980;**44**:657–667.
15. Sharma S, Devine W, Anderson RH, Zuberbuhler JR. The determination of atrial arrangement by examination of appendage morphology in 1842 heart specimens. *Br Heart J* 1988;**60**:227–231.
16. Anderson C, Devine WA, Anderson RH, Debich DE, Zuberbuhler JR. Abnormalities of the spleen in relation to congenital malformations of the heart: a survey of necropsy findings in children. *Br Heart J* 1990;**63**:122–128.
17. Van Praagh R, Van Praagh S. Atrial isomerism in the heterotaxy syndromes with asplenia, or polysplenia, or normally formed spleen: an erroneous concept. *Am J Cardiol* 1990;**66**:1504–1506.
18. Rubino M, Van Praagh S, Kadoba K, Pessetto R, Van Praagh R. Systemic and pulmonary venous connections in visceral heterotaxy with asplenia: diagnostic and surgical considerations based on seventy-two autopsied cases. *J Thorac Cardiovasc Surg* 1995;**110**:641–650.
19. Uemura H, Ho SY, Devine WA, Kilpatrick LL, Anderson RH. Atrial appendages and venoatrial connections in hearts from patients with visceral heterotaxy. *Ann Thorac Surg* 1995;**60**:561-569.
20. Campbell M, Deuchar DC. Absent inferior vena cava, symmetrical liver, splenic agenesis and situs inversus and their embryology. *Br Heart J* 1967;**29**:268–275.
21. Chandra RS. Biliary atresia and other structural anomalies in congenital polysplenia syndrome. *J Pediatr* 1974;**85**:649–655.
22. Lev M. Pathologic diagnosis of positional variations in cardiac chambers in congenital heart disease. *Lab Invest* 1954;**3**:71–82.
23. Van Praagh R, David I, Wright GB, Van Praagh S. Large RV plus small LV is not single RV. *Circulation* 1980;**61**:1057–1058.
24. Van Praagh R, Vlad P. Dextrocardia, mesocardia, and levocardia: the segmental approach to diagnosis in congenital heart disease. In: Keith JD, Rowe RD, Vlad P (eds). *Heart Disease in Infancy and Childhood*, 3rd ed. New York: Macmillan. 1978: pp 638–697.
25. Uemura H, Ho SY, Devine WA, Anderson RH. Analysis of visceral heterotaxy according to splenic status, appendage morphology, or both. *Am J Cardiol* 1995;**76**:846–849.
26. Van Mierop LHS, Wiglesworth FW. Isomerism of the cardiac atria in the asplenia syndrome. *Lab Invest* 1962;**11**:1303–1315.
27. Dickinson DF, Wilkinson JL, Anderson KR, Smith A, Ho SY, Anderson RH. The cardiac conduction system in situs ambiguus. *Circulation* 1979;**59**:879–885.
28. Ho SY, Seo J, Brown NA, Cook AC, Fagg NLK, Anderson RH. Morphology of the sinus node in human and mouse hearts with isomerism of the atrial appendages. *Br Heart J* 1995;**74**:437–442.

29. Pohanka I, Vitek B. The conducting system of the heart in the syndrome of visceral symmetry. *Folia Morphol (Praha)* 1978;**26**:379–388.
30. Stumper OFW, Sreeram N, Elzenga NJ, Sutherland GR. Diagnosis of atrial situs by transesophageal echocardiography. *J Am Coll Cardiol* 1990;**16**:442–446.
31. Deanfield JE, Leanage R, Stroobant J, Chrispin AR, Taylor JFN, Macartney FJ. Use of high kilovoltage filtered beam radiographs for detection of bronchial situs in infants and young children. *Br Heart J* 1980;**44**:577–583.
32. Huhta JC, Smallhorn JF, Macartney FJ. Two dimensional echocardiographic diagnosis of situs. *Br Heart J* 1982;**48**:97–108.
33. Uemura H, Ho SY, Anderson RH, Devine WA, Smith A, Shinohara T, Yagihara T. The surgical anatomy of coronary venous return in hearts with isomeric atrial appendages. *J Thorac Cardiovasc Surg* 1995;**110**:436–444.
34. Bharati S, Lev M. The course of the conduction system in dextrocardia. *Circulation* 1978;**57**:163–171.
35. De Tommasi SM, Daliento L, Ho SY, Macartney FJ, Anderson RH. Analysis of atrioventricular junction, ventricular mass and ventriculoarterial junction in 43 specimens with atrial isomerism. *Br Heart J* 1981;**45**:236–247.
36. Caruso G, Becker AE. How to determine atrial situs? Considerations initiated by 3 cases of absent spleen with a discordant anatomy between bronchi and atria. *Br Heart J* 1979;**41**:559–567.
37. Britz-Cunningham S, Shan M, Zuppan C, Fletcher W. Mutations of the connexin 43 gap junction gene in patients with heart malformations and defects of laterality. *N Engl J Med* 1995;**332**:1323–1329.
38. Penman Splitt M, Burn J, Goodship J. Connexin 43 mutations in sporadic and familial defects of laterality. Letter. *New Engl J Med* 1995;**333**:941–942.
39. Gobbia M, Towbin JA, Casey B. Failure to detect connexin 43 mutations in 38 cases of sporadic and familial heterotaxy. *Circulation* 1996;**94**:1909–1912.
40. Layton WM, Jr., Manasek FJ. Cardiac looping in early iv/iv mouse embryos. In: Van Praagh R, Takao A (eds). *Etiology and Morphogenesis of Congenital Heart Disease*. Mount Kisco, New York: Futura Publishing Company. 1980: pp 109–126.
41. Seo JW, Brown NA, Ho SY, Anderson RH. Abnormal laterality and congenital cardiac anomalies: relations of visceral and cardiac morphologies in the iv/iv mouse. *Circulation* 1992;**86**:642–650.
42. Meno C, Saijoh Y, Fujii H, Ikeda M, Yokoyama T, Yokoyama M, Toyoda Y, Hamada H. Left-right asymmetric expression of the TGFb-family member lefty in mouse embryos. *Nature* 1996;**381**:151–156.
43. Lowe L, Supp DM, Sampath K, Yokoyama T, Wright CVE, Potter SS, Overbeek P, Kuehn MR. Conserved left/right asymmetry of nodal expression and alternations in mouse situs inversus. *Nature* 1996;**381**:158–161.
44. Bellomo D, Brown NA. Morphological and cellular asymmetries in the embryonic mouse heart that precede looping. *Dev Dynamics* 1997; in press.

Chapter 4

Tetralogy of Fallot

INTRODUCTION

In 1888, Etienne-Louis Arthur Fallot published an account describing the unifying pathologic features of patients with "la maladie bleue".[1] Up till the present day his observations have proven to be valid, and the eponym "Fallot" is used world-wide. Fallot's observations, based on clinicopathological correlations, established a combination of anatomical derangements as the underlying disorder; his tetralogy was made up of pulmonary arterial stenosis, an interventricular communication, deviation of the aorta to the right, and concentric hypertrophy of the right ventricle (Fig. 1).

From a pathophysiological viewpoint, the hallmark of the condition is obstruction within the right ventricular outflow tract, downstream to a ventricular septal defect, with biventricular connection of the aorta. This creates the unique setting such that the overriding aortic valvar orifice will receive a mix of saturated blood from the left and unsaturated blood from the right ventricle, with the degree of mixing being determined by the extent of narrowing within the right ventricular outflow tract. It is the anatomic features, therefore, which determine the presence or absence of cyanosis. Indeed,

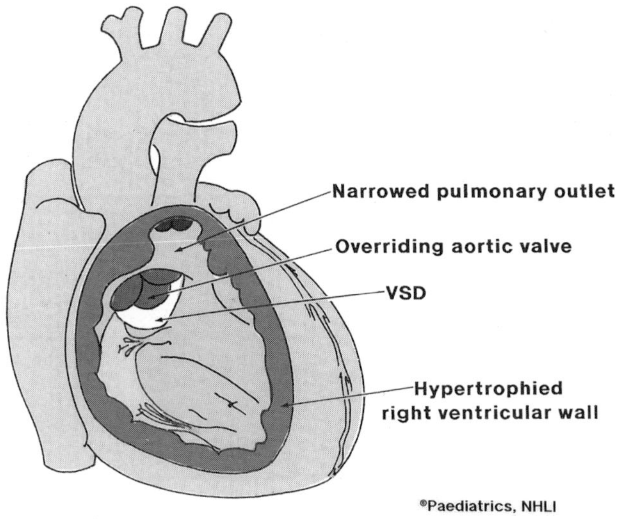

Fig. 1 The basic configuration of the cardiac malformation which Etienne-Louis Fallot identified as the commonest cause of "la maladie bleue".

cyanosis is not necessarily present at birth, and can be a relatively late phenomenon, dictated by ventricular remodelling with increasing right ventricular hypertrophy and progressive narrowing of the stenotic right ventricular outflow tract. From the anatomical point of view, the hallmark of the condition is an antero-cephalad disposition of the muscular septum which separates the subpulmonary and subaortic outflow tracts coupled with marked hypertrophy of septoparietal trabeculations, the muscular structures combining to produce the characteristic subpulmonary obstruction (Fig. 2). This is seen together with the characteristic "malalignment" of interventricular communication, and with the leaflets of the overriding and dextroposed aortic valve connected in both the right and left ventricles. Within this framework of unifying anatomic features, nonetheless, there can exist a wide range of anatomical variables.[2] These relate most commonly to the morphology of the ventricular septal defect, the precise degree of aortic override, the specific morphology of the structures narrowing the subpulmonary infundibulum, the occurrence of anomalies in origin and course of coronary arteries, and the presence of peripheral pulmonary arterial stenosis. Simply because there is such a wide range of anatomical variables, it is to be expected that some will give rise to controversy. Following a recapitulation of the unifying pathology of Fallot's tetralogy, therefore, in which we will emphasize those morphologic

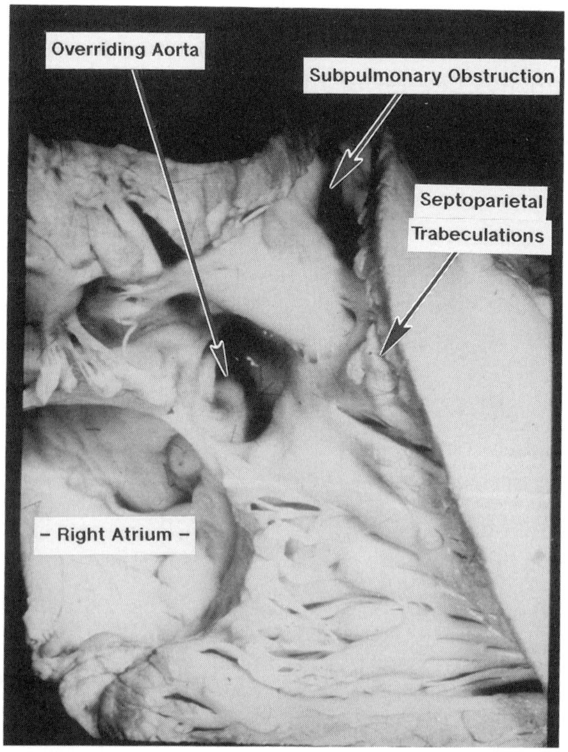

Fig. 2 It is the antero-cephalad deviation of the muscular outlet septum, coupled with hypertrophy of the septoparietal trabeculations, which produces the characteristic subpulmonary obstruction.

features which remain contentious, we will focus on the other remaining controversial aspects.

UNIFYING PATHOLOGY

As discussed above, the obvious anatomic hallmark of Fallot's tetralogy (Fig. 2) is antero-cephalad insertion of the septal attachment of the muscular outlet (infundibular or conal) septum relative to the anterior limb of the septomarginal trabeculation (septal band). This arrangement in itself, however, is not sufficient to narrow the subpulmonary infundibulum. A directly comparable antero-cephalad insertion of the muscular septum relative to the septomarginal trabeculation (Fig. 3) can be seen in the so-called "Eisenmenger" ventricular septal defect.[3] In this lesion, however, despite the antero-cephalad position of the outlet septum, the pulmonary outflow tract is widely patent.[4] The unobstructed flow of blood to the lungs promotes the early development of pulmonary vascular disease (the so-called Eisenmenger reaction). Something over and beyond the malalignment of the outlet septum

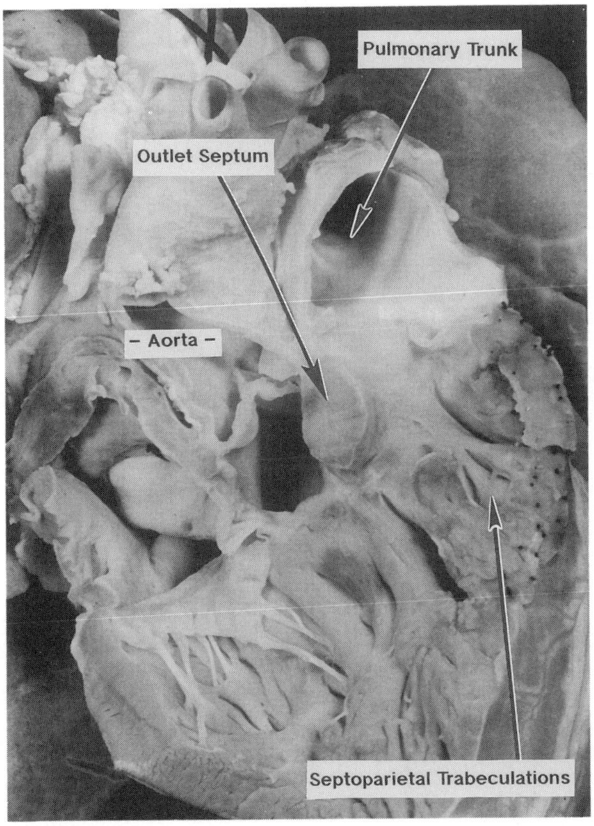

Fig. 3 This right anterior oblique section across a heart with a so-called "Eisenmenger" ventricular septal defect shows that mere deviation of the outlet septum does not narrow the subpulmonary infundibulum even in the presence of hypertrophied septoparietal trabeculations.

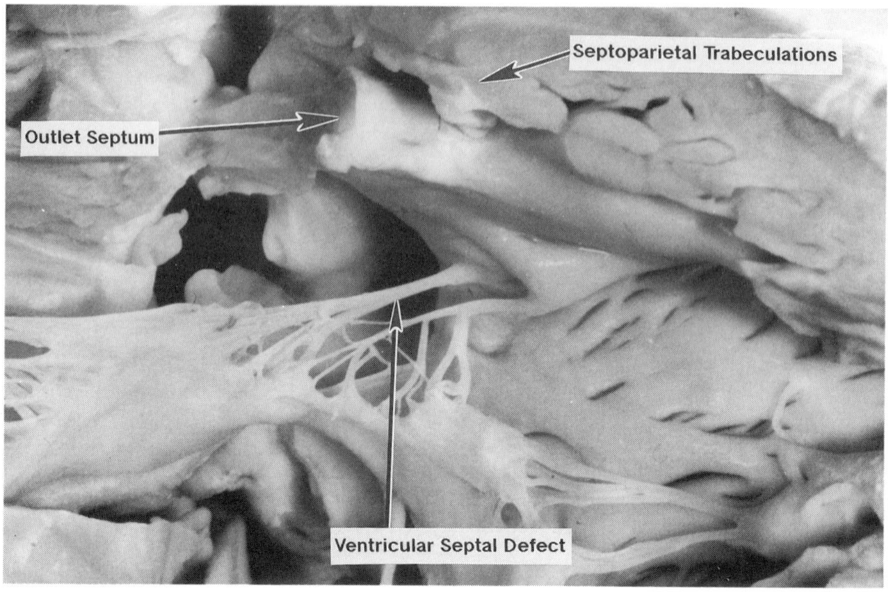

Fig. 4 The muscular ring produced by the outlet septum and the septoparietal trabeculations which narrows the subpulmonary infundibulum is excacerbated by fibrous accretions in this heart.

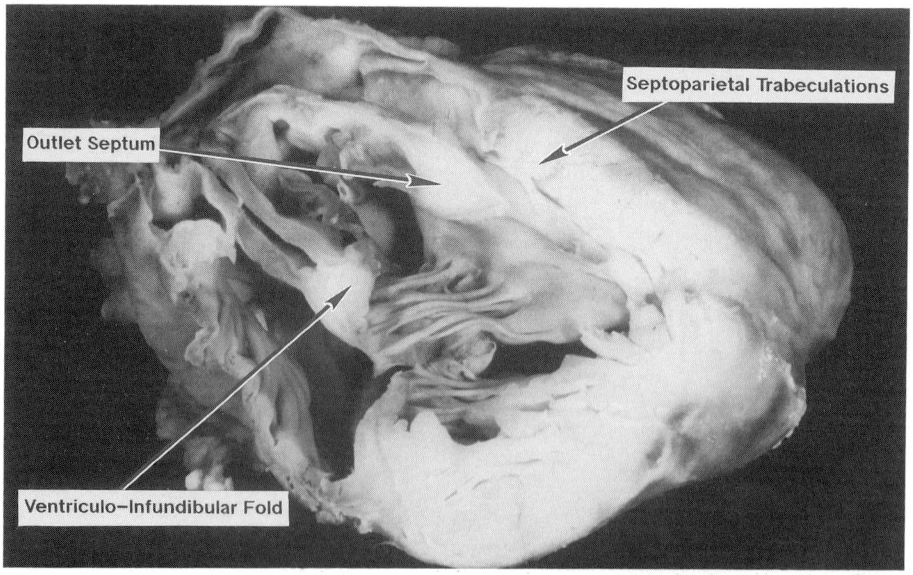

Fig. 5 This oblique subcostal equivalent section (compare with Fig. 3) shows the muscular bundles which bound the ventricular septal defect and the subpulmonary infundibulum in tetralogy of Fallot.

is needed, therefore, to produce the pathognomonic arrangement of Fallot's tetralogy. This additional feature is the presence of a stenosing muscular ring at the entrance to the subpulmonary infundibulum which incorporates hypertrophied septoparietal trabeculations (Figs. 4, 5). The septoparietal trabeculations are a feature of the normal right ventricular muscular architecture, running to the parietal wall of the ventricle from the anterior margin of the septomarginal trabeculation as a serried array of individual muscular bundles (Fig. 6).[5] The trabeculations are also seen, and can be hypertrophied, along the anterior margin of the infundibulum in the Eisenmenger ventricular septal defect. But, in this situation, they do not produce obstruction (Fig. 3). The key feature of the arrangement in tetralogy, therefore, is the anatomic "squeeze" produced by the union of the extensions of the outlet septum and the septoparietal trabeculations. The union of these muscular structures produces a discrete and characteristic entrance to the smooth and extensive subpulmonary infundibulum which, with time, can become exacerbated by the laying down of fibrous tissue (Fig. 7).

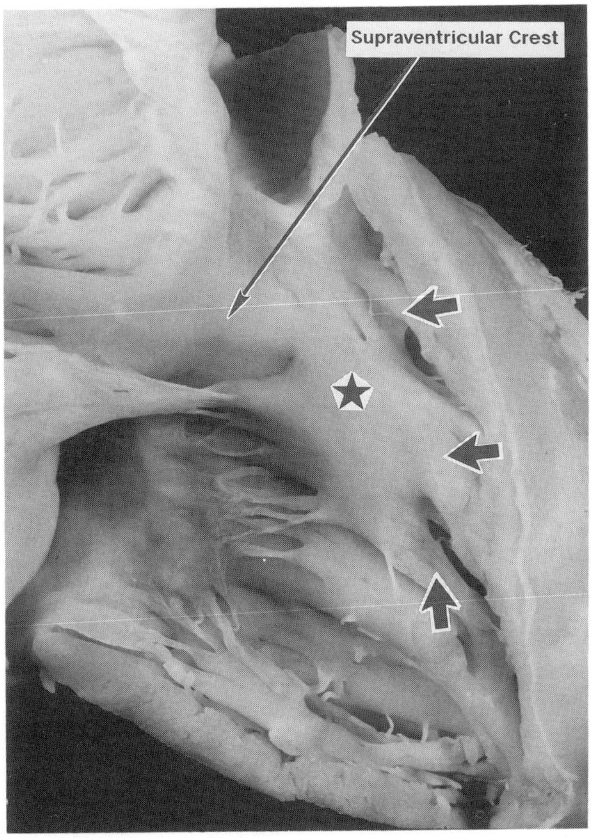

Fig. 6 In this normal heart, it is easily seen how the supraventricular crest inserts between the limbs of the septomarginal trabeculation (septal band – star). Note the array of septoparietal trabeculations which extend from the anterior border of the septomarginal trabeculation (arrowed).

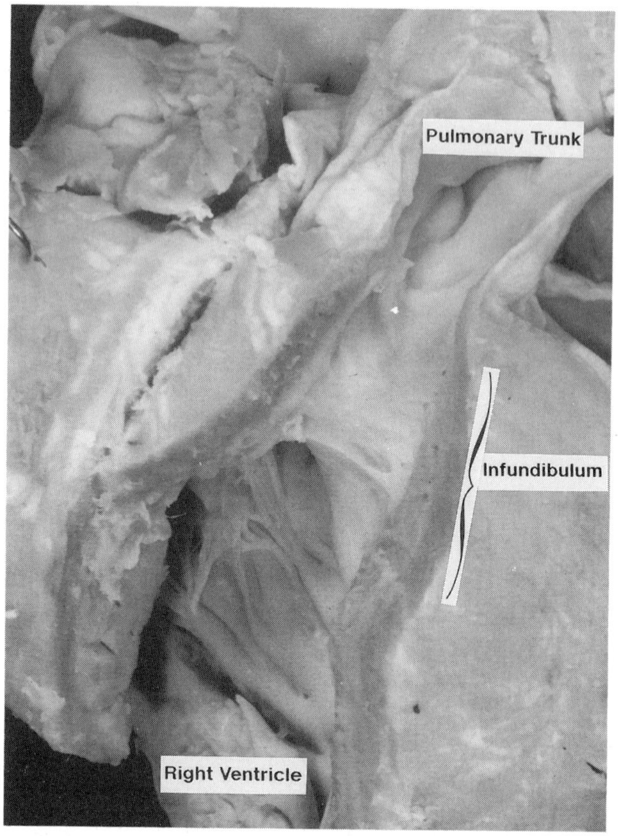

Fig. 7 The subpulmonary infundibulum has been revealed by removal of its parietal wall. It is extensive and smooth-walled. Note the fibrous ridge at its mouth.

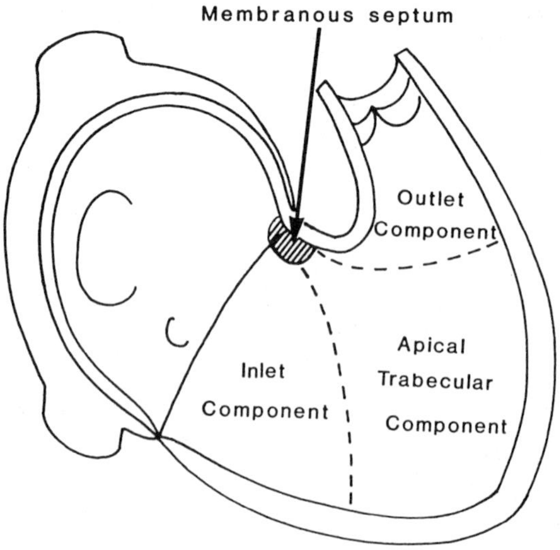

Fig. 8 In the initial classification of ventricular septal defect proposed by Soto and colleagues[6] we divided the muscular ventricular septum as shown in the diagram into inlet, apical trabecular, and outlet components. We now know that most of the area depicted as outlet septum is made up of the free-standing subpulmonary infundibulum.

The antero-cephalad location of the outlet septum is a crucial feature, nonetheless, in that it bears upon the presence of the ventricular septal defect. In the normal heart, it is not possible to separate different components of the muscular ventricular septum, simply to distinguish its membranous and muscular segments. The area which, in the past, we had thought to represent the "outlet septum" we now know to be made up largely of the free-standing subpulmonary infundibulum. An understanding of this morphology is crucial in adjudicating several of the controversies which surround the morphology of tetralogy of Fallot. Thus, when, together with Soto, we first proposed a classification for ventricular septal defects,[6] we divided the normal ventricular septum into inlet, apical trabecular and outlet components (Fig. 8). Our view, at that time, was that all the "septal" surface of the right ventricle seen distal to a vertical line drawn at the level of the medial papillary muscle was made up of the outlet septum. We now know that this interpretation was incorrect, because the larger part of this apparent "septal" musculature is, in reality, a free-standing sleeve of infundibular musculature (Fig. 9). When this area is removed in the normal hearts, then rather than entering the subaortic outlet of the left ventricle, which would be the result were the tissue truly to represent a muscular outlet septum, the dissection reveals the aortic sinuses (Fig. 10).

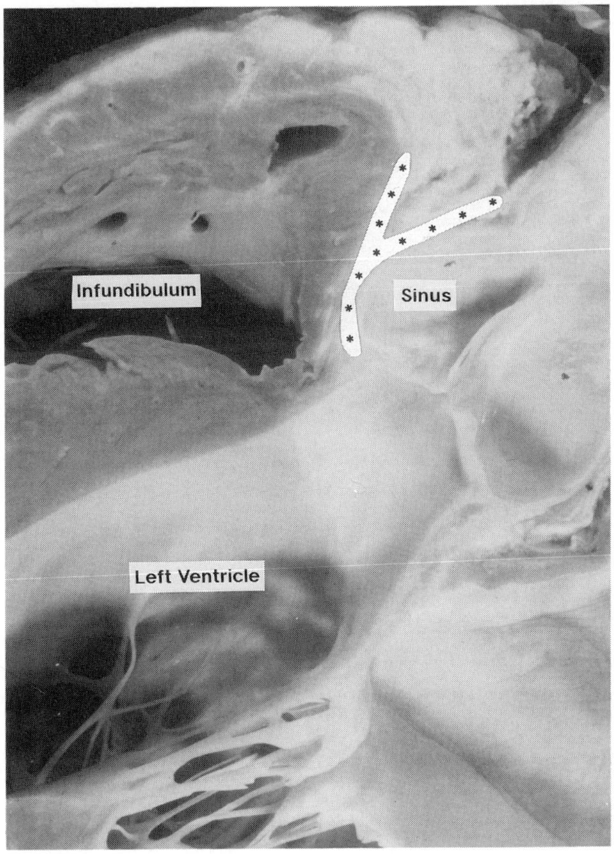

Fig. 9 In the normal heart, the right coronary aortic sinus overlies the cavity of the infundibulum of the right ventricle, but the two cavities are separated by a fibrofatty tissue plane (stars) continuous with the extracardiac space.

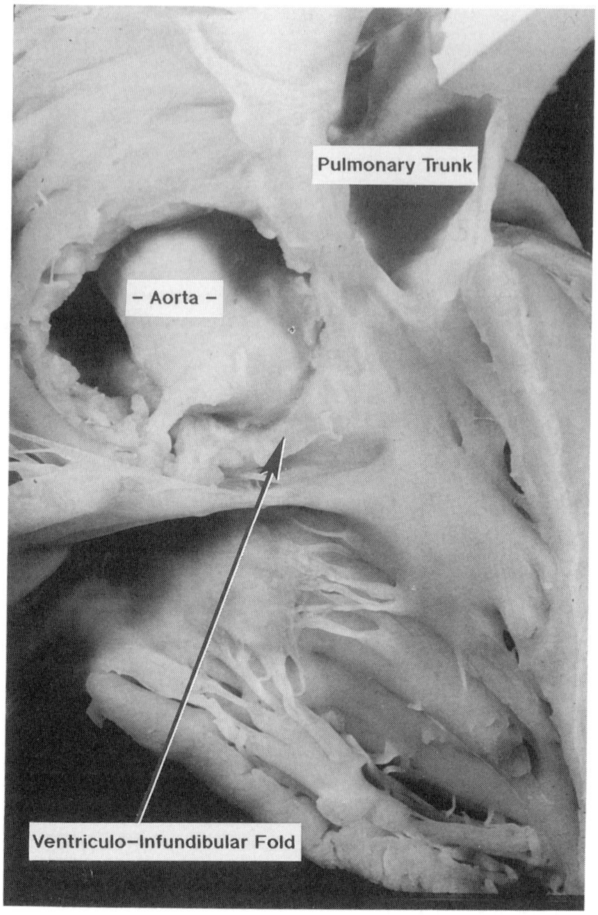

Fig. 10 This dissection of the heart shown in Fig. 6 reveals that the greater part of the supraventricular crest is made up of the parietal wall of the heart between the hingepoints of the leaflets of the tricuspid and pulmonary valves. This is the structure we identify as the ventriculo-infundibular fold.

Thus, the posterior margins of the subpulmonary infundibulum in the area of the supraventricular crest (crista supraventricularis) separate the cavity of the right ventricle from the fibrofatty tissue plane which interposes between the muscular infundibulum and the facing sinuses of the aortic root (Fig. 11). As already discussed, it is not possible in the normal heart to distinguish any part of this muscular supraventricular crest specifically as a muscular outlet septum. Only the most medial part of the crest is positioned between the cavities of the right and left ventricles (Fig. 12). The remainder, and greater part, of the crest separates the hingepoints of the leaflets of the tricuspid and pulmonary valves. This part is the ventriculo-infundibular fold, and represents the inner heart curvature.

In tetralogy of Fallot, because of the disordered architecture, these building blocks of the right ventricular outflow tract have sprung apart (Fig. 13). The outlet septum now becomes visible in its own right as the muscular structure interposed between the subaortic and subpulmonary outlets. But, once more, because of the presence of a sleeve of free-standing subpulmonary infundibulum,

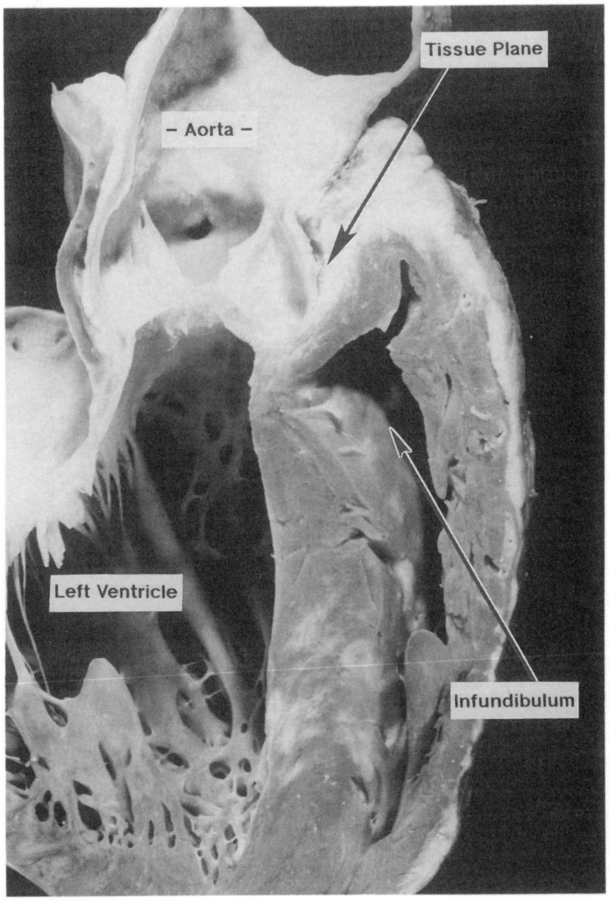

Fig. 11 A further section across the outflow tracts of the normal heart shows the tissue plane which interposes between the aortic sinuses and the subpulmonary infundibulum.

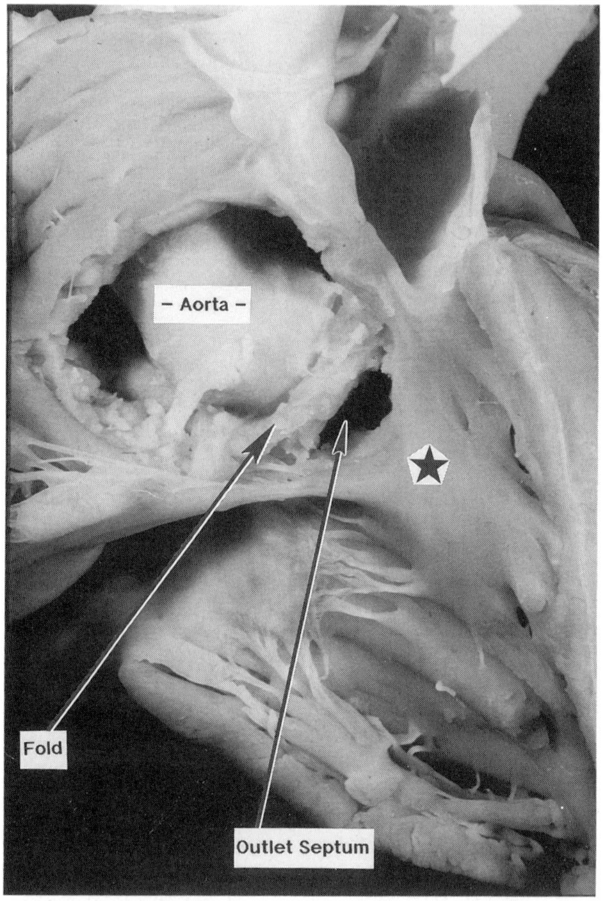

Fig. 12 Further dissection of the normal heart shown in Figs. 6 and 10 shows the very small part of the muscular ventricular septum which interposes between the subaortic and subpulmonary outflow tracts. Star – septomarginal trabeculation.

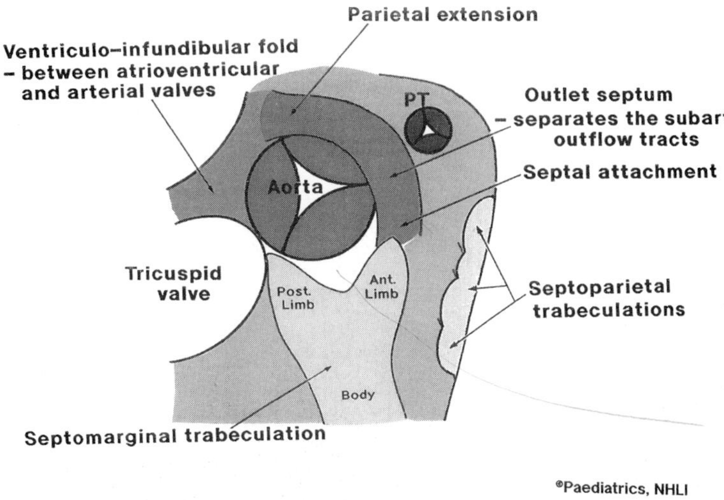

Fig. 13 This diagram, based on the heart shown in Fig. 2, demonstrates the position and definition of the muscle bundles which surround the ventricular septal defect in tetralogy of Fallot. See also Fig. 5.

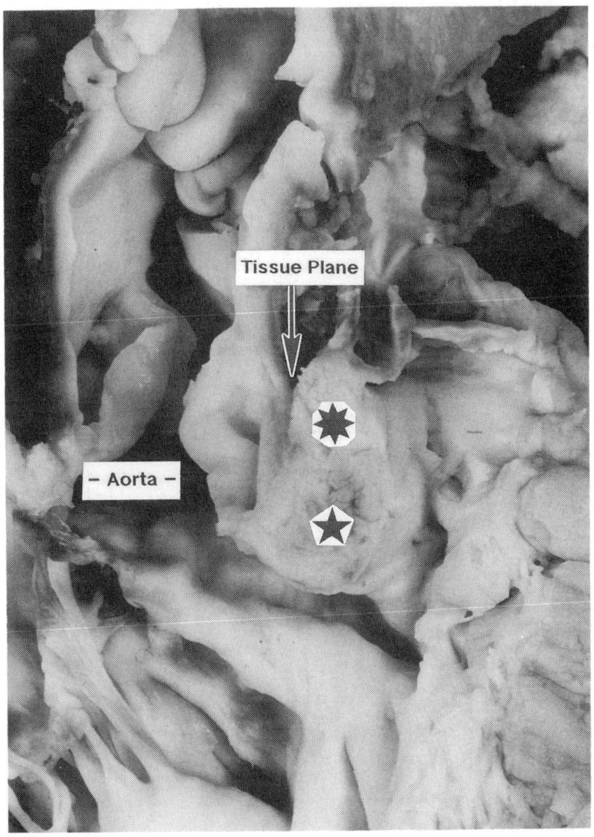

Fig. 14 This section across the ventricular outflow tracts in tetralogy of Fallot shows the distinction between the muscular outlet septum within the cavity of the right ventricle (five-pointed star) and the free-standing and hypertrophied infundibular sleeve (eight-pointed star) which is separated by a fibro-fatty tissue plane from the aortic valvar sinus.

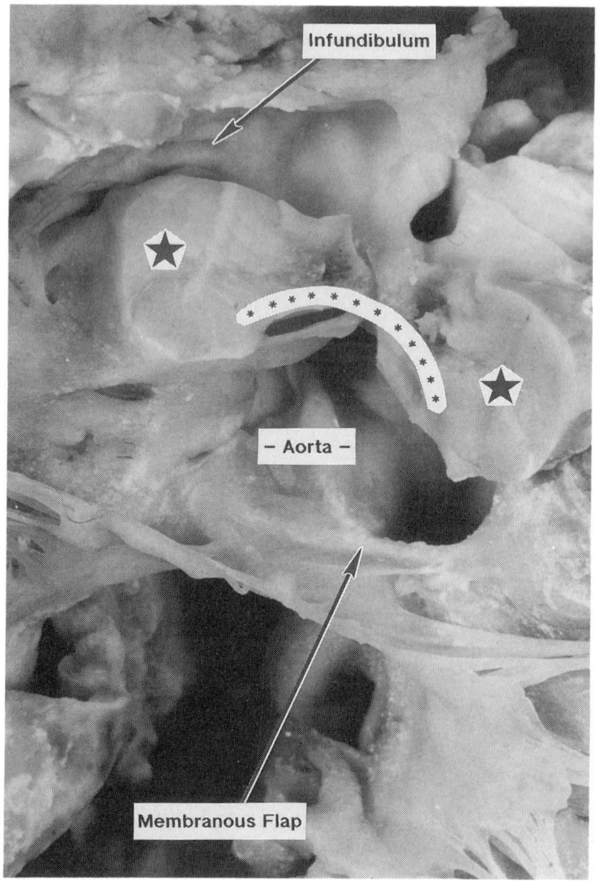

Fig. 15 Another heart, with a section across a more extensive outlet septum (large stars – compare with Fig. 14), in which the tissue plane bordering the sleeve of free-standing subpulmonary infundibulum has been shown with a line of small stars.

the septum is not as extensive as would be imagined from viewing the infundibulum from its pulmonary aspect (Fig. 7). The true outlet septum, which is now exclusively a right ventricular structure by virtue of its deviation relative to the septomarginal trabeculation, hangs down like a teardrop into the ventricular cavity. Its extent on its posterior surface is limited by the semilunar hingepoints of the leaflets of the aortic valve, with small parts of the musculature being incorporated within the aortic sinuses of Valsalva (Fig. 14). On its anterior surface, however, the septum merges directly with the sleeve of infundibular musculature, the sleeve then supporting the entirety of the hingepoints of the leaflets of the pulmonary valve. Only the lower part of the extensive subpulmonary infundibulum, therefore, is formed by the muscular outlet septum (Fig. 15). As we will see, this part can vary markedly in size, as can the length of the sleeve of infundibular musculature (compare Figs. 14 and 15). As with the normal heart, dissection through the more distal part of the muscular wall would lead to the fibrofatty tissue plane separating the infundibulum from the aortic sinuses (Fig. 14).

The leaflets of the aortic valve itself are connected to the bases of both ventricles (Fig. 16). This arrangement differs markedly from that of the normal heart in which the leaflets of the aortic valve are, of necessity, attached exclusively within the left ventricle. The aortic sinuses supporting the valvar leaflets adjacent to the pulmonary trunk, however, bulge so that the cavity of the sinus is related to the cavity of the right ventricle, but with a fibrofatty tissue plane interposed between the right and left ventricular structures (Fig. 11). Some investigators have described this arrangement as "aortic overriding".[7] We find this very confusing. The aortic sinus is related in space to the cavity of the right ventricle, but the two are separated by the discrete fibrofatty tissue plane which is continuous with, and part of, the extracardiac space (Fig. 17). This arrangement is fundamentally different from the situation produced in presence of a perimembranous ventricular septal defect. Then, because the ventricular septum comes apart, as it were, between the muscular and membranous components (Fig. 18), the aortic valvar leaflets take direct attachment from right ventricular structures, namely the tricuspid valvar leaflets (Fig. 19). When the aorta stays connected predominantly within the left ventricle, there is very minimal overriding of the muscular septum by the aortic valvar orifice. In tetralogy of Fallot, in contrast, the valvar orifice is positioned so that the aortic leaflets are supported much more extensively by right ventricular structures (Fig. 20). Because of this, a cone of space is subtended between the crest of the ventricular septum and the overriding leaflets of the aortic valve (Fig. 21). Many of the controversies which relate to classification of tetralogy of Fallot, which we will discuss shortly, reflect failure of agreement on which of the borders of this cone of space, or which of the planes within

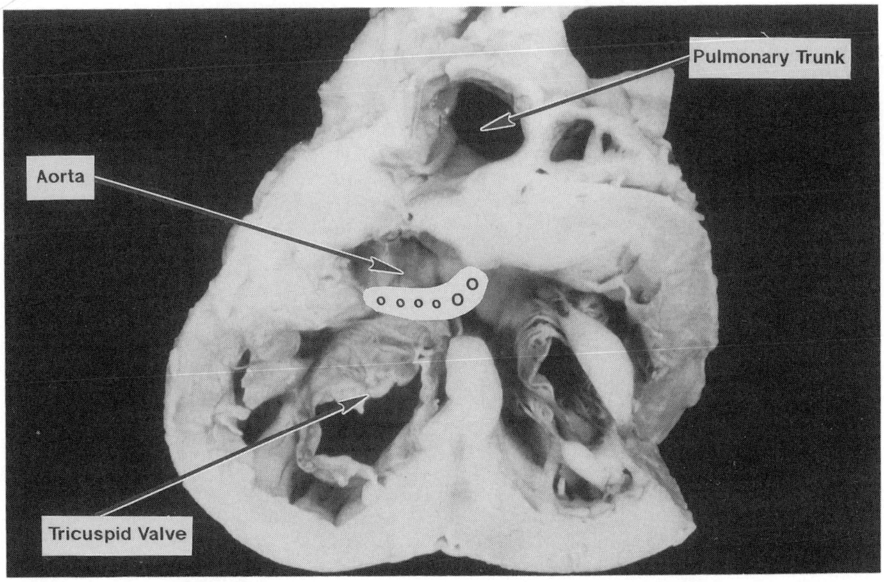

Fig. 16 This short-axis section of the heart with tetralogy of Fallot is viewed from beneath. The small circles indicate the proportion of the aortic valvar leaflets connected within the right ventricle. Note that this is greater than the proportion connected within the left ventricle (large circles).

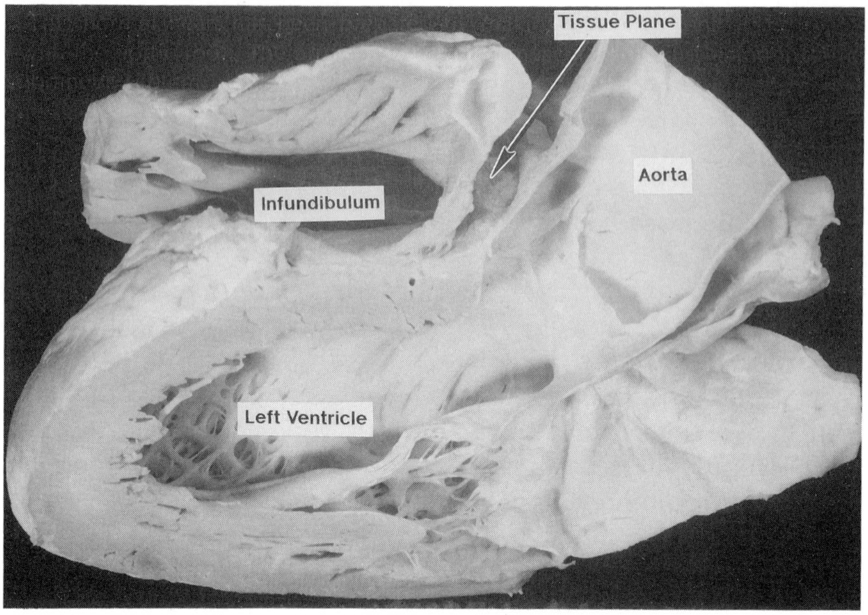

Fig. 17 In the normal heart, revealed here by a parasternal long-axis section equivalent, the aortic valvar leaflets are exclusively connected within the left ventricle, and it is the aortic valvar sinuses which are related to the subpulmonary infundibulum, albeit separated by an extensive fibro-fatty tissue plane, which has been cleaned in this specimen.

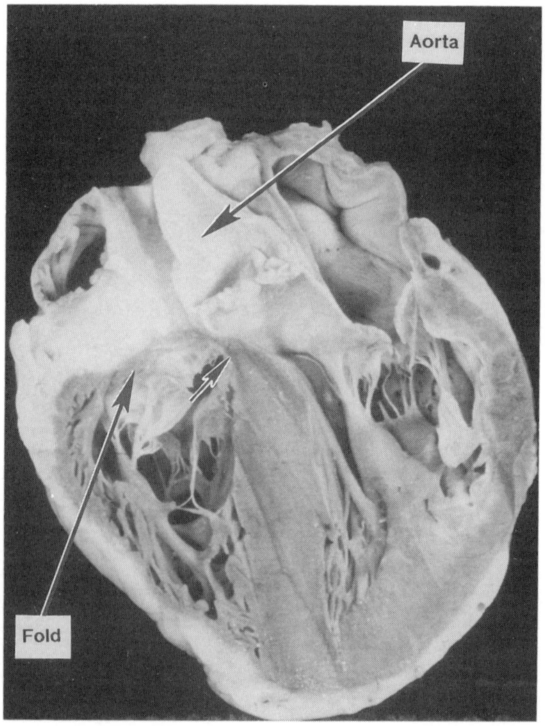

Fig. 18 This normal heart has been prepared by making an equivalent of the four-chamber section with the aortic root. The arrow points to the muscular fold just anterior to the area of the membranous septum.

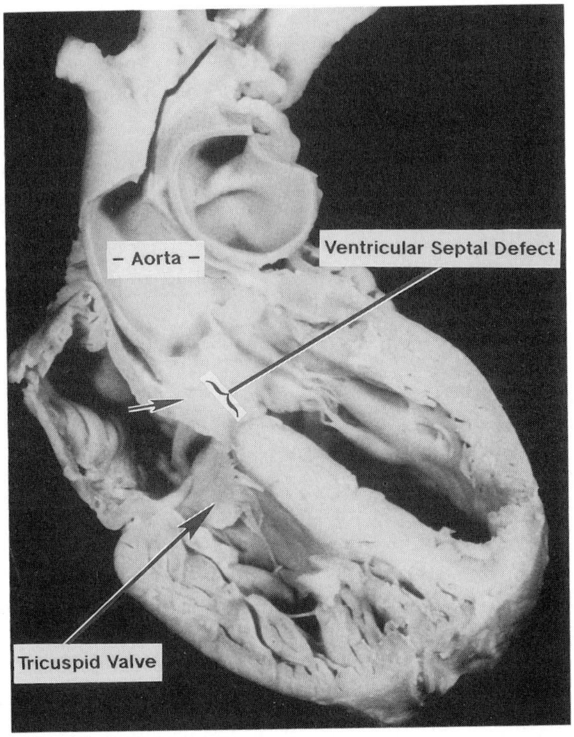

Fig. 19 In hearts with perimembranous ventricular septal defects, the septum comes apart, as it were, between the membranous and muscular components, as revealed in this four-chamber section equivalent. The leaflets of the aortic valve are then attached, in part, to the leaflets of the tricuspid valve within the right ventricle (arrow).

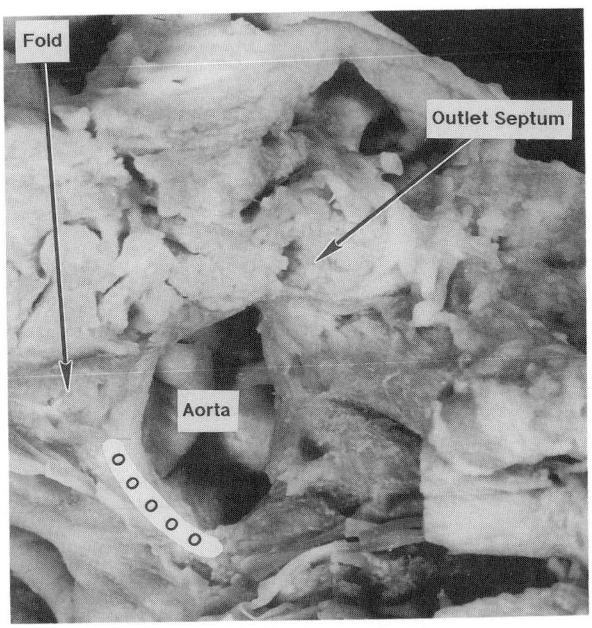

Fig. 20 In tetralogy of Fallot with perimembranous ventricular septal defect, the leaflets of the aortic valve, in consequence of its biventricular connection, achieve a much greater attachment within the right ventricle, shown here by the circles.

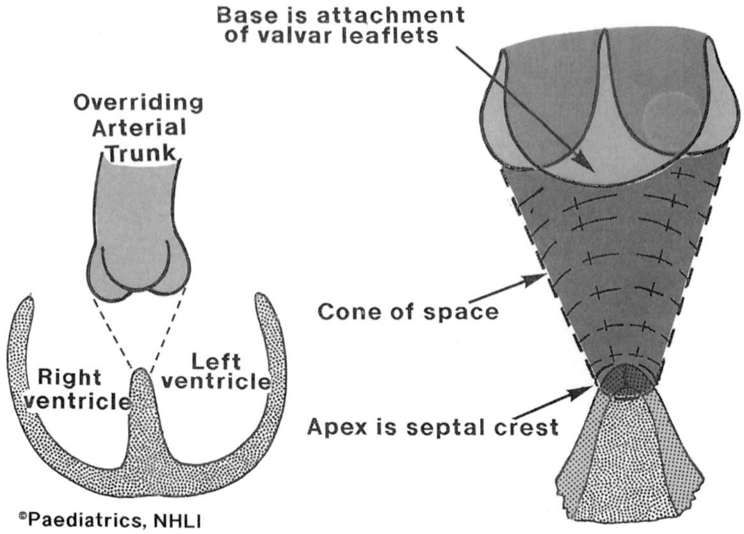

Fig. 21 When the aortic valve has a biventricular connection, as in tetralogy of Fallot, then a cone of space is subtended from the circumference of the valvar leaflets to the crest of the ventricular septum.

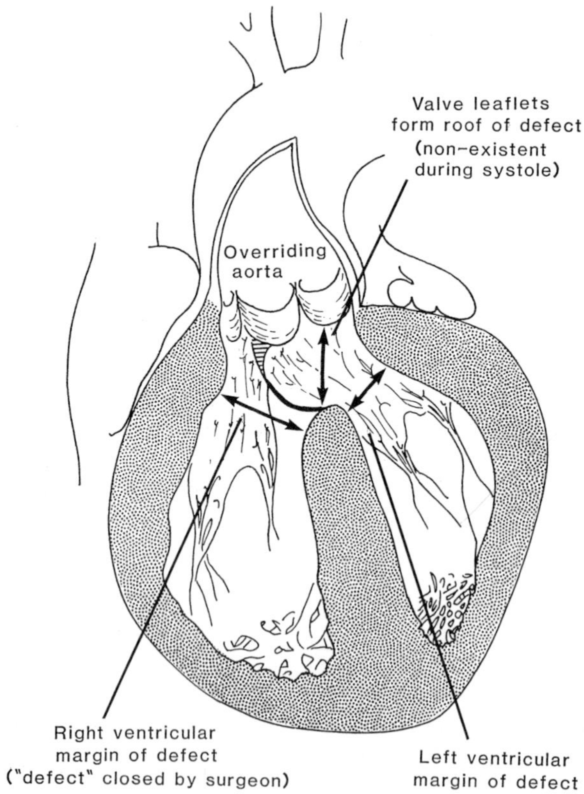

Fig. 22 Within the cone of space illustrated in Fig. 21, any plane can be nominated as a septal defect. As shown in this drawing, three are particularly important — the right and left ventricular borders and the direct upward extension of the long axis of the muscular septum. The latter plane abuts on the leaflets of the aortic valve during diastole, but not in systole when the aortic valve is open.

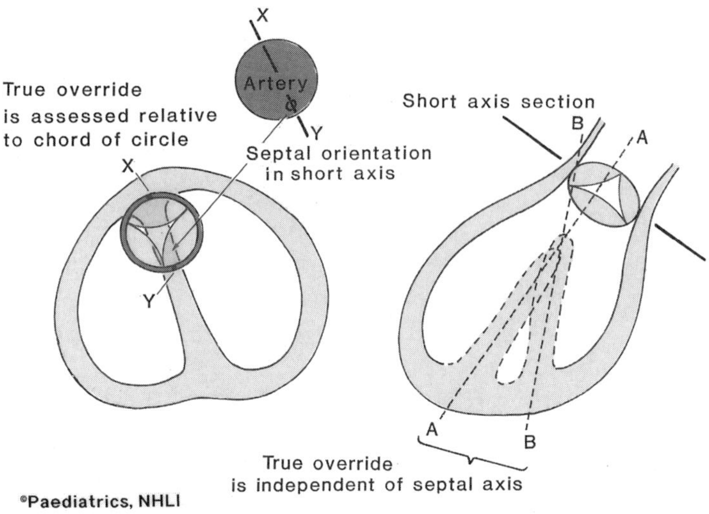

Fig. 23 The degree of override of an arterial valve is judged most accurately in the short axis by assessing the chord formed by the muscular septum relative to the orifice of the valve. Taking the long axis of the septum is more likely to introduce artefact.

it, should be considered to represent the septal defect.[8,9] In reality, any of the planes within the cone can be nominated as a septal defect (Fig. 22). The important one for the surgeon is the right ventricular border, since this is the location of the patch which will be placed to reconnect the aorta to the left ventricle. The left ventricular border is also important, since this will become the outlet from the left ventricle once the surgical repair is complete. The other important plane, nonetheless, is that represented by the direct continuation of the long axis of the ventricular septum. This plane will, of necessity, transect the undersurface of the aortic valvar leaflets when they are closed during ventricular diastole. Many echocardiographers consider this plane to represent the ventricular septal defect. It is certainly the plane of the interventricular communication. It is not the locus, however, around which the surgeon will place the patch used for correction. Nor is it the ideal plane to be used so as to arbitrate the degree of aortic override (Fig. 23). For all of these reasons, we prefer to nominate the right ventricular margin of the cone of space as the septal defect for the purposes of our classification (see below).

If we summarize the anatomy described thus far, an extensive interventricular communication is present in subaortic position in tetralogy of Fallot because of malalignment of the muscular outlet septum, the malaligned septum combining with hypertrophied septoparietal trabeculations to produce subpulmonary muscular obstruction. Rightward deviation of the aortic orifice, such that its valvar leaflets override the crest of the muscular septum to become attached in both ventricles, completes the characteristic morphology. Hypertrophy of right ventricular myocardium, the fourth part of the original tetralogy, is merely an adaptive phenomenon occurring consequent to the systemic afterload shared by both left and right ventricles.

Accurate and comparable description of this anatomy in the past has been bedevilled by different uses of the so-called "crista". As we have demonstrated, the supraventricular crest ("crista") of the normal right ventricle represents in its greater part the parietal myocardium supporting the leaflets of the pulmonary valve. The outlet septum cannot be distinguished as such in the normal heart, and the part of the crest which interposes between the ventricular cavities is insignificant compared to the contributions of the ventriculo-infundibular fold. The septomarginal trabeculation, or "septal band", is a muscular strap which reinforces the septal surface of the morphologically right ventricle. It cannot, under any circumstances, be considered to be supraventricular. The use of the components of the "crista supraventricularis" as descriptive terms, therefore, is problematic even for hearts having normal outflow tracts.

In Fallot's tetralogy, the problems are hugely magnified (Fig. 24). When the presumed components of the enigmatic crista were first used in this setting, by Kjellberg and his colleagues,[10] it was the outlet septum and the septoparietal trabeculations, together forming the ring at the mouth of the subpulmonary infundibulum, which were correlated with the septal and parietal bands. Subsequently, however, Van Praagh[11] described the septomarginal trabeculation as the septal band, considering the outlet (or conal) septum to be representative of the parietal band. The situation was further complicated when others[12] identified the persisting ventriculo-infundibular fold between the leaflets of the tricuspid and aortic valves as "parietal band 2", distinguishing this structure from the outlet septum, which was held to represent "parietal band 1". It was because of this confusion and disagreement that we suggested restriction of the term "crista supraventricularis", or supraventricular crest, to the description of the muscular roof of the right ventricle as seen in the normal heart.[13] We argued that it was much less confusing to describe the building blocks of the outflow tracts as seen in tetralogy of Fallot in their own right, specifying their names according to their locations (Figs. 5, 13). Thus, the ventriculo-infundibular fold was considered to represent any muscular structure interposing between the attachments of the leaflets of the atrioventricular and arterial valves. The outlet septum was the muscular structure interposed between the leaflets of the arterial valves. The

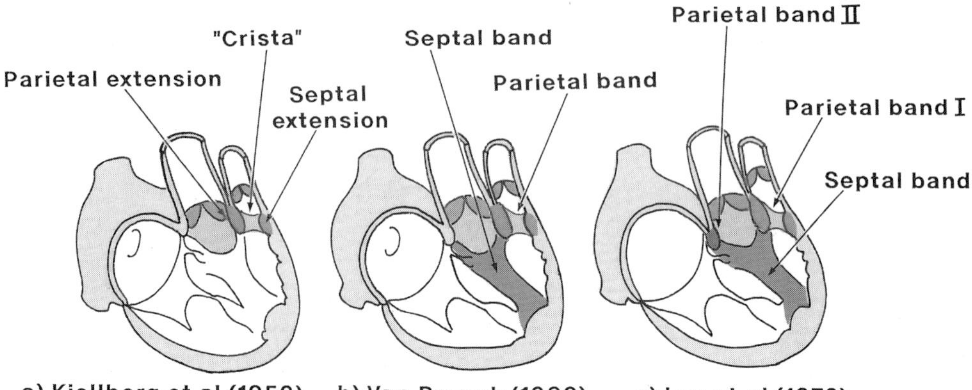

Fig. 24 The different names given by various investigators to the muscular structures which produce the mouth of the subpulmonary infundibulum (see Figs. 5, 13).

septomarginal trabeculation was defined as the extensive strap reinforcing the right ventricular aspect of the ventricular septum. We see no reason to change these initial definitions but, in addition to them, we now recognize the need also to define the septoparietal trabeculations along with the free-standing sleeve of subpulmonary infundibular musculature.

VARIATIONS IN THE CHARACTERISTIC ANATOMY

We have already intimated that the variations to be encountered can involve all aspects of tetralogy. The significant ones are related to the margins of the interventricular communication as seen from the right ventricular aspect, the morphology of the subpulmonary obstruction, the variations in connection of the leaflets of the overriding aortic valve, and the coronary arterial supply.

We have also described already the basic position of the ventricular septal defect, and indicated the problems which exist in defining which particular plane of space is to constitute the defect. It is recognition of different planes by different groups for the purposes of classification that accounts for some apparent conflicts existing within the literature. Thus, within the initial classification proposed by Soto *et al.*,[6] a defect was considered to be perimembranous when its border, as viewed from the right ventricular aspect, was made up in part by fibrous continuity between the leaflets of the aortic and tricuspid valves (Fig. 25). In the subsequent approach recommended by Soto and different colleagues,[14] a perimembranous defect was held to be one bordered by the leaflets of the aortic valve, but the defect defined in this fashion was considered to represent the continuation of the long axis of the ventricular septum. Thus, a different plane of space is defined as the defect in these two systems. It is hardly surprising, therefore, that discrepancies in description now exist between them. The beauty of the initial system proposed by Soto *et al.*[6] is that it is valid with or without the presence of overriding valves, and that it permits the surgeon accurately to predict the location of the atrioventricular conduction axis. Thus, in the setting of tetralogy of Fallot, as with any other defect, the defining criterion for it to be considered perimembranous is the presence of aortic-tricuspid valvar continuity along its margin as viewed from the right ventricle (Fig. 25). The major danger area for the surgeon along this right ventricular border is the area of aortic-tricuspid valvar continuity, since the conduction axis penetrates at this point to pass from the apex of the triangle of Koch into the left ventricular outflow tract (Fig. 26). Having penetrated, the bundle usually branches below the crest of the ventricular septum (Fig. 27). On occasion, however, branching can occur directly astride the septal crest.[15,16] This then increases the vulnerability of the bundle during surgical correction (Fig. 28). In most of these perimembranous defects, the postero-inferior fibrous margin of the defect is reinforced by a flap of fibrous tissue derived from the membranous septum (Fig. 25).[17,18] This membranous flap can be used to anchor sutures, but care is needed not to pass the sutures too deeply within the fibrous tissue, since the flap overlies directly the location of the penetrating atrioventricular bundle (Fig. 27). Perimembranous defects of this type are found in approximately four-fifths of

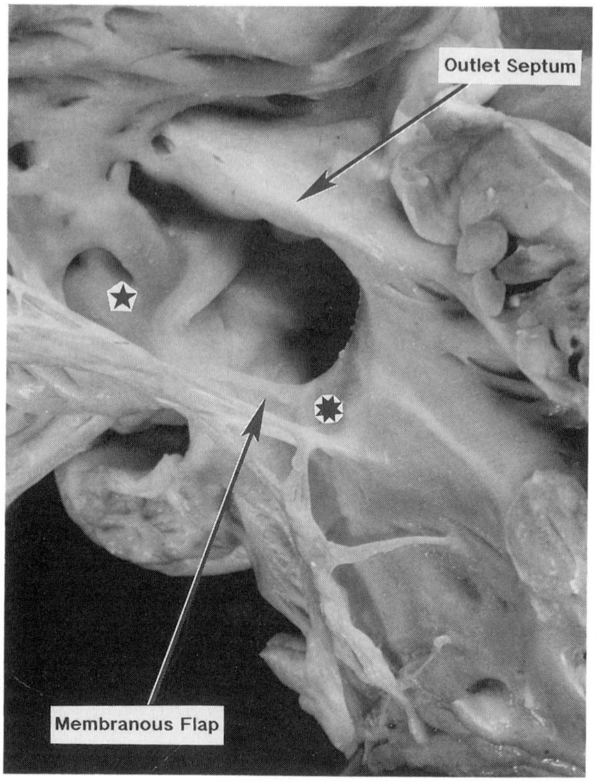

Fig. 25 This ventricular septal defect is described as being perimembranous because of the extensive part of the right ventricular border which is formed by fibrous continuity between the leaflets of the tricuspid and aortic valves between the posterior limb of the septomarginal trabeculation (eight-pointed star) and the ventriculo-infundibular fold (five-pointed star). Note the membranous flap.

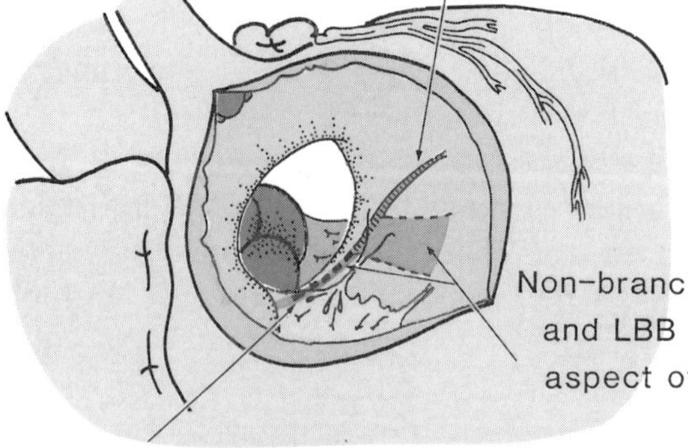

Fig. 26 The view of the location of the atrioventricular conduction axis (orange) as it would be seen by the surgeon working through a right ventriculotomy. RBB, LBB, right and left bundle branches.

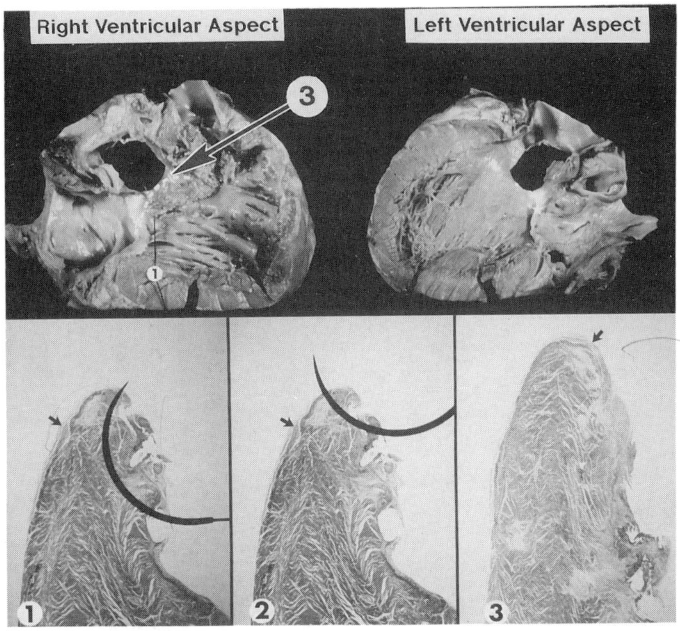

Fig. 27 This ventricular septum, from a specimen of tetralogy of Fallot with a perimembranous ventricular septal defect, is shown from the right and left ventricular aspects. It was then sectioned to produce the histological sections shown in panels 1–3. The conduction axis, which is arrowed, is carried on the left ventricular aspect of the septum at points 1 and 2, and is safe from the sutures. The right bundle branch, however, is astride the septum at point 3. Reproduced by kind permission of Prof. Hiromi Kurosawa, Jikei University, Tokyo, Japan.

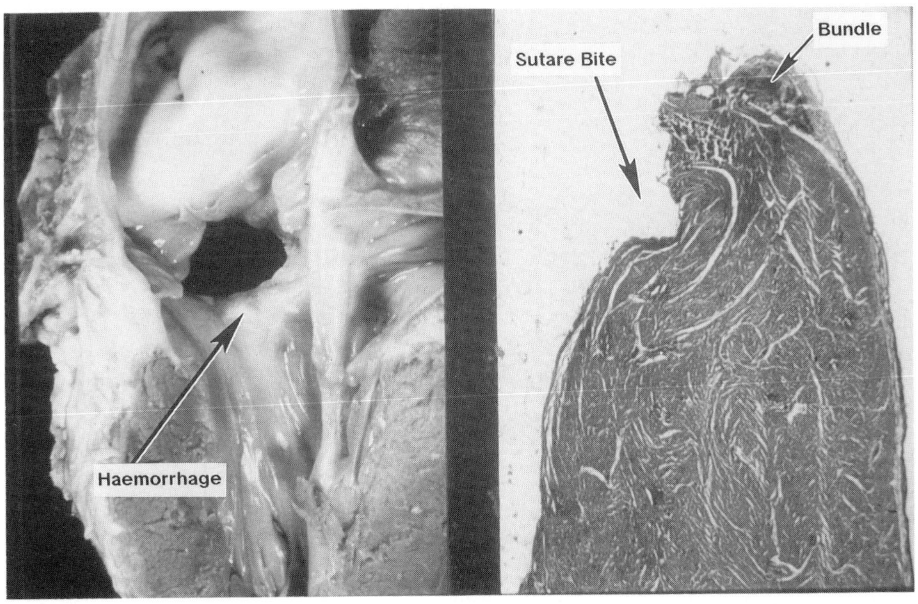

Fig. 28 In this case, the conduction axis was positioned directly astride the crest of the muscular ventricular septum. The left-hand panel shows a view of the left ventricular aspect, and shows the haemorrhage produced by a suture placed in the septal crest. The right-hand panel shows how the stitch has passed directly round the conduction axis. Reproduced by kind permission of Mr James Monro, Wessex Cardiothoracic Centre, Southampton, United Kingdom.

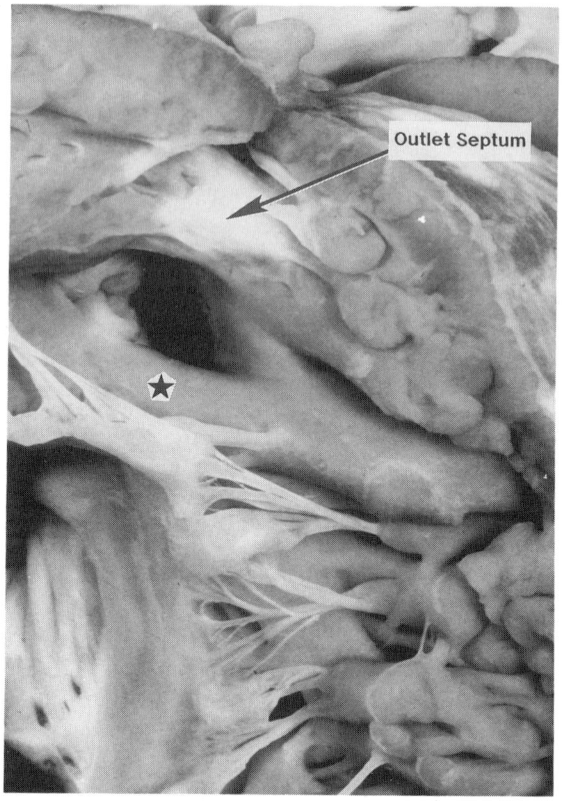

Fig. 29 The variant of ventricular septal defect in tetralogy of Fallot in which fusion of the ventriculo-infundibular fold with the posterior limb of the septomarginal trabeculation (star) produces a muscular postero-inferior border between the leaflets of the aortic and tricuspid valves.

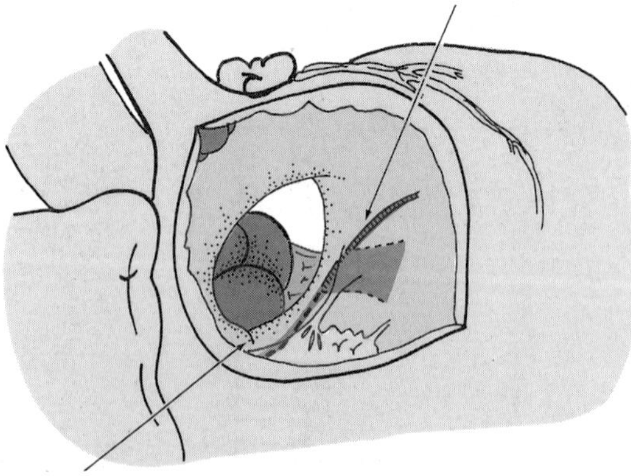

Fig. 30 The view of the defect with a muscular postero-inferior rim as seen by the surgeon working through a right ventriculotomy. The muscular border protects the conduction axis (orange).

patients with tetralogy of Fallot seen in the western world.[2] In most of the remaining patients, a fundamental variation is found in the structure of the postero-inferior margin of the border of the defect as seen from the right ventricle. Instead of this border being formed by fibrous tissue, as is the case with the perimembranous defect, the posterior limb of the septomarginal trabeculation fuses with the ventriculo-infundibular fold (Fig. 29). This fusion of the two muscular structures produces a muscular postero-inferior rim between the leaflets of the tricuspid valve and aortic valves (Fig. 30). This protects the point of penetration of the atrioventricular conduction axis, so that, provided the muscular border is of sufficient size, stitches can be placed within it without fear of damaging the conduction pathways.

In a small proportion of patients seen in the west, but in a larger proportion of those seen in the Far East or South America,[19–21] there is then a further variation in the structure of the right ventricular margin of the cone of space beneath the overriding aortic valve. This occurs when there is complete absence of the muscular outlet septum, along with the margins of the subpulmonary infundibulum which usually interpose between the right

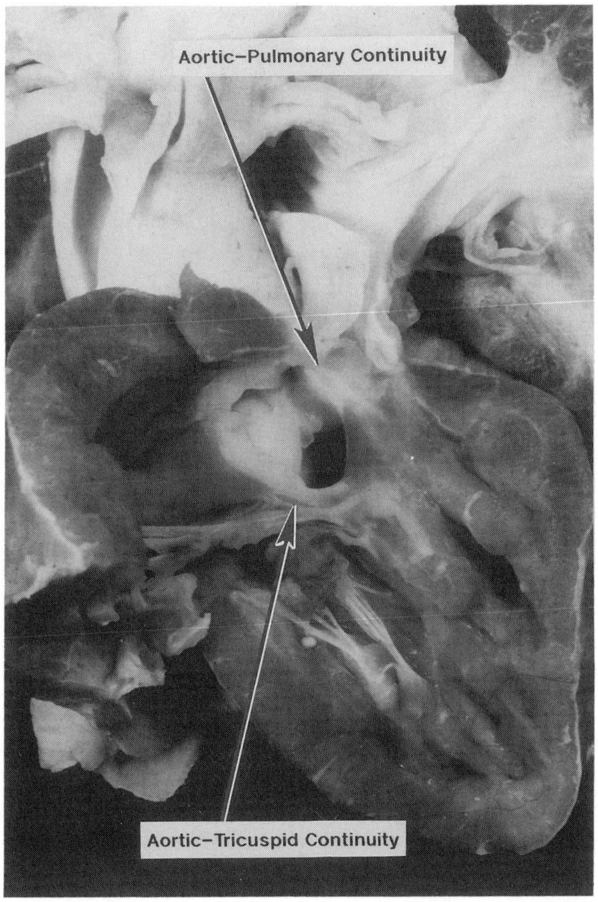

Fig. 31 In this heart, there is absence of the muscular outlet septum and the "septal" components of the subpulmonary infundibulum. The ventricular septal defect is perimembranous and doubly committed and juxta-arterial.

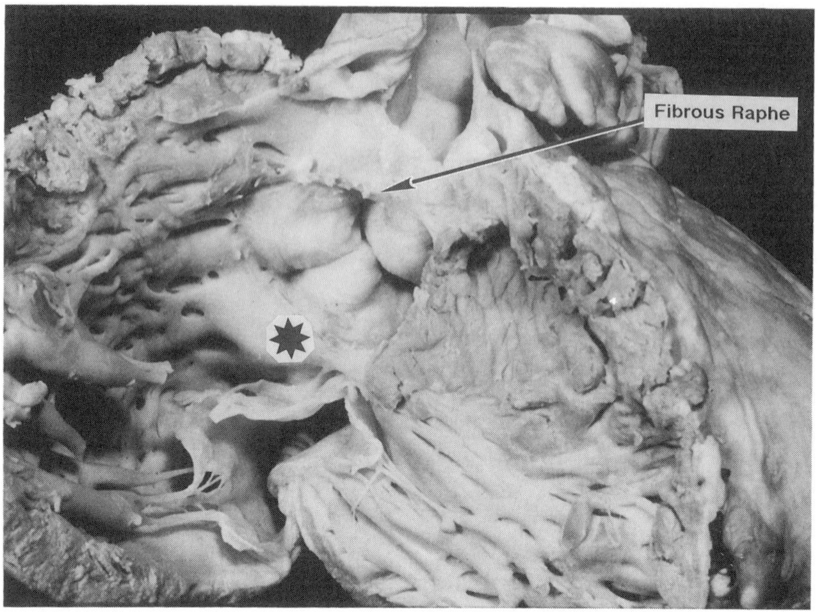

Fig. 32 In this heart, a muscular postero-inferior rim (star) interposes between the leaflets of the tricuspid and pulmonary valves, although the defect is doubly committed and juxta-arterial.

ventricle and the aortic valvar sinuses. This means that the facing leaflets of the aortic and pulmonary valves are in fibrous continuity in the roof of the defect (Fig. 31). Such presence of fibrous continuity between the arterial valvar leaflets was the criterion used for distinguishing defects as being doubly committed in the original classification of Soto *et al.*[6] We continue to describe these defects in this way. According to the nature of the posterior margin of the right ventricular border, the doubly committed defects can extend to become perimembranous (Fig. 31) or can have a muscular postero-inferior rim (Fig. 32). It is the morphology in this postero-inferior margin which determines the location of the atrioventricular conduction axis. Others describe these doubly committed defects as being subpulmonary.[19]

Another obvious area of variation is in the extent of attachment, and support, of the aortic valvar leaflets within the two ventricles. In the majority of cases, the leaflets are connected predominantly within the left ventricle, with extensive fibrous continuity between the leaflets of the aortic and mitral valves. The right coronary aortic leaflet, however, is also in fibrous continuity with the antero-superior leaflet of the tricuspid valve, this feature emphasizing the connection of the overriding aortic valve within the right ventricle (Fig. 16). Even when the ventriculo-infundibular fold interposes between the leaflets of the aortic and tricuspid valves, four chamber (Fig. 33) and short axis sections show that the aortic leaflets are attached to right ventricular structures. On occasion, even when the aorta is predominantly connected within the left ventricle (Fig. 34), the ventriculo-infundibular fold can persist as a muscular structure separating the aortic leaflets from those of the mitral valve. The outflow tract morphology, nonetheless, is unequivocally that of tetralogy. Equally, with typical outflow tract morphology, but with fibrous continuity between the leaflets of aortic, mitral, and tricuspid valves, the aorta can be positioned such that over 90% of its circumference is attached within the right ventricle. This means that a heart with the morphology of tetralogy of Fallot co-exists with double outlet ventriculo-arterial connections.[22,23]

Still further variation then exists in the nature of the obstruction to flow of blood to the lungs. We have emphasized that the essential part of this obstruction is a squeeze between the deviated outlet septum and the septoparietal trabeculations. This muscular stenosis is then usually further excacerbated by valvar stenosis, occurring in most cases in the setting of a valve with two leaflets (Fig. 35). Still further stenosis can occur in the peripheral branches of the pulmonary trunk. Stenosis can also be found within the body of the right ventricle, when excessive hypertrophy of the apical component of the body of the septomarginal trabeculation produces so-called "two-chambered right ventricle". The major variation, nonetheless, is seen at the muscular mouth of the subpulmonary infundibulum, with fibrous tissue often accreting round this area to worsen the situation (Fig. 36). On occasion, this thickening can be so severe as to produce atresia at the orifice of the infundibulum, or else the pulmonary valve can become imperforate, again producing tetralogy of Fallot with pulmonary atresia (Fig. 37).

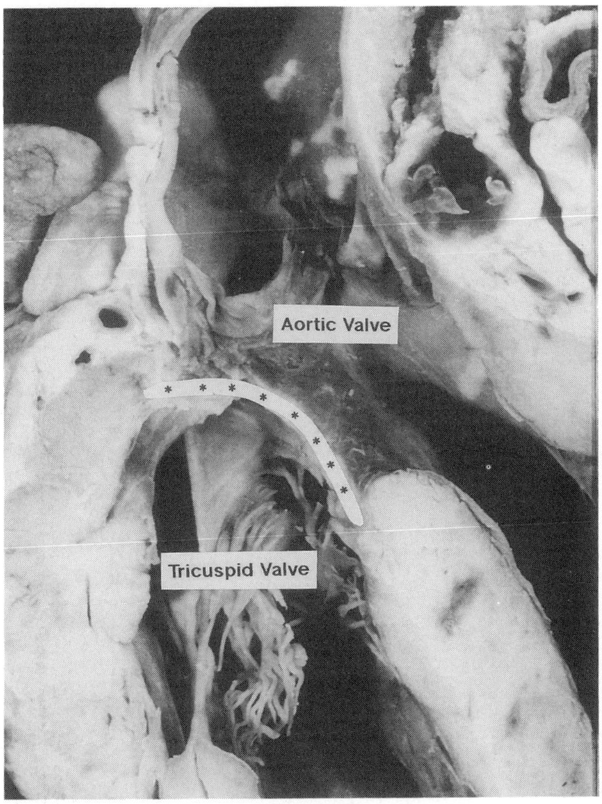

Fig. 33 The muscular rim interposes between the leaflets of the tricuspid and aortic valves, but the aortic valve is shown by this four-chamber section to be connected predominantly to right ventricular structures.

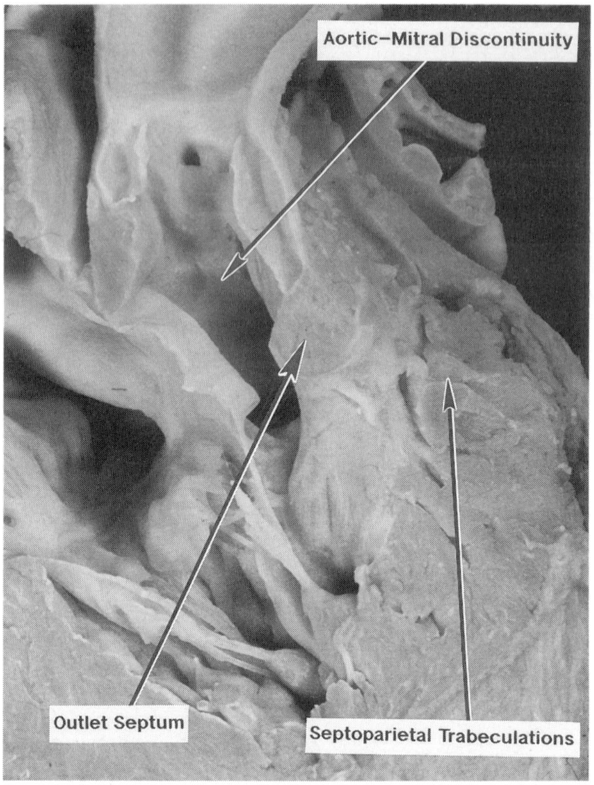

Fig. 34 In this heart, with overriding and biventricular connection of the aortic valve, and the typical subpulmonary infundibular morphology of tetralogy of Fallot, the persisting ventriculo-infundibular fold produces discontinuity between the leaflets of the aortic and mitral valves.

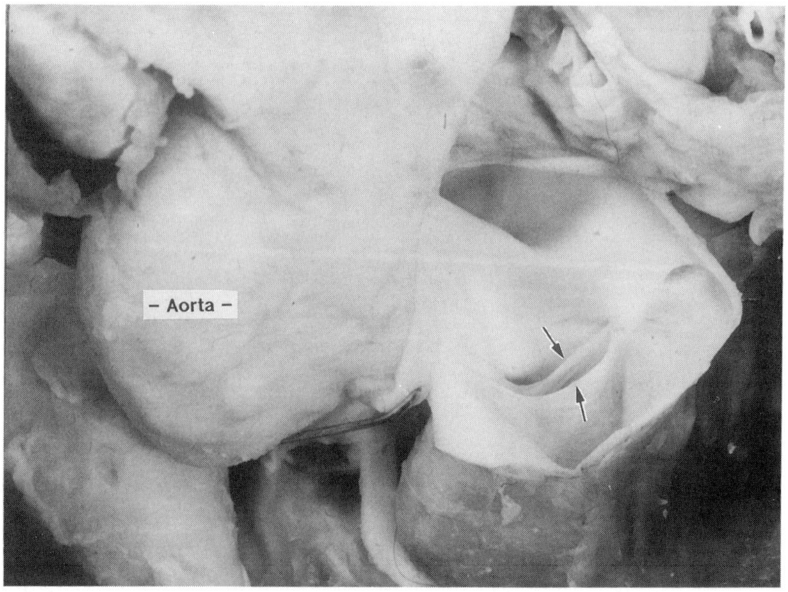

Fig. 35 The pulmonary valve in this specimen of tetralogy of Fallot has only two leaflets.

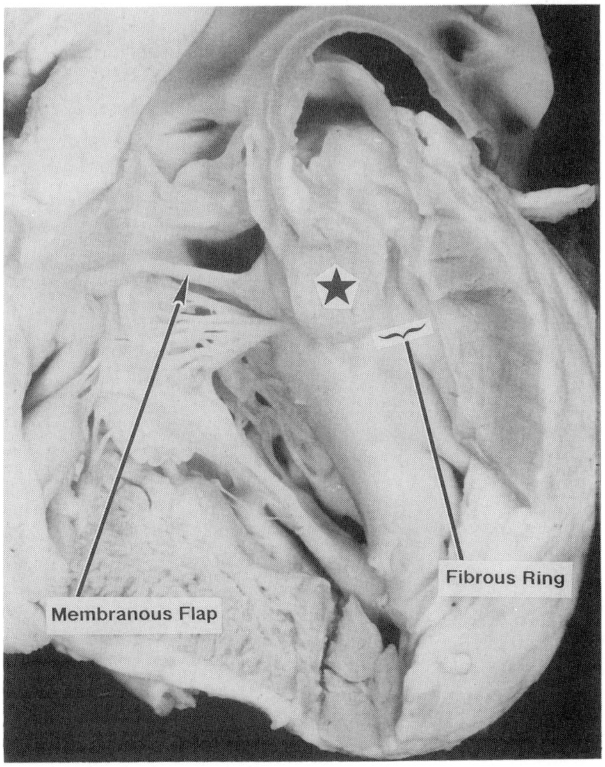

Fig. 36 This oblique subcostal equivalent section shows a fibrous ring accentuating the obstruction at the mouth of the subpulmonary infundibulum. Note the membranous flap forming the postero-inferior border of the perimembranous ventricular septal defect.

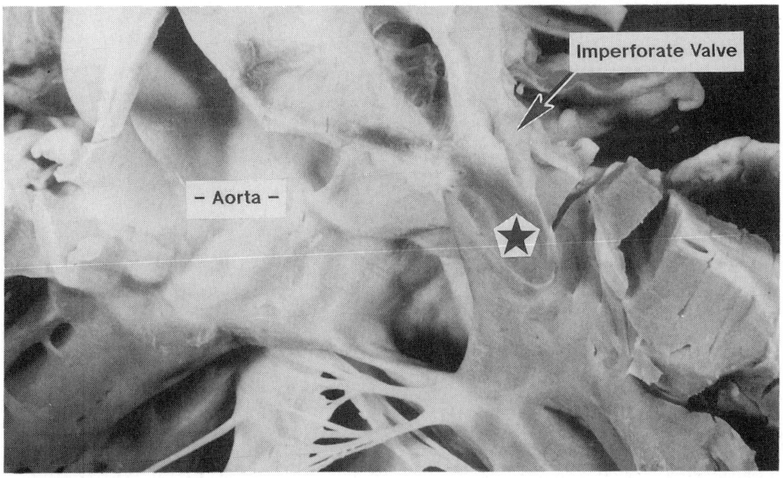

Fig. 37 In this specimen, with the typical antero-cephalad deviation of the outlet septum (star), the pulmonary valve is imperforate.

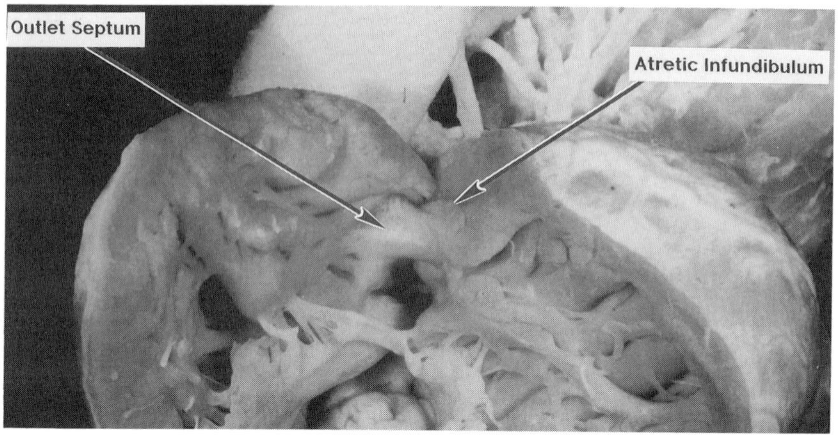

Fig. 38 The typical intracardiac anatomy of tetralogy of Fallot with perimembranous ventricular septal defect is seen in this heart with co-existing muscular pulmonary atresia.

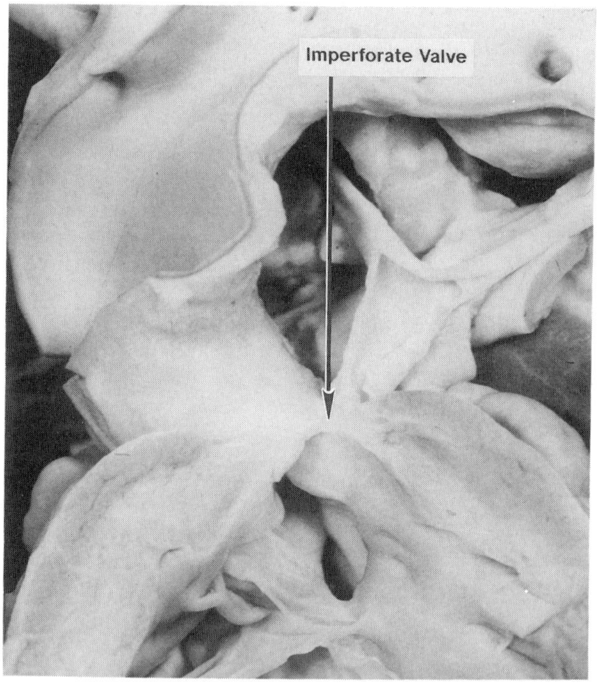

Fig. 39 In this heart with tetralogy of Fallot and pulmonary atresia, the ventricular septal defect is doubly committed and juxta-arterial, extending to the undersurface of the imperforate pulmonary valve in absence of the muscular outlet septum (compare with Fig. 31).

This association has itself been the source of contention, with many preferring to describe the combination as pulmonary atresia with ventricular septal defect. We cannot cavil at the accuracy of this designation, since the hearts clearly have both pulmonary atresia and a ventricular septal defect. But so do many other hearts, such as those with the segmental connections of complete or corrected transposition, yet those latter specimens do not have the intracardiac morphology of tetralogy of Fallot. In the presence of an atretic infundibular mouth, or an imperforate valve (Fig. 37), there can be no question concerning the hallmarks of tetralogy. Similarly, in the majority of patients with muscular atresia at the ventriculo-pulmonary junction, the intracardiac anatomy is unmistakenly that of tetralogy (Fig. 38). Even those with absence of a blind-ending muscular infundibulum can be interpreted to represent atresia in the setting of tetralogy with a doubly committed and juxta-arterial defect (Fig. 39). All of this is significant because, almost without exception, cases with pulmonary arterial supply derived from systemic-to-pulmonary collateral arteries are found only when the intracardiac anatomy is that of tetralogy or one of its variants. This is why, in our opinion, it is preferable to include these cases within the overall spectrum as examples of tetralogy with pulmonary atresia rather than stenosis.

CONTROVERSIAL ASPECTS

The right ventricular outflow tract or infundibulum

The right ventricular outflow tract, or infundibulum, in Fallot's tetralogy is the tubular sleeve of right ventricular myocardium which supports the leaflets of the pulmonary valve. As we have seen, only a part of the infundibulum is formed by the true outlet septum. In other words, the essence of Fallot's tetralogy is not simply malpositioning of the outlet septum, but rather abnormal formation of the entire infundibulum, including the hypertrophied septoparietal trabeculations. It is the subpulmonary infundibulum , therefore, which is narrow and obstructive in Fallot's tetralogy. But is it also short? According to Van Praagh and his colleagues,[24] this structure is, indeed, "too short, too narrow and too shallow" in tetralogy of Fallot. The narrowed infundibulum, in their opinion, is underdeveloped in all three of its dimensions. This concept, however, is based largely on embryological premises, with lack of conal growth being advanced as the major underlying developmental error. As far as we know, measurements have not been carried out in autopsied hearts by Van Praagh and his associates so as to substantiate the hypothesis. We have had great difficulties with this statement from the very start. Our own morphometric studies of a series of hearts with Fallot's tetralogy, conducted over twenty years ago, showed that the infundibular length, compared to the subpulmonary infundibulum of the normal heart, certainly was not "too short". Rather, it was more extensive.[25] In normal hearts, when we measured the length of the infundibular sleeve and expressed the value relative to the total length of the right ventricular outflow tract measured from the apex to pulmonary valve, the mean ratio was 0.28. In hearts with Fallot's tetralogy, the average of the ratio was 0.36 (Fig. 40). These findings were subsequently confirmed in more extensive studies.[26] These data, therefore, obtained by simple observation and measurement, show that it is not the case that, in hearts with Fallot's tetralogy, the infundibulum is "too short, too narrow and too shallow". The situation reminds us of the statement attributed to Bertrand Russell "Aristotle could have avoided the mistake of thinking that women have fewer teeth than men by the simple device of asking Mrs. Aristotle to open her mouth".

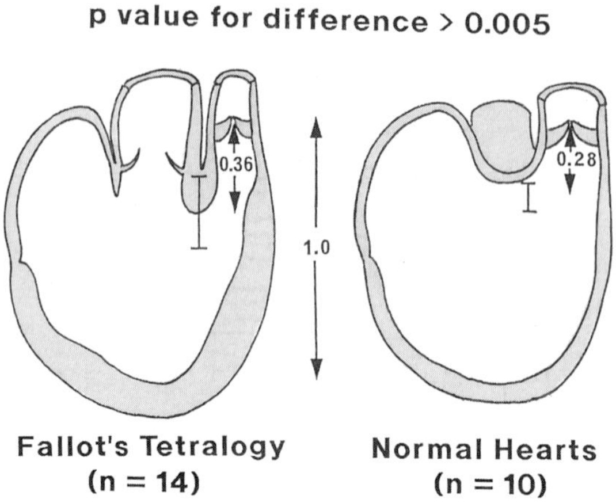

Fig. 40 This diagram shows the values for the length of the subpulmonary infundibulum in tetralogy of Fallot and in the normal heart from the study of Becker *et al.*[25]

This, of course, should not be construed to suggest that there is no such thing as a "short infundibulum" in Fallot's tetralogy. On the contrary, the length of the infundibulum is highly variable, and hearts with extremely short infundibulums certainly exist (Fig. 41). As a matter of fact, as we have demonstrated, this infundibular hypoplasia may reach the stage where the "septal" component is lacking, along with the outlet septum, giving rise to the doubly committed and juxta-arterial ventricular septal defect (Fig. 31). It is then arguable as to whether hearts with these doubly committed and juxta-arterial defects should be included within the spectrum of tetralogy. We have indicated that the hallmark of the condition is antero-cephaled deviation of the outlet septum, coupled with hypertrophied septoparietal trabeculations. Yet the outlet septum, and part of the subpulmonary infundibulum, are lacking in the hearts with doubly committed defects. The septoparietal trabeculations, in contrast, are present and remain hypertrophied. Furthermore, the outlet septum and sleeve of infundibular musculature can vary to being very long or very short when they are present. It is not unreasonable, therefore, to consider absence of the muscular outlet septum as the end of a spectrum of diminishing size. And, should an outlet septum be considered to represent the raphe usually present between the hingepoints of the leaflets of the aortic and pulmonary valves, the typical anatomy of tetralogy would be restored. Indeed, this effect can sometimes inadvertently be created during surgical repair, with residual stenosis ensuing if attention has not been given to resection of the septoparietal trabeculations. For all these reasons, one of us (AEB) has always considered it appropriate to include this lesion within the category of tetralogy.[2] The other (RHA) was initially sceptical,[27] but has been convinced by the force of the arguments outlined above. Hypoplasia of the subpulmonary infundibulum, therefore, can certainly occur in the setting of a malformed heart which in any other respect is that of tetralogy of Fallot, but it is the exception rather than the rule. It is the structure of the subpulmonary infundibulum, not its length, which is the hallmark of the malformation.

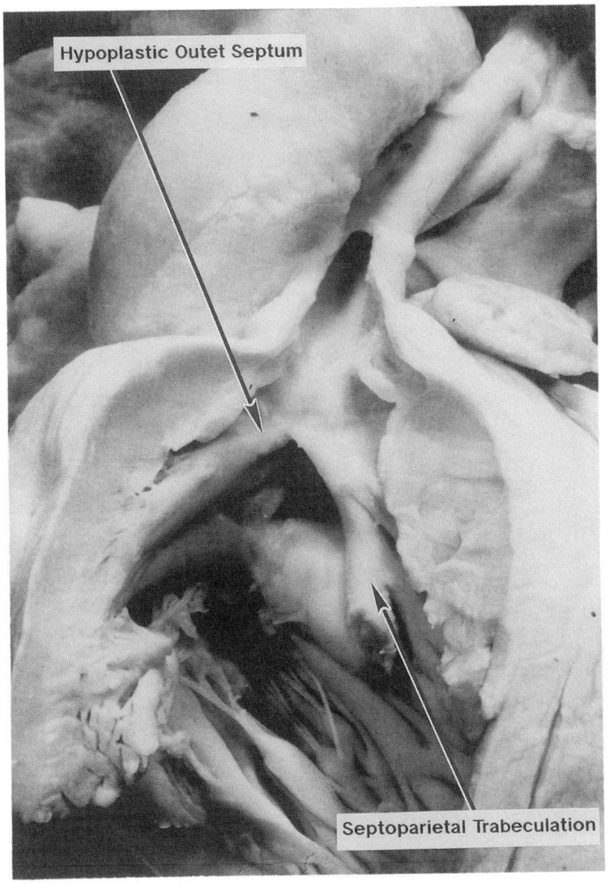

Fig. 41 The subpulmonary infundibulum is not always extensive in tetralogy of Fallot, as shown in this specimen (compare with Fig. 7). As shown by the measurements in Fig. 40, nonetheless, the infundibulum is longer than normal in most hearts.

Fallot's tetralogy versus double outlet right ventricle

All agree that one of the classical anatomic features of Fallot's tetralogy is a large ventricular septal defect associated with overriding of the aorta. As we emphasized at the outset, from the pathophysiological viewpoint this makes Fallot's tetralogy a heart in which both right and left ventricles eject blood into the aorta. The right ventricle, of course, also has another outlet, albeit narrowed, into the pulmonary trunk. Hence, in all hearts, to some extent, there is double outlet from the right ventricle. But very few hearts with tetralogy of Fallot exhibit bilateral infundibulums (conuses). This remains a source of major contention. To put this in perspective, it is necessary to consider the roots of terminology in congenital heart disease. Double outlet right ventricle is the perfect example of the situation which might be considered as "spotlight" terminology, the spotlight being the double outlet from the right ventricle. The question arises, however: at what stage of override of the aorta does the ventricle achieve its double outlet? This may sound "spooky", until it is realized that, with increasing connection of the aortic valve to the right ventricle, it is the ventriculo-arterial connection that changes, and not the ventricle. Fallot's tetralogy perfectly exemplifies this point. We have shown how, in tetralogy of Fallot, the degree of aortic override may vary considerably. Indeed, in some hearts which otherwise show all the characteristics of Fallot's tetralogy, the aorta is connected within the right ventricle for 90%, or more, of its circumference. We have always followed the general principle that the specific pattern of a ventriculo-arterial connection will change at the stage where more than 50% of an arterial trunk overrides,[28] and see no reason to change this rule for Fallot's tetralogy.[29] With more than 50% attachment of the aortic valve in the right ventricle, therefore, it is the ventriculo-arterial *connection* which is categorized as double outlet. This is no reason to exclude such a heart from the category of Fallot's tetralogy. Similarly, there is no reason to exclude hearts from the category of Fallot's tetralogy simply because *dis*continuity exists between the leaflets of the mitral and aortic valves (Fig. 34). The key to the resolution of this semantic argument is to appreciate that the double outlet condition represents the ventriculo-arterial connection, whereas Fallot's tetralogy exists because of a particular morphologic arrangement of the right ventricular outflow tract.

So, if the question is posed: "are all tetralogies of Fallot also double outlet right ventricles?" the answer is no. Only those with more than half of the aortic valve connected within the right ventricle have a double outlet ventriculo-arterial connection and, as such, could be categorized among other hearts classified as double outlet right ventricle. Similarly, if the question is then: "are all double outlet right ventricles also examples of Fallot's tetralogy?" the answer is no again. Only those hearts with the characteristic morphology of the outflow tracts fit this category. The majority of hearts with double outlet right ventricle have nothing in common with Fallot's tetralogy. The apparent controversy, in our opinion, is basically a matter of indoctrination. If conventional wisdom dictates that double outlet right ventricle is a specific entity, then there is a problem. But those who might promote such a concept must admit that the so-called entity contains a large variety of hearts which share as their common feature only the double outlet ventriculo-arterial connection from the right ventricle. In other aspects, the hearts may be quite different. For instance, the so-called Taussig-Bing heart, creating controversy in its own right,[11,30] unequivocally belongs to the class of hearts with double outlet right ventricle. There is no morphological similarity whatsoever between the Taussig-Bing malformation and Fallot's tetralogy. Reiterating our initial point, the spotlight terminology of double outlet right ventricle is based on the notion that the ventriculo-arterial connection is double outlet rather than anything else. Extending this point, if another condition is associated with double outlet right ventriculo-arterial connection, it could then be argued that the heart should either be classified as "double outlet right ventricle" or "whatever the other condition might be". Take, for example, the association of an atrioventricular septal defect with common atrioventricular junction and double outlet right ventricle. This combination promotes little discussion. It is widely accepted that the two abnormalities may coexist. Why, then, should there be controversy in the case of Fallot's tetralogy when the pathognomonic abnormality of the right ventricular outflow tract coexists with such a degree of aortic override that the ventriculo-arterial connection becomes double outlet? It is high time that this controversy is put to rest.

DEVELOPMENTAL CONSIDERATIONS

It is clear that the factory for the production of tetralogy of Fallot lies in the outlet component of the developing heart tube. It is equally clear from the morphologic findings outlined in this chapter that the abnormal development involves the entirety of the outlet component, and is not simply a matter of malposition of the septal component within otherwise normally developing outlets. The measurements produced by the Leiden group,[4] when they showed that the position of the outlet septum was comparable in hearts with the Eisenmenger variant of ventricular septal defect and in tetralogy of Fallot (compare Figs. 2, 3), provide strong evidence that the abnormal growth involves the entirety of the subpulmonary infundibulum. This, indeed, was very much the hypothesis advanced by Van Praagh and his colleagues[24] under the banner of differential conal growth. Their argument was that the entire subpulmonary infundibulum was under-developed, being "too short, too narrow and too shallow". The subpulmonary infundibulum is certainly of lower volume than normal, and is too narrow and shallow. As we have demonstrated, however, it is not too short. All the measurements of which we are aware show that, in fact, the subpulmonary infundibulum is longer in tetralogy of Fallot than in the normal heart. The muscular outlet septum is much better represented in the abnormal situation, not being recognizable as a discrete entity when development occurs in normal fashion. The resolution of the morphogenetic problems, therefore, will come when we understand the origin of the free-standing sleeve of subpulmonary infundibulum, and how this is derived from the structures which septate the outlet component of the developing heart tube. It is well established that the outlet segment is the distal extent of the ascending limb of the ventricular loop. Initially, the entire arterial segment, or the aortic sack, is supported by the outlet component above the developing right ventricular apex, which is also derived from the distal limb of the ventricular loop.[31] During the process of normal development, the aortic sack is divided so that the fourth aortic arches are placed in continuity with the aortic half of the outlet component, while the sixth aortic arches are placed in continuity with the subpulmonary outlet. This is achieved by division of the aortic sack by the aortopulmonary septum, with cells in this area being derived initially from the neural crest, and fusion of this septum with the ridges or swellings which septate the outlet component of the heart tube itself. The elegant studies of Patterson and his colleagues in Keeshond dogs have shown that the outlet ridges are abnormally located in animals developing tetralogy of Fallot,[32] but it is still not known why the ridges should be malpositioned. Nor is it known how the mesenchymal ridges are transformed into the muscular subpulmonary infundibulum. This change, in which the septal ridges which initially divide a common outflow tract become, in part, a free-standing sleeve of right ventricular infundibulum is, perhaps, the key to development. Conventional wisdom dictates that the outflow ridges, having fused, also

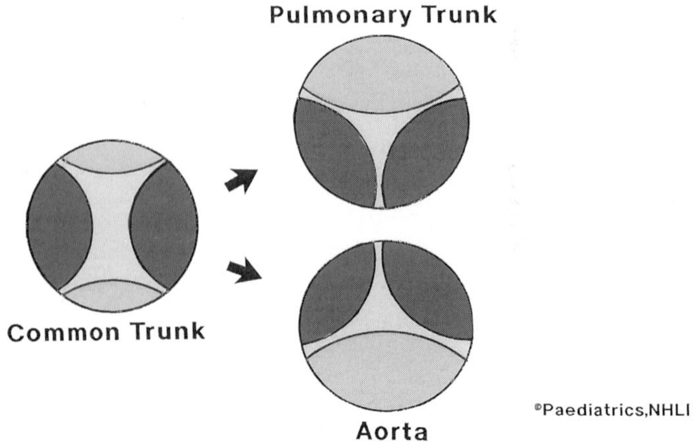

Fig. 42 Most concepts of embryology, as far as we are aware, contend that the ridges and cushions which septate the common arterial trunk which exist during early developmental stages (left-hand panel) give rise to the facing valvar leaflets of the aorta and pulmonary trunk (right-hand panel). The concepts fail to address the fact that, in the definitive heart, the two valves are separated by the free-standing muscular subpulmonary infundibulum (see Fig. 17).

give rise to four of the sinuses of the arterial trunks and the arterial valvar leaflets they contain (Fig. 42). This process is not quite as simple as might be imagined, because this developmental event is also complicated by formation of the subpulmonary infundibulum. Thus, at the end of development, the leaflets of the pulmonary valve are separated from those of the aortic valve by the full extent of the subpulmonary infundibulum, with the long axes of the two normal ventricular outlets being almost at right angles to each other. This process, that of formation of the subpulmonary infundibulum, has failed to occur in hearts with doubly committed and juxta-arterial defects. These hearts, in effect, are examples of a common ventricular outlet but with separate arterial valves and trunks, analogous to the so-called ostium primum defect in the setting of a common atrioventricular junction. Thus, when we know the precise mechanisms involved in the formation of the free-standing sleeve of subpulmonary muscular infundibulum, we will not only be in a better position to understand the morphogenesis of tetralogy of Fallot, but also to relate it to hearts with doubly committed juxta-arterial defects and, in addition, common arterial trunk.

REFERENCES

1. Fallot A. Contribution a l'anatomie pathologique de la maladie bleue (cyanose cardiaque). *Mar Med* 1888;**25**:77–403.
2. Becker AE. Tetralogy of Fallot: from unifying pathology to variables. In: Yacoub M, Pepper JR (eds). *Annals of Cardiac Surgery.* London: Current Science. 1992: pp 81–91.
3. Eisenmenger V. Die angeborenen Defecte der Kammerscheidewand des Herzens. *Ztschr Klin Med* 1897;**32**:1–28.

4. Oppenheimer-Dekker A, Gittenberger-De-Groot AC, Bartelings MM, Wenink ACG, Moene RJ, Van der Harten JJ. Abnormal architecture of the ventricles in hearts with an overriding aortic valve and a perimembranous ventricular septal defect ("Eisenmenger VSD"). *Int J Cardiol* 1985;**9**:341–355.
5. Goor DA, Lillehei CW. *Congenital Malformations of the Heart.* New York: Grune and Stratton. 1975: pp 1–37.
6. Soto B, Becker AE, Moulaert AJ, Lie JT, Anderson RH. Classification of ventricular septal defects. *Br Heart J* 1980;**43**:332–343.
7. Kleinert S, Geva T. Echocardiographic morphometry and geometry of the left ventricular outflow tract in fixed subaortic stenosis. *J Am Coll Cardiol* 1993;**22**:1501–1508.
8. Anderson RH, Becker AE, Tynan M. Description of ventricular septal defects — or how long is a piece of string? Editorial review. *Int J Cardiol* 1986;**13**:267–278.
9. Baker E, Leung MP, Anderson RH, Fischer DR, Zuberbuhler JR. The cross-sectional anatomy of ventricular septal defects: a reappraisal. *Br Heart J* 1988;**59**:339–351.
10. Kjellberg SR, Mannheimer E, Rudhe U, Jonsson B. *Diagnosis of Congenital Heart Disease,* 2nd ed. Chicago: Year Book Medical Publishers, 1959.
11. Van Praagh R. What is the Taussig-Bing malformation? *Circulation* 1968;**38**:445–449.
12. Lev M, Bharati S, Meng CCL, Liberthson RR, Paul MH, Idriss F. A concept of double-outlet right ventricle. *J Thorac Cardiovasc Surg* 1972;**64**:271–281.
13. Anderson RH, Becker AE, Van Mierop LHS. What should we call the "crista"? *Br Heart J* 1977;**39**:856–850.
14. Soto B, Ceballos R, Kirklin JW. Ventricular septal defects: a surgical viewpoint. *J Am Coll Cardiol* 1989;**14**:1291–1297.
15. Titus JL, Daugherty GW, Kirklin JW, Edwards JE. Lesions of the atrioventriular conduction system after repair of ventricular septal defect. Relation to heart block. *Circulation* 1963;**28**:82–88.
16. Anderson RH, Monro JL, Ho SY, Smith A, Deverall PB. Les voies de conduction auriculo-ventriculaires dans le tetralogie de Fallot. *Coeur* 1977;**8**:793–807.
17. Kurosawa H, Imai Y, Becker AE. Surgical anatomy of the atrioventricular conduction bundle in tetralogy of Fallot. New findings relevant to the position of the sutures. *J Thorac Cardiovasc Surg* 1988;**95**:586–591.
18. Kurosawa H, Becker AE. *Atrioventricular Conduction in Congenital Heart Disease. Surgical Anatomy.* Tokyo: Springer-Verlag. 1987: pp 97–144.
19. Ando M. Subpulmonary ventricular septal defect with pulmonary stenosis. Letter to Editor. *Circulation* 1974;**50**:412–410.
20. Neirotti R, Galindez E, Kreutzer G, Coronel AR, Pedrini M, Becú L. Tetralogy of Fallot with sub-pulmonary ventricular septal defect. *Ann Thorac Surg* 1978;**25**:51–56.
21. Vargas FJ, Kreutzer GO, Pedrini M, Capelli H, Corone AR. Tetralogy of Fallot with subarterial ventricular septal defect. Diagnostic and surgical considerations. *J Thorac Cardiovasc Surg* 1986;**92**:908–912.
22. Wilcox BR, Ho SY, Macartney FJ, Becker AE, Gerlis LM, Anderson RH. Surgical anatomy of double-outlet right ventricle with situs solitus and atrioventricular concordance. *J Thorac Cardiovasc Surg* 1981;**82**:405-417.
23. Edwards WD. Double-outlet right ventricle and tetralogy of Fallot. Two distinct but not mutually exclusive entities. *J Thorac Cardiovasc Surg* 1981;**82**:418–422.
24. Van Praagh R, Van Praagh S, Nebesar RA, Muster AJ, Sinha SN, Paul MH. Tetralogy of Fallot: underdevelopment of the pulmonary infundibulum and its

sequelae. Report of a case with cor triatriatum and pulmonary sequestration. *Am J Cardiol* 1970;**26**:25–33.
25. Becker AE, Connor M, Anderson RH. Tetralogy of Fallot: a morphometric and geometric study. *Am J Cardiol* 1975;**35**:402–412.
26. Howell CE, Ho SY, Anderson RH, Elliott MJ. Variations within the fibrous skeleton and ventricular outflow tracts in tetralogy of Fallot. *Ann Thorac Surg* 1990;**50**:450–457.
27. Griffin ML, Sullivan ID, Anderson RH, Macartney FJ. Doubly committed subarterial ventricular septal defect: new morphological criteria with echocardiographic and angiocardiographic correlation. *Br Heart J* 1988;**59**:474–479.
28. Tynan MJ, Becker AE, Macartney FJ, Quero-Jimenez M, Shinebourne EA, Anderson RH. Nomenclature and classification of congenital heart disease. *Br Heart J* 1979;**41**:544–553.
29. Kirklin JW, Pacifico AD, Bargeron LM, Soto B. Cardiac repair in anatomically corrected malposition of the great arteries. *Circulation* 1973;**48**:153–159.
30. Hinkes P, Rosenquist GC, White RIJ. Roentgenographic re-examination of the internal anatomy of the Taussig-Bing heart. *Am Heart J* 1971;**81**:335–339.
31. de Jong S, Viràgh S, Moorman AFM. Cardiac development: a morphologically integrated molecular approach. *Cardiol Young* 1997;**7**:228–240.
32. Patterson DF, Pyle RL, Van Mierop L, Melbin J, Olson M. Hereditary defects of the conotruncal septum in Keeshond dogs: pathologic and genetic studies. *Am J Cardiol* 1974;**34**:187–205.

Chapter 5

Hearts with Univentricular Atrioventricular Connection

INTRODUCTION

As we discussed in our opening chapter, the hearts which have either double inlet ventricle or atrioventricular valvar atresia have given us as many problems over our combined experience as the other congenitally malformed hearts put together. As we will explain, it was the recognition that these hearts are unified because they exhibit a univentricular atrioventricular connection, rather than being univentricular hearts, which clarified the situation for us, and enabled us to describe the overall group in an entirely logical manner.[1,2] We should emphasize from the outset that, even now, we never describe any individual heart as having a "univentricular atrioventricular connection". There are much more precise ways of describing the individual lesions themselves. The concept of the univentricular connection is simply a means of grouping together hearts with comparable morphologies across the atrioventricular junctions, and separating them from the much larger group of hearts which have biventricular atrioventricular connections. It is also the case that a small proportion of the hearts described as having a univentricular atrioventricular connection will also have a solitary chamber within the ventricular mass. The greatest majority, in contrast, have one big and one small ventricle, with the atrial chambers either being exclusively or predominantly connected to the big ventricle. It has been the desire, over the years, to describe these hearts with imbalance of the chambers within the ventricular mass as "univentricular", or "single ventricle", or variations on these themes,[3,4] which has created problems. In the old days, when it was often difficult precisely to recognize the morphologic make-up of the ventricular mass during life, and diagnosis was more often made on the basis of inference, there were extenuating circumstances which supported this approach. Nowadays, when it is possible to show exactly the structure of the ventricular myocardium, and its relationship to the atrioventricular valves (Fig. 1), there can be no excuse for using terms which are either illogical or imprecise. All the problems are resolved when different terms are used to describe the arrangement of the atrioventricular junction as opposed to the morphology of the chambers within the ventricular mass.

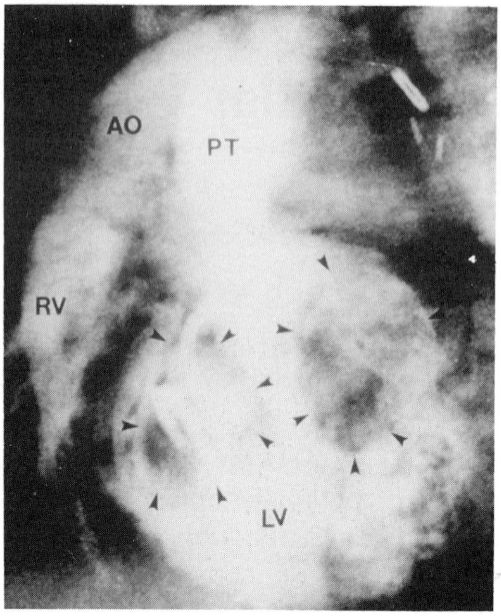

Fig. 1 This angiogram shows that the heart with double inlet left (LV) ventricle has a big left (LV) and a small right (RV) ventricle. The two atrioventricular valves connected to the big ventricle are shown by the arrows. The ventriculo-arterial connections are discordant (AO-aorta; PT-pulmonary trunk). Reproduced by kind permission of Dr Michael Rigby, Royal Brompton Hospital, London.

THE ATRIOVENTRICULAR JUNCTIONS

As we discussed extensively in Chapter 2, the normal heart has two atrioventricular junctions, around which the segments of atrial myocardium are inserted into the vestibules of the mitral and tricuspid valves (Fig. 2). These arrangements produce biventricular atrioventricular connections. The essence of the overall group of hearts which have univentricular atrioventricular connections is that the segments of atrial myocardium are connected to only one chamber within the ventricular mass. The exemplar of this situation is seen with double inlet atrioventricular connection (Fig. 3). In the setting of double inlet, the segments of right-sided and left-sided atrial myocardium can both be connected to a dominant left ventricle (Fig. 3), to a dominant right ventricle (Fig. 4), or to a solitary and indeterminate ventricle (Fig. 5). A univentricular connection across the atrioventricular junctions is also produced when one of the atrioventricular connections is completely absent, the muscular floor of the involved atrial chamber then being separated from the ventricular mass by the fibro-fatty tissues of the atrioventricular groove. This second type of univentricular connection can be found when the absent connection is right-sided (Fig. 6) or left-sided (Fig. 7). These arrangements can also be found with the patent atrioventricular junction connected to a dominant left, a dominant right, or to a solitary and indeterminate ventricle (Fig. 8).

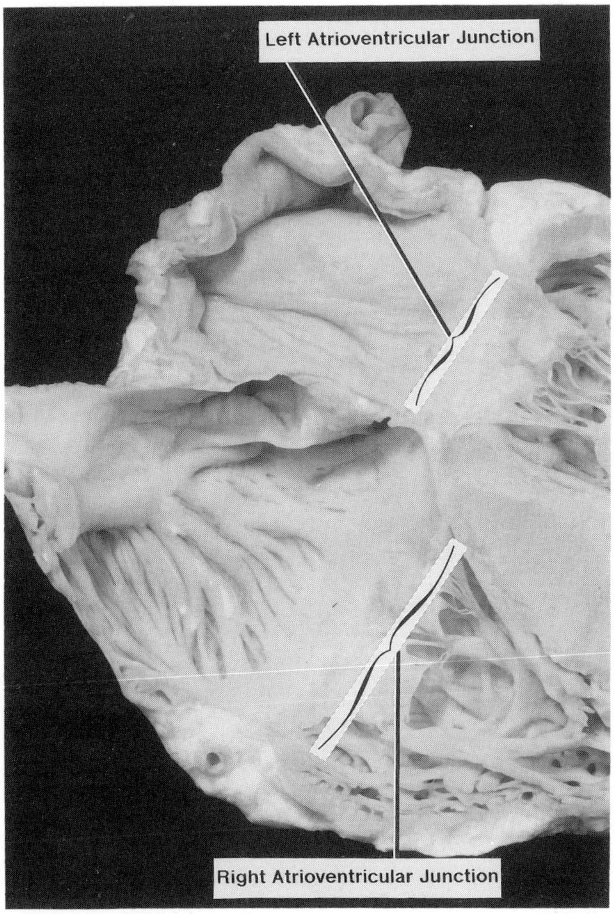

Fig. 2 The normal heart has two atrioventricular junctions, each guarded by a separate atrioventricular valve.

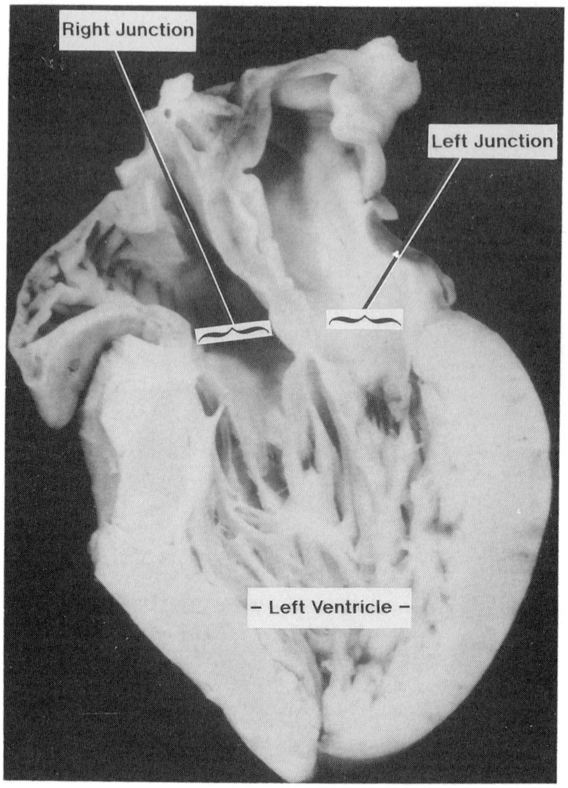

Fig. 3 In this heart, both atrioventricular junctions are connected to the same ventricle, which is of left ventricular morphology, through two atrioventricular valves.

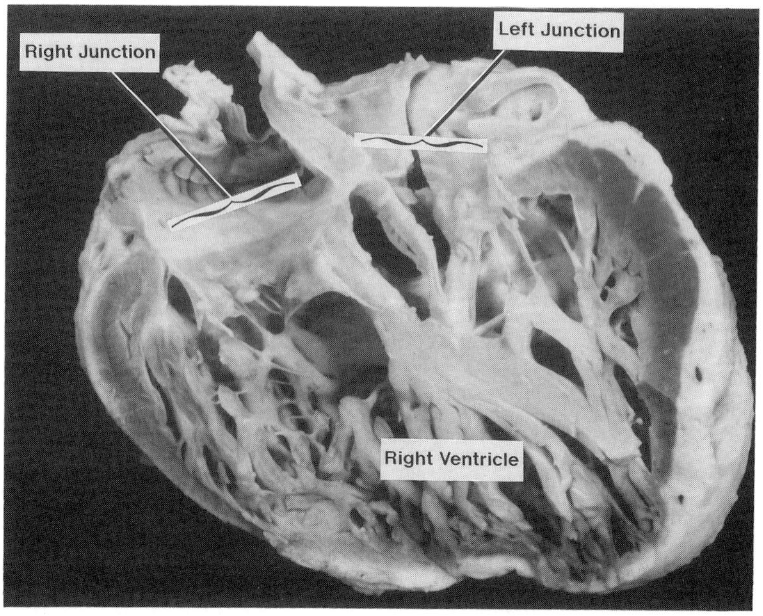

Fig. 4 This illustration shows double inlet, again through two atrioventricular valves, to a right ventricle.

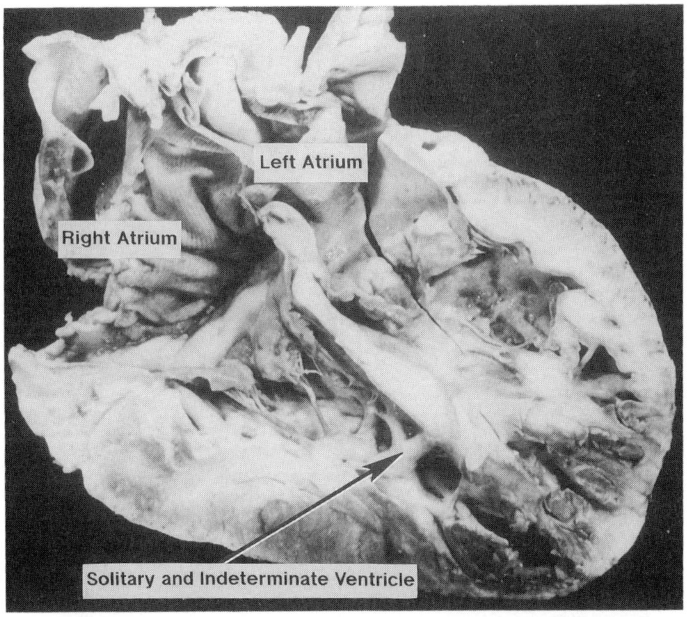

Fig. 5 The ventricle to which both atriums are connected in this heart, again through separate atrioventricular valves, is of neither right nor left ventricular morphology. It is a solitary ventricle of indeterminate morphology.

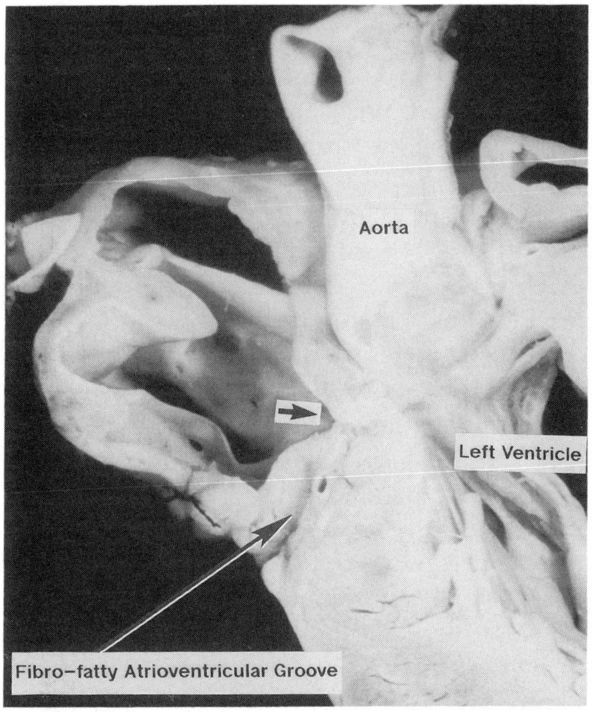

Fig. 6 This heart has been sectioned in four-chamber plane through the atrioventricular junctions. The right junction is completely absent, the muscular atrial floor being separated from the ventricular mass by the fibro-fatty right atrioventricular groove. Note that the dimple in the atrial floor points to the outflow tract of the dominant left ventricle (arrowed).

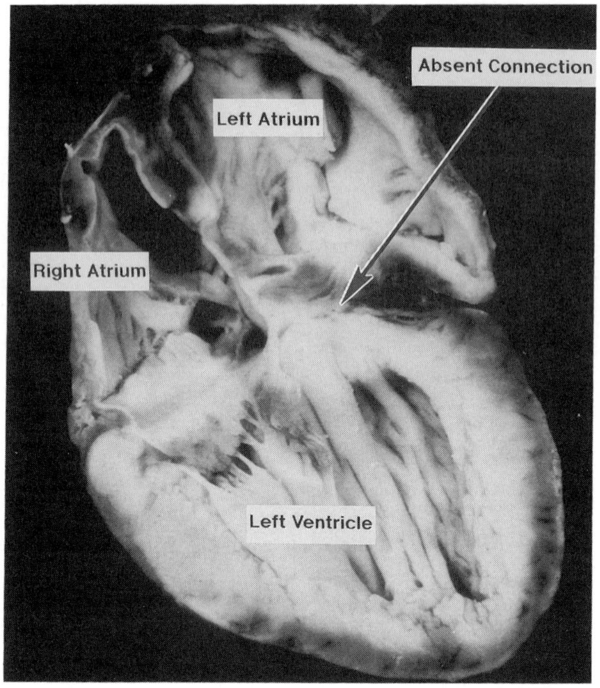

Fig. 7 In this heart, again prepared by four-chamber section, it is the left atrioventricular connection which is absent. The right atrium is connected to a dominant left ventricle.

Since the atrioventricular connections reflect only the way in which the atrial myocardium is joined with the ventricular mass, the junctional morphology is independent of the structure of the valvar tissue which guards the univentricular connection. Thus, in the setting of double inlet ventricle (Fig. 9), the two junctions joining to the same ventricle can be guarded by two atrioventricular valves (Figs. 3–5), one of which may be imperforate (Fig. 10), by a common valve (Fig. 11), or by a valvar orifice which overrides the ventricular septum (Fig. 12). Hearts with overriding valvar orifices are of particular interest because, in terms of the junctional morphology, they are intermediate between the groups of hearts having biventricular as opposed to univentricular atrioventricular connections (Fig. 13). In a heart with one big and one small ventricle, as long as the greater part of the overriding atrioventricular junction is connected to the big ventricle, then the connection across the atrioventricular junctions of the heart with a straddling atrioventricular valve is effectively double inlet. In contrast, when a minority of the overriding junction is connected to the ventricle which already receives the other atrioventricular junction, then the arrangement is effectively biventricular. Thus, when the specific atrioventricular connection is adjudicated as changing at the mid-point of this spectrum, this approach is entirely valid for categorization of the atrioventricular connections.[5] This was not the case when we used the degree of valvar override to adjudicate the state of the chambers within the ventricular mass. In our old system,[6] we described a chamber receiving greater than half of the circumference of an overriding valve as a ventricle, whereas a chamber receiving less than half the overriding atrioventricular junction was denied ventricular status. This was despite the fact that, irrespective of the degree of overriding, the morphology of the ventricular apical trabecular component was the same (Figs. 14, 15). This approach was justifiably criticized by Van Praagh and his colleagues as being non-morphologic.[7] The lack of logic in this system, particularly describing the "non-ventricle" as being of right or left ventricular morphology, was then emphasized by Brandt.[8] The obvious validity of these criticisms brought home to us the realization that, within the hearts described, it was the atrioventricular connection which shifted from being univentricular to biventricular. This realization, in turn, prompted the shift to our current approach as described herein. As we will see, this is now entirely logical, unambiguous, and descriptive.[1,2]

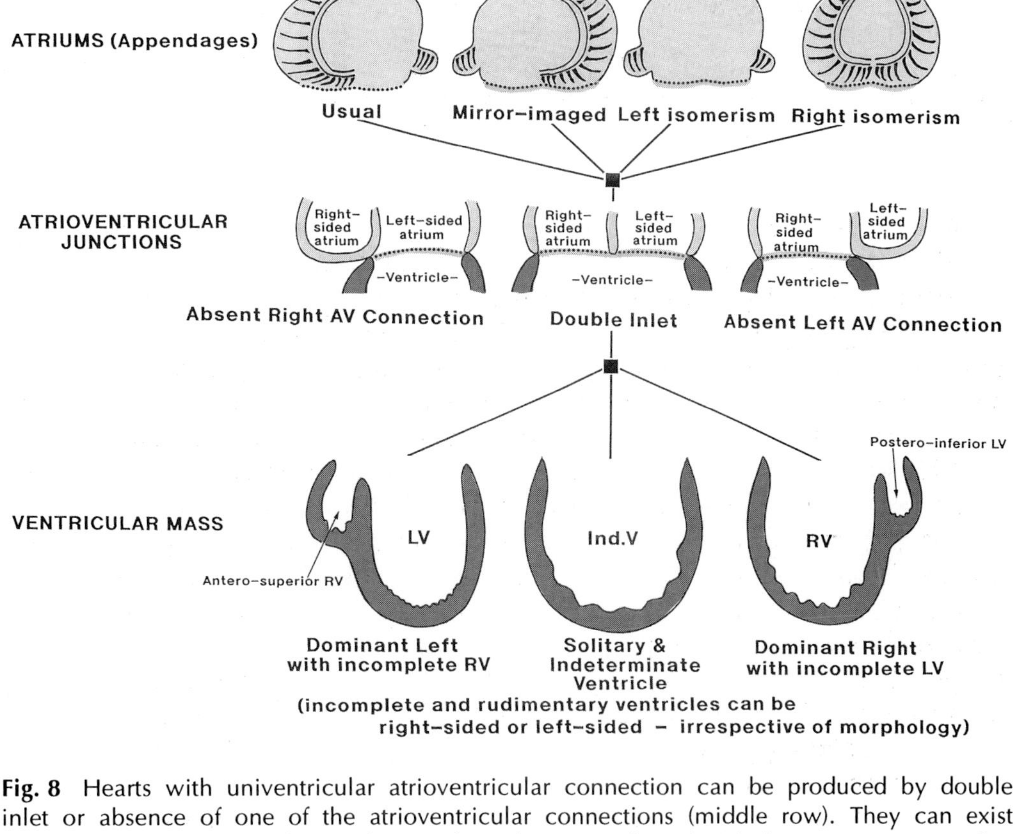

Fig. 8 Hearts with univentricular atrioventricular connection can be produced by double inlet or absence of one of the atrioventricular connections (middle row). They can exist with any arrangement of the atrial appendages (upper row), and with the atrium connected to a dominant left, a dominant right, or a solitary and indeterminate ventricle (bottom row). Only the hearts with indeterminate ventricles are univentricular. The diagram does not account for variations in ventricular relationships, ventriculo-arterial connections, or associated malformations. Reproduced by kind permission of the Editors and Publishers of Cardiology in the Young.[5]

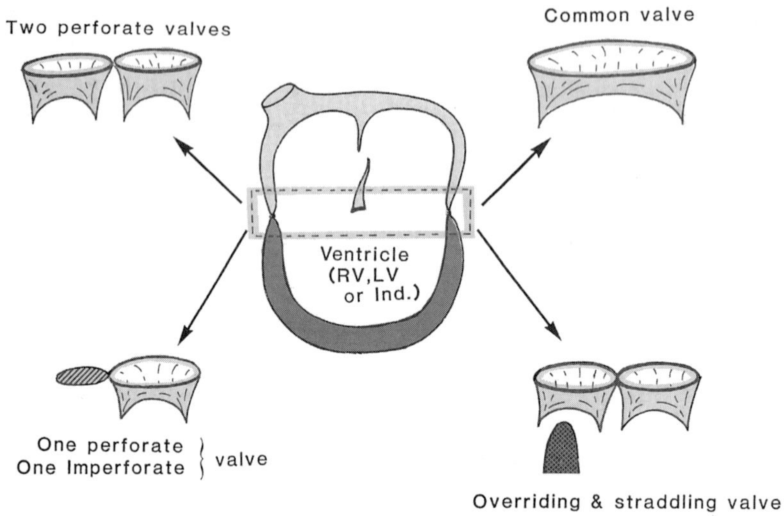

Fig. 9 When both atriums are connected to the same ventricle, the double inlet connection can be guarded by various arrangements of the atrioventricular valves which, as shown, are independent of the atrioventricular connection.

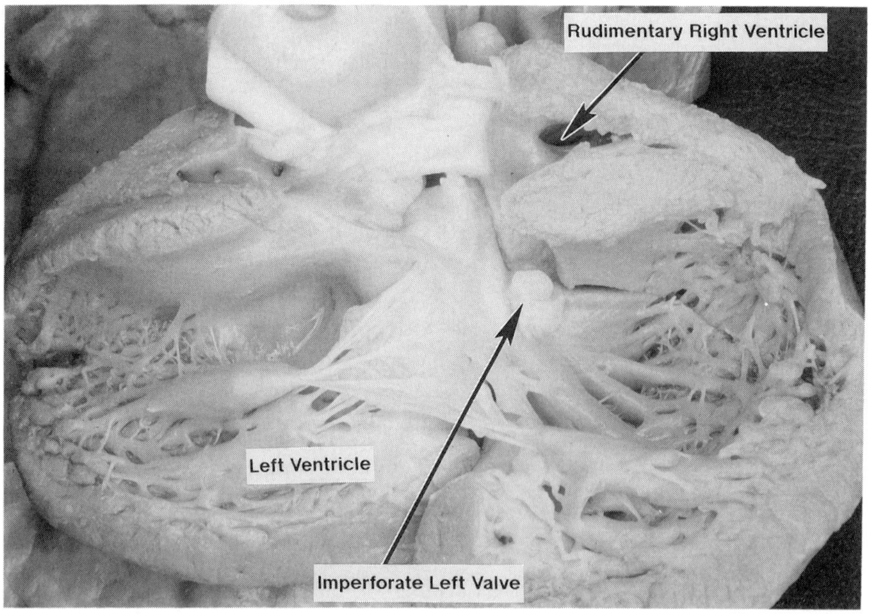

Fig. 10 In this heart with double inlet left ventricle, the left atrioventricular valve (arrowed) is imperforate.

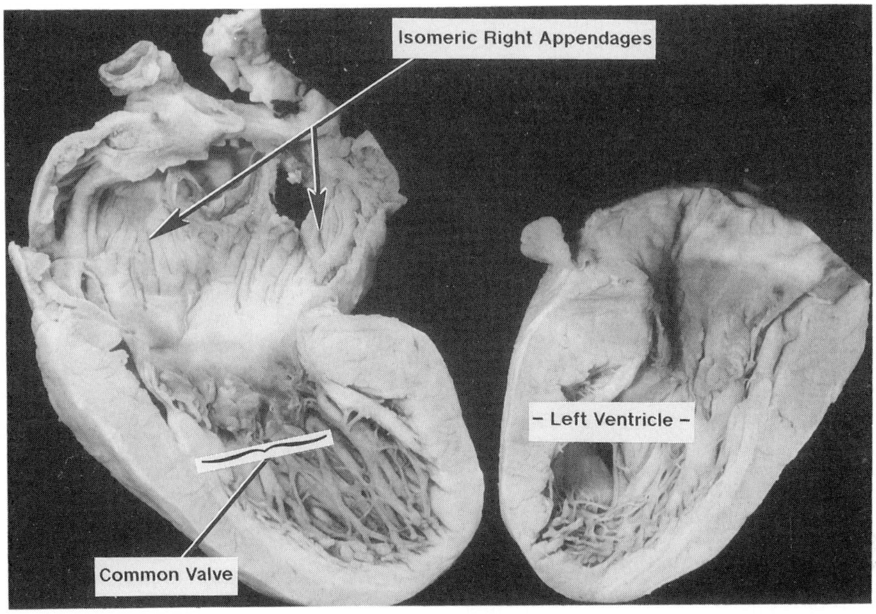

Fig. 11 This heart, with isomerism of the right atrial appendages and double inlet left ventricle, has both atrioventricular junctions guarded by a common valve.

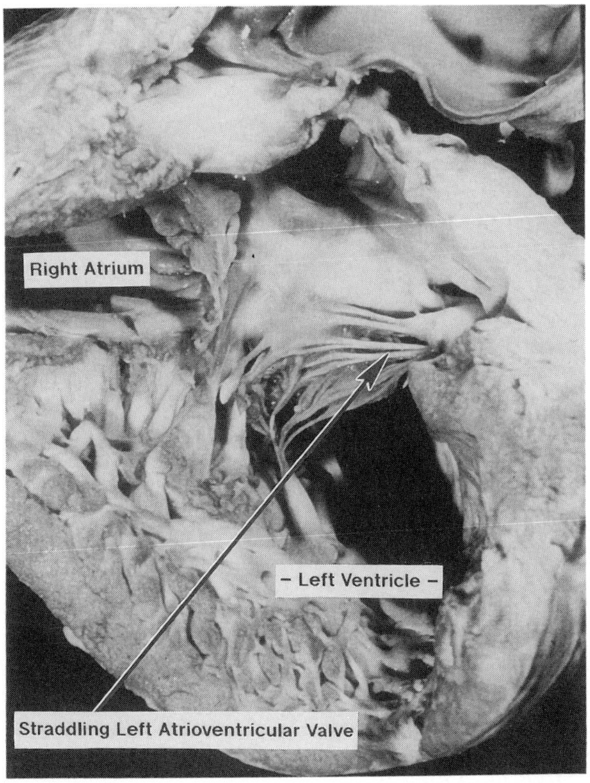

Fig. 12 In this heart, with dominant left and rudimentary right ventricle, the right atrioventricular valve straddles and overrides, but the minimal override into the rudimentary ventricle means that the atrioventricular connection remains one of double inlet.

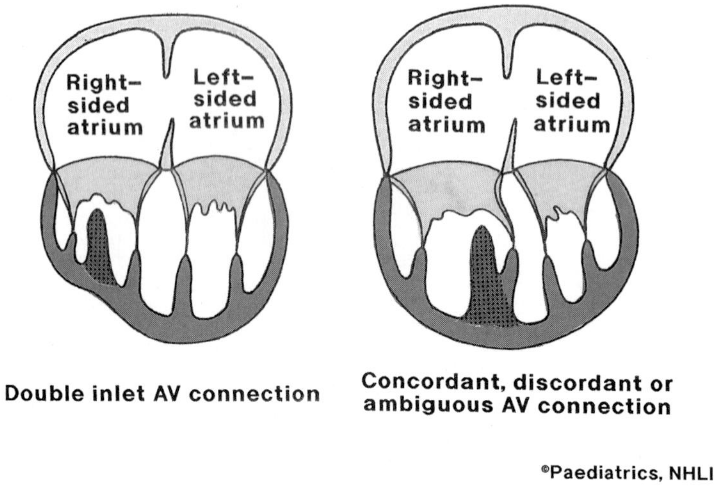

Fig. 13 In the presence of an overriding atrioventricular junction, the connection changes from being biventricular to univentricular as more of the overriding junction is committed to the dominant ventricle. The heart remains biventricular, however, in all variants. The ventricular septum is the stippled area.

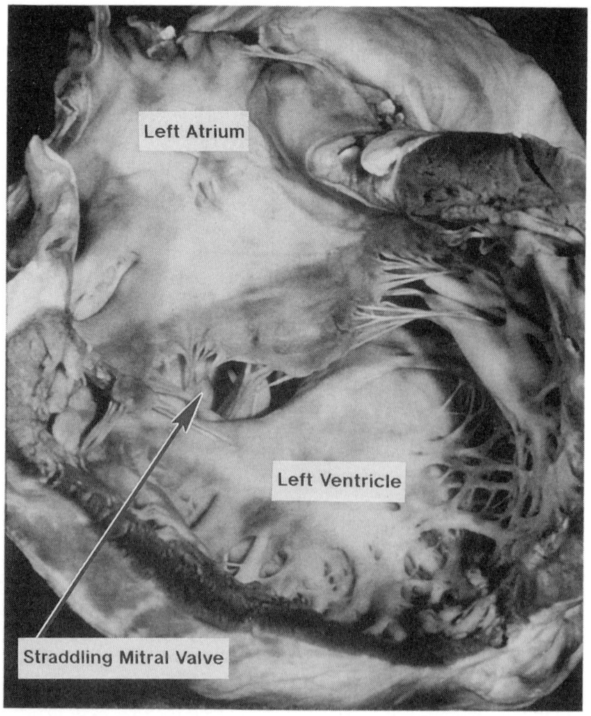

Fig. 14 This heart has straddling of the mitral valve with concordant atrioventricular connections.

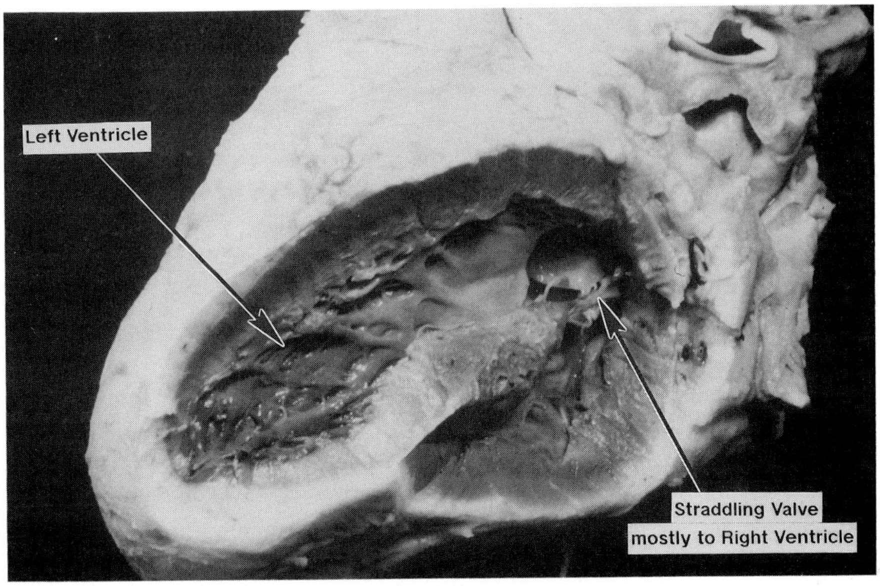

Fig. 15 In this heart, the overriding mitral valvar orifice is connected mostly to the dominant right ventricle (double inlet connection). The rudimentary ventricle, however, is still unequivocally a left ventricle, albeit lacking its outlet and the greater part of its inlet component (compare with Fig. 14).

The appreciation of the precise nature of atrioventricular junctional morphology, and its relationship to ventricular structure, is also crucial in understanding the differences of opinion which have existed concerning atrioventricular valvar atresia.[9–12] The term "atresia" simply means blockage of a natural communication within some part of the body. In the setting of the atrial chambers, this blockage of the communication to the ventricles can

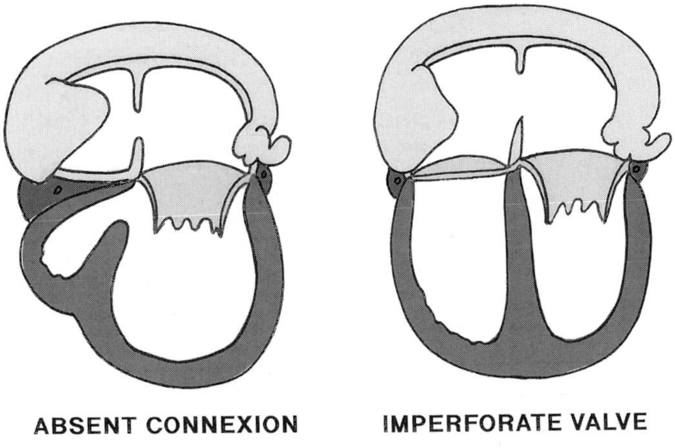

Fig. 16 There is a fundamental difference in junctional morphology between tricuspid atresia as produced by absence of the right atrioventricular connection when compared to an imperforate right atrioventricular valve. The same variation can be found for mitral atresia, and for several other segmental combinations.

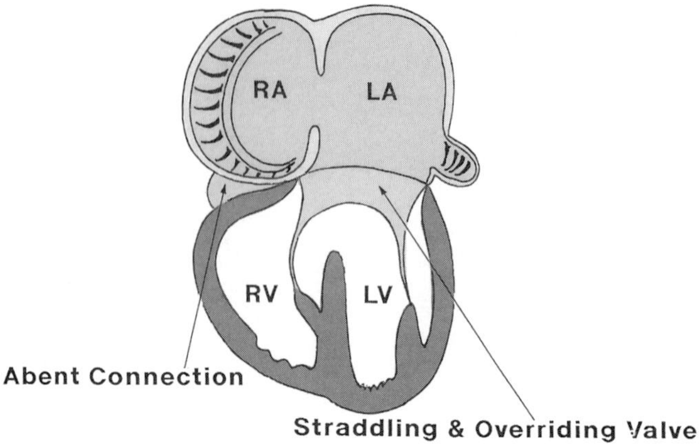

Fig. 17 When the solitary atrioventricular valve found in hearts with absence of one atrioventricular connection is straddling and overriding, the atrioventricular connection is uniatrial but biventricular. Both ventricles (RV, LV) are rudimentary to variable extent. The same situation is produced when the left atrioventricular connection is absent and the right valve straddles and overrides. RA – right atrium; LA – left atrium. Reproduced by kind permission of the Editors and Publishers of Cardiology in the Young.[5]

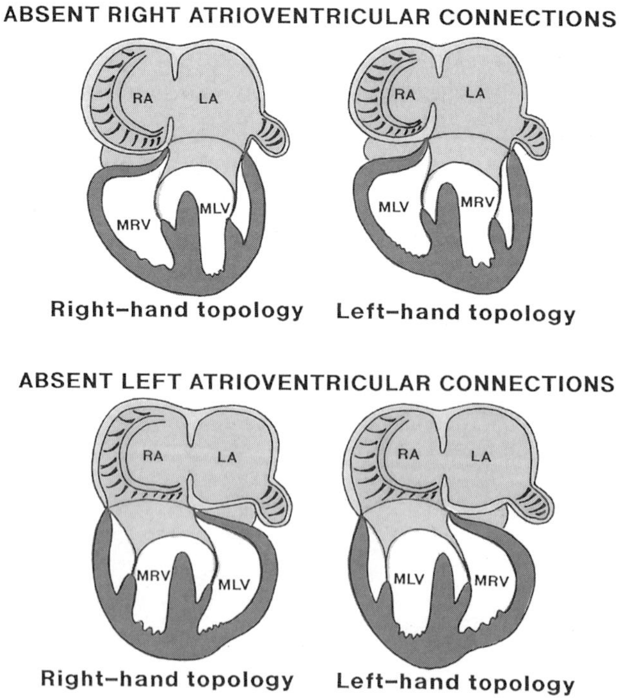

Fig. 18 The uniatrial but biventricular connection can exist in various guises depending upon the ventricular topology and which atrioventricular connection is absent. RA – right atrium; LA – left atrium; MRV – morphologically right ventricle; MLV – morphologically left ventricle. Reproduced by kind permission of the Editors and Publishers of Cardiology in the Young.[5]

exist either because an atrioventricular valve is imperforate, or because the entire atrioventricular connection is absent (Fig. 16). As discussed above, the absence of one atrioventricular connection itself constitutes a specific arrangement across the atrioventricular junction. Just as with double inlet ventricle (see above), the atrioventricular connection which remains patent in these hearts can be committed to a dominant left ventricle, to a dominant right ventricle, or to a solitary and indeterminate ventricle (Fig. 8). The variation in morphology of the valve which guards the atrioventricular connection in this setting is limited when compared to the variation possible with double inlet (Fig. 8). The solitary atrioventricular valve found in hearts with absence of one atrioventricular connection can either be exclusively connected within the dominant or solitary ventricle, or else can override so as to be shared between the right and left ventricles (Fig. 17). The variant of straddling atrioventricular valve co-existing with absence of an atrioventricular connection then, in itself, produces a specific group of atrioventricular connections which is uniatrial but biventricular. Variation within the group depends on which atrioventricular connection is absent, and on the topology and relationships of the chambers within the ventricular mass (Fig. 18). We will consider this arrangement in greater detail below.

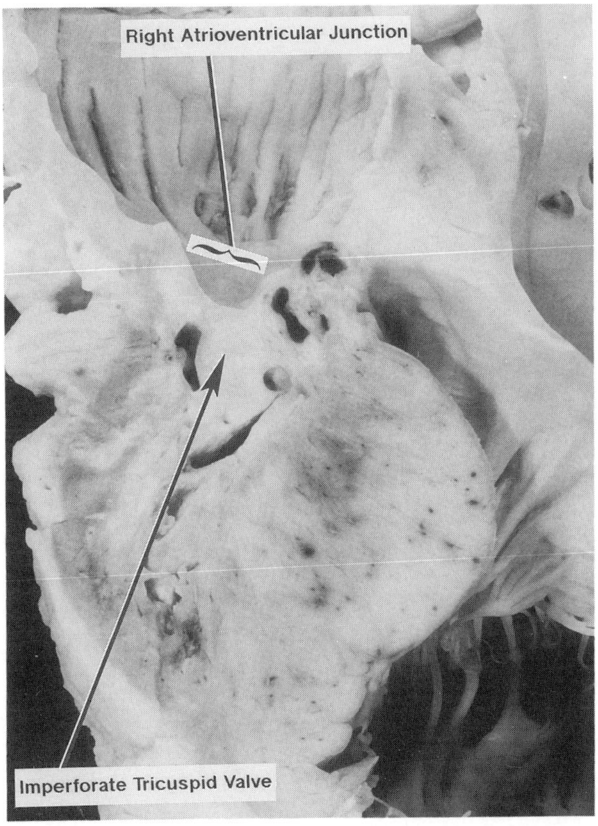

Fig. 19 This imperforate tricuspid valve is from a heart which has pulmonary atresia with intact ventricular septum and concordant atrioventricular connections. Note that it blocks the right atrioventricular connection, which is present (compare with Fig. 6).

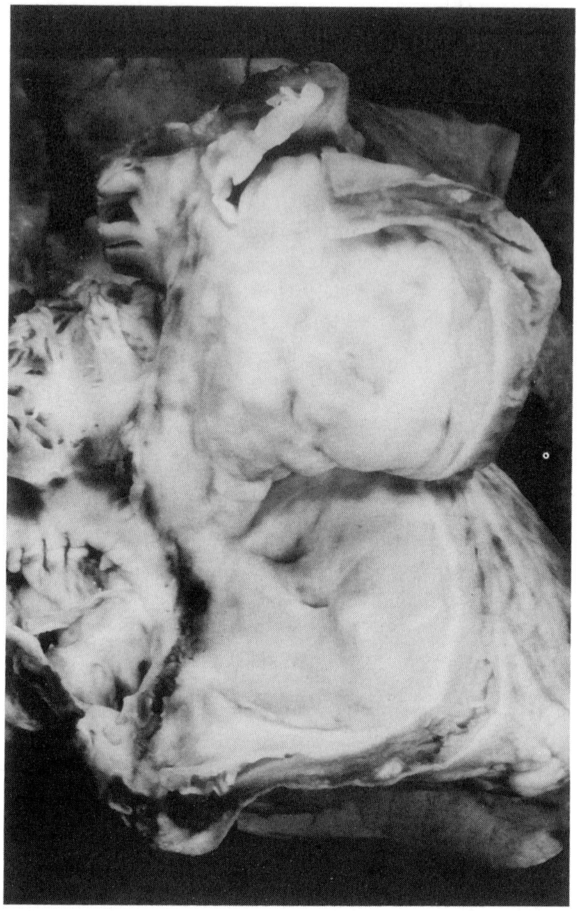

Fig. 20 This imperforate tricuspid valve, from a heart with concordant atrioventricular connections, also exhibits Ebstein's malformation. Note that the inlet component of the right ventricle is smooth and lacks trabeculations.

The variant of atrioventricular valvar atresia produced by an imperforate atrioventricular valve can also show marked variation according to the junctional morphology. Thus, we have already illustrated a heart in which an imperforate valve was found in the setting of double inlet ventricle (Fig. 10). Such imperforate valves can produce either right-sided or left-sided atrioventricular valvar atresia. But imperforate valves, either on the right side or the left side, can also be found with concordant (Fig. 19), discordant, or ambiguous and biventricular atrioventricular connections. When seen in the setting of concordant atrioventricular connections, the valve which is imperforate often shows the additional features of Ebstein's malformation (Fig. 20). All these variants of atrioventricular valvar atresia found with biventricular atrioventricular connections are beyond the scope of this chapter. Suffice it to say that it is difficult, if not impossible, to account for all this morphological variation within the simple headings of tricuspid and mitral atresia.

DESCRIPTION OF VENTRICULAR MORPHOLOGY

It is in the description of the ventricular mass that most controversies have been generated concerning the morphology of hearts unified because the atrial chambers are connected to only one ventricle. The majority of such hearts, as we have already discussed, possess one big and one small ventricle. Yet, for many years, it was conventional to describe these hearts as "single ventricle" when they possessed a double inlet atrioventricular connection.[13–15] At the same time, it was accepted that hearts with atrioventricular valvar atresia should be excluded from this univentricular category.[10,13–15] The controversies stemming from these conventions impinge on two unrelated premises. The first is exclusively semantic. Can a logical argument be constructed to justify the description of hearts with two chambers in their ventricular mass as "univentricular" or "single ventricle"? The answer to this question is that logic can be achieved only when the smaller chamber is disqualified, on arbitrary grounds, from ventricular status, thus validating the use of the otherwise illogical description. This was our initial approach to this group of hearts[6] which we now recognize to have been misplaced.[1,2] The second consideration is morphological, and concerns the structure of the small ventricle in lesions such as double inlet left ventricle when compared with the structure of the similar chamber seen in tricuspid atresia produced by absence of the right-sided atrioventricular connection in hearts with usual atrial arrangement and with the left atrium connected to a dominant left ventricle.

Returning to our first premise, the deficiencies in our initial semantics were well summarized by Van Praagh and his colleagues when they criticized our initial use of "univentricular heart". It is worth citing their arguments in full, because we recognize their validity, and they bear particularly on subsequent descriptions of these lesions. They argued, at that time, that: "Cardiac chambers should be identified, designated and classified in terms of their myocardial morphologic characteristics, because these are virtual constants in congenital heart disease." They went on to state "each variable should be defined primarily in terms of itself, not primarily in terms of any other variable".[7] We accept the force of both these arguments. It was because of such arguments that we discontinued our use of "univentricular heart" to describe those malformations having one big and one small ventricle. It was similarly the strength of such arguments which pointed to the myocardial morphologic characteristics of the atrial appendages as being the arbiters of isomerism within the atrial segment of the heart (see Chapter 3). Having accepted the principles proposed by Van Praagh *et al.*,[7] it was clear that we could no longer distinguish between ventricles and non-ventricles in hearts with double inlet atrioventricular connection. All hearts are now described as having a dominant ventricle and a rudimentary and incomplete ventricle, the incomplete ventricle being rudimentary because it lacks one or more of its component parts. An advantage of this approach is that the communication between the big and small ventricles can be described as the ventricular septal defect. In hearts with double inlet left ventricle (Fig. 21), the right ventricle is incomplete and rudimentary (Fig. 22) either because it lacks its inlet component, which is connected to the dominant ventricle (Fig. 21), or because it lacks both inlet and outlet components (Fig. 23) when the dominant left ventricle is not only connected to both atriums, but also supports both ventricular outlets (Fig. 24). In these circumstances, the anterior rudimentary chamber is recognized as being right ventricular because of the nature of its apical trabeculations (Figs. 22, 23). Such recognition follows precisely the principle of myocardial morphologic characteristics proposed by Van Praagh and his colleagues.[7] In similar fashion, when both atriums are connected exclusively, or in their greater part, to the dominant right ventricle (Fig. 25), the second ventricle is rudimentary and incomplete, but still recognizable as being left ventricular on the basis of its apical trabecular pattern (Fig. 26). There is no longer any need, therefore, or any justification, for describing hearts with either double inlet left or double inlet right ventricles as "univentricular" or "single ventricle". As argued by Brandt,[8] it is more sensible and descriptive to specify the nature of the hearts on the basis of their atrioventricular junctional arrangements. Only those hearts which possess a solitary and indeterminate ventricle (Fig. 27) are accurately described as being univentricular. Even in this setting, it is more specific to state the indeterminate nature of the solitary ventricle. Hearts which have huge ventricular septal defects, with a persisting rim of apical trabecular septum (Fig. 28), should similarly not be considered univentricular. In these, it is possible to identify biventricular atrioventricular connections because of the nature of the ventricular myocardium on either side of the septal remnant.

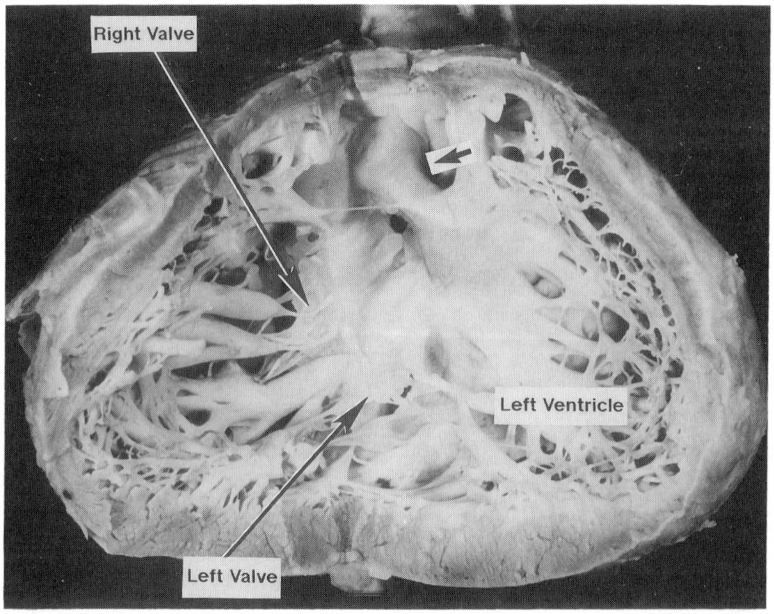

Fig. 21 Both atrioventricular valves are connected in their entirety to the dominant ventricle, which supports the pulmonary trunk. The ventricular septal defect (arrowed) leads to the rudimentary and incomplete right ventricle (see Fig. 22).

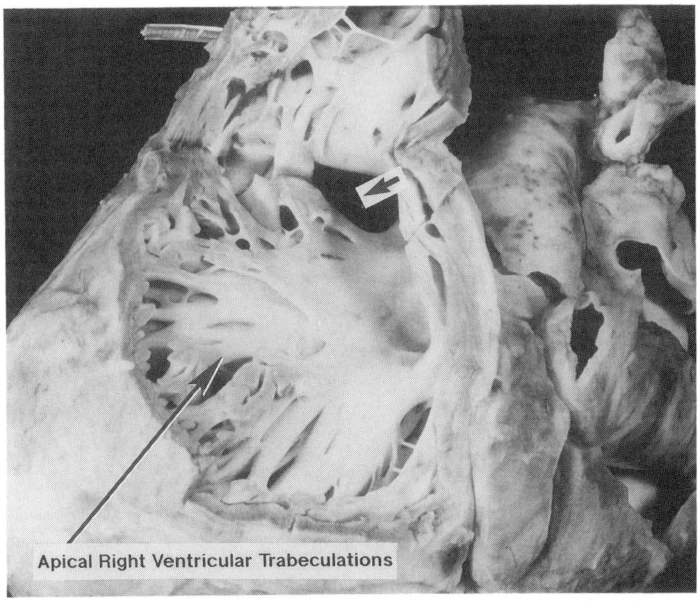

Fig. 22 The left-sided rudimentary ventricle from the heart shown in Fig. 21 has unmistakable apical trabeculations of right ventricular morphology and gives rise to the aorta. It receives its blood through the ventricular septal defect (arrowed).

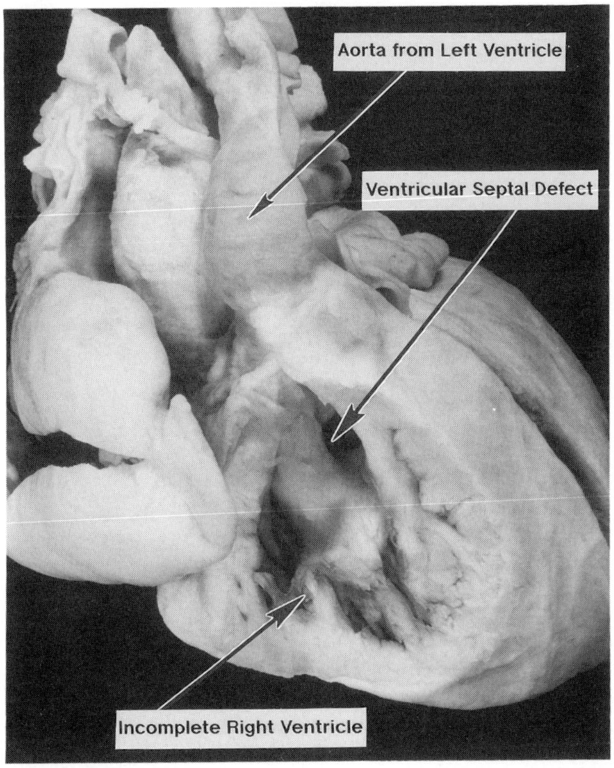

Fig. 23 This incomplete and rudimentary right ventricle lacks its inlet and its outlet, but can still be recognized as right ventricular on account of its apical trabeculations (the myocardial morphologic method).

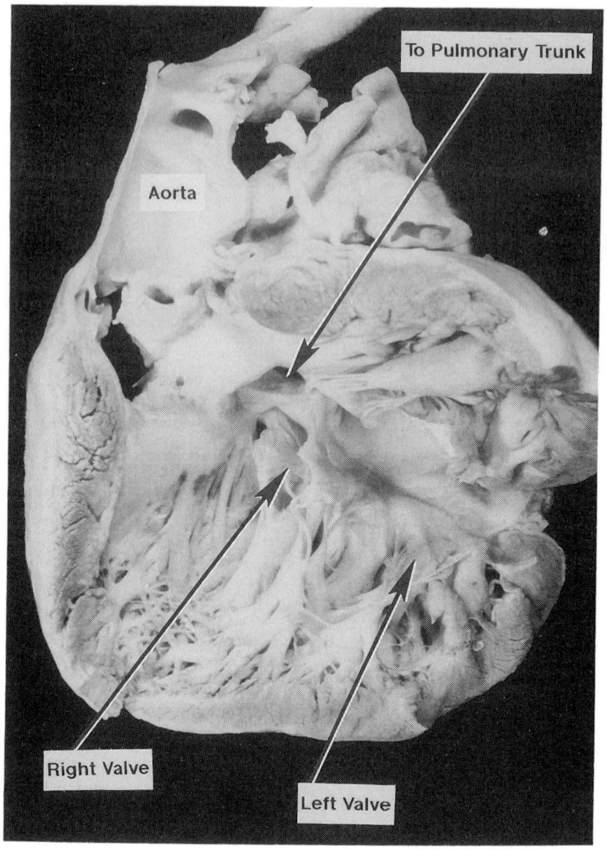

Fig. 24 In the heart shown in Fig. 23, the dominant left ventricle receives both atrioventricular valves and gives rise to both arterial trunks (double inlet and double outlet left ventricle).

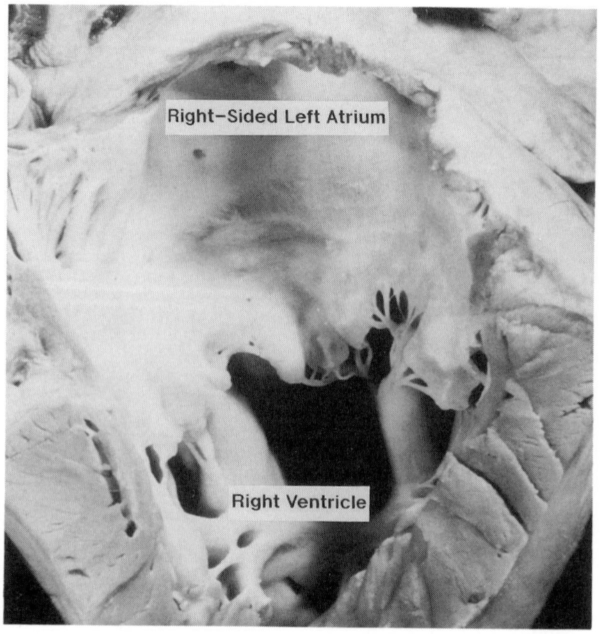

Fig. 25 The right-sided left atrium in this heart with mirror imaged atrial appendages is connected to the right ventricle.

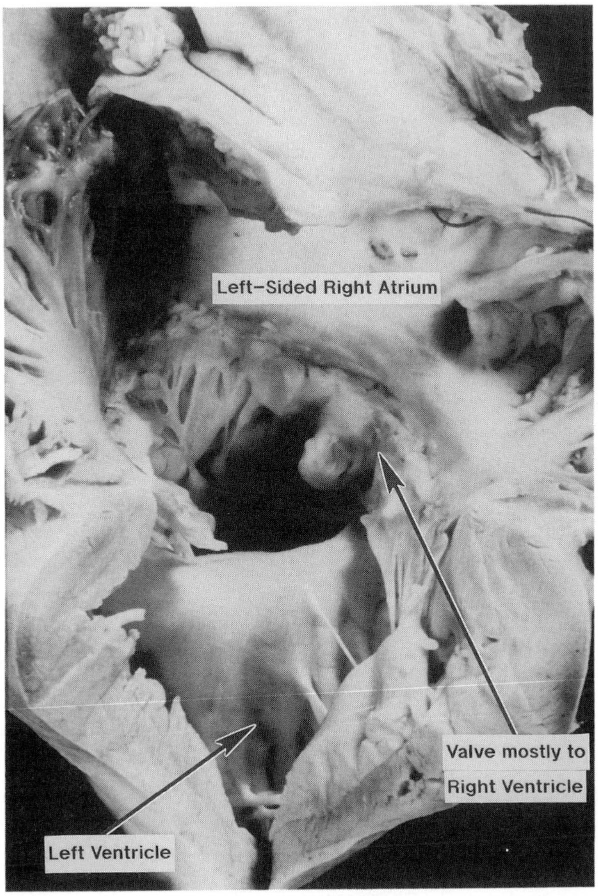

Fig. 26 The left-sided morphologically right atrium is shown from the heart illustrated in Fig. 25. The left-sided atrioventricular junction is also connected predominantly to the dominant right ventricle (double inlet right ventricle). The rudimentary and incomplete left ventricle is left-sided (right-hand topology).

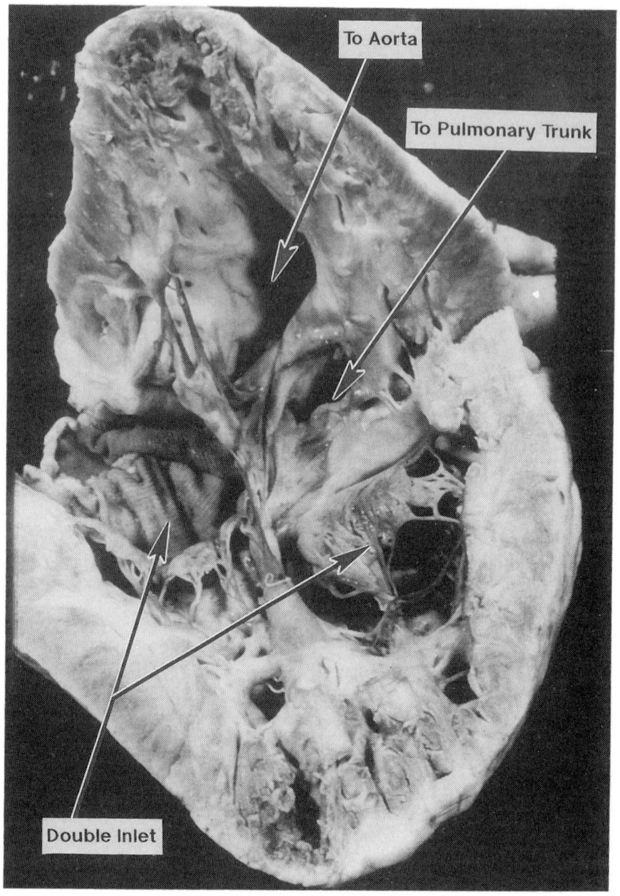

Fig. 27 This solitary and indeterminate ventricle, with particularly coarse apical trabeculations, receives both atrioventricular valves and gives rise to both arterial trunks (double inlet and double outlet).

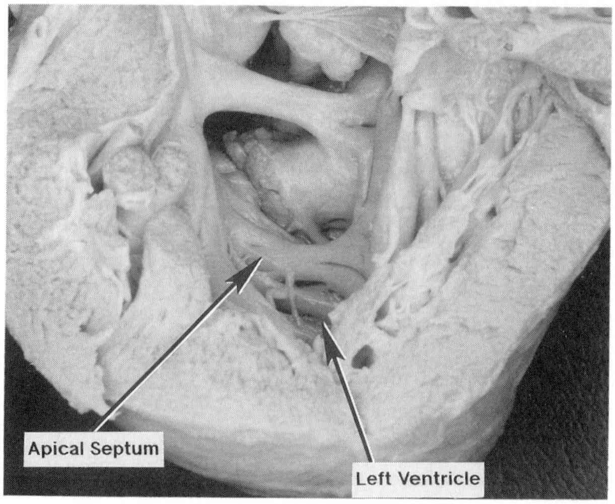

Fig. 28 In this heart with a huge ventricular septal defect, the remnant of the ventricular septum separates the apical trabecular component of left morphology from the right ventricle. The heart has concordant atrioventricular connections, and is not univentricular.

What, then, of the morphological premise, namely the relationship between the rudimentary and incomplete ventricles present in hearts with double inlet ventricle and those in hearts with atrioventricular valvar atresia due to absence of one atrioventricular connection? It was the remarkable similarity between the anterior ventricular chamber as seen in double inlet left ventricle with concordant ventriculo-arterial connections (the so-called "Holmes heart", Fig. 29, right) and the small right ventricle in classical tricuspid atresia (Fig. 29, left) which first drew our attention to the potential morphological affinities between these lesions.[16] It would have been much better if, from the outset, having recognized these similarities, we had argued that both double inlet left ventricle and tricuspid atresia had biventricular hearts, but in the setting of univentricular atrioventricular connections. Unfortunately, we did not,[10] accepting the opinion prevailing at the time[13,14] that the double inlet was the best criterion for definition of "single ventricle". Our inappropriate application, at that time, of the adjective "univentricular" to the heart rather than to the atrioventricular connection does not in any way disguise the comparability of the rudimentary and incomplete right ventricle in the two situations. When Deanfield and colleagues[17] measured a series of hearts with, on the one hand, double inlet left ventricle and, on the other hand, classical tricuspid atresia, they showed that whatever differences existed between the right ventricles reflected not the atrioventricular but the ventriculo-arterial connections (Fig. 30). Thus, when the Holmes heart is compared to hearts with classical tricuspid atresia and concordant ventriculo-arterial connections (Fig. 29), or when double inlet left ventricle with a right-sided rudimentary right ventricle supporting the aorta (Fig. 31) is compared to classical tricuspid atresia as seen with discordant ventriculo-arterial connections (Fig. 32), the similarities in ventricular morphology are obvious.

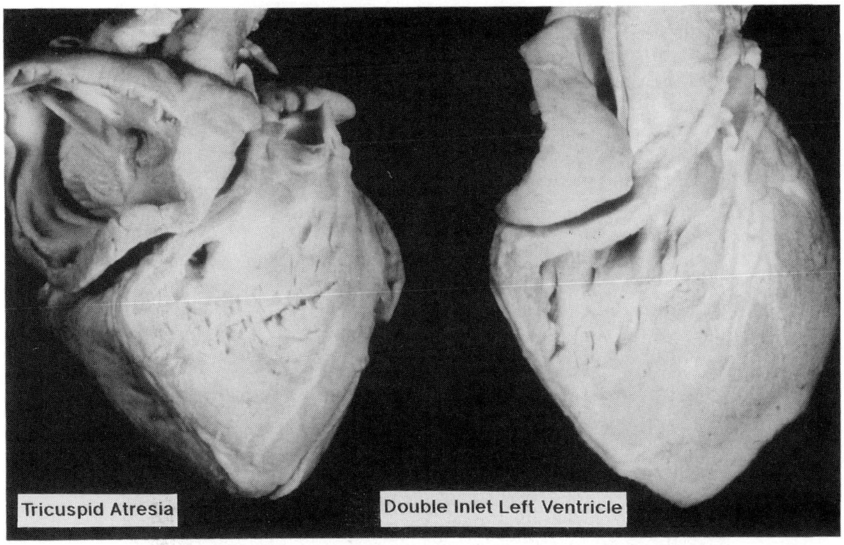

Fig. 29 These hearts have classical tricuspid atresia (left) and double inlet left ventricle (right). The morphology of the rudimentary right ventricle is virtually identical, the ventriculo-arterial connections being concordant in both hearts.

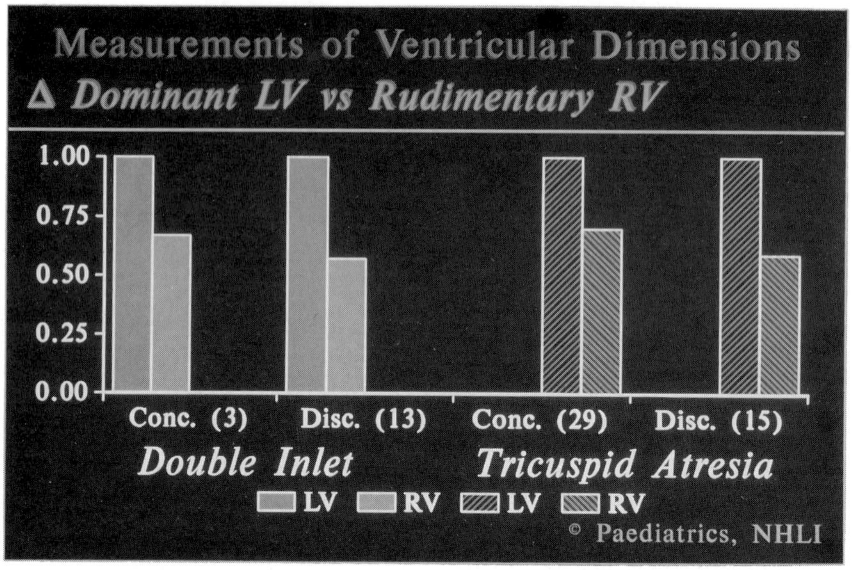

Fig. 30 The measurements made by Deanfield and colleagues[17] showed that it was the ventriculo-arterial connections (concordant [con.] versus discordant [disc.]) which altered the proportions of the dominant left (LV) and rudimentary right (RV) ventricles, not the atrioventricular connections (double inlet versus tricuspid atresia). The numbers show the hearts studied in each group. The results were statistically significant – $p>0.5$.

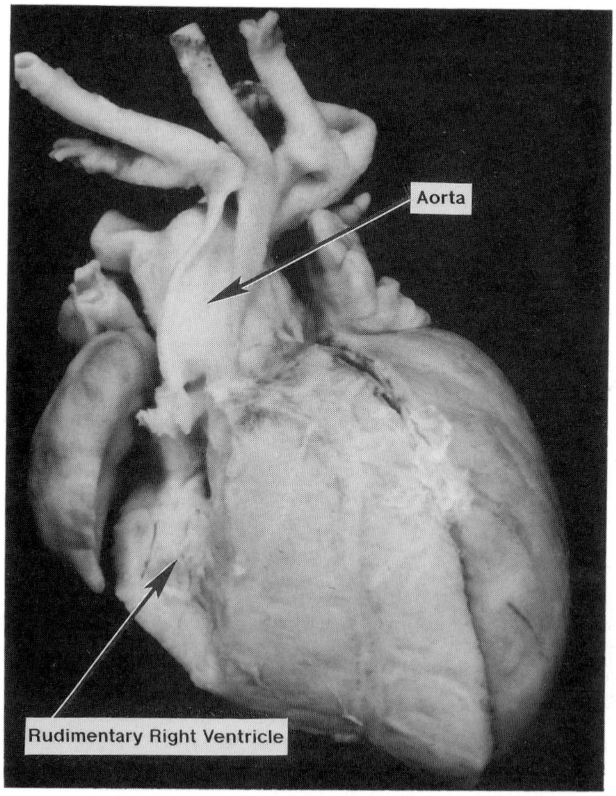

Fig. 31 The right-sided rudimentary right ventricle is shown from a heart with double inlet left ventricle and discordant ventriculo-arterial connections.

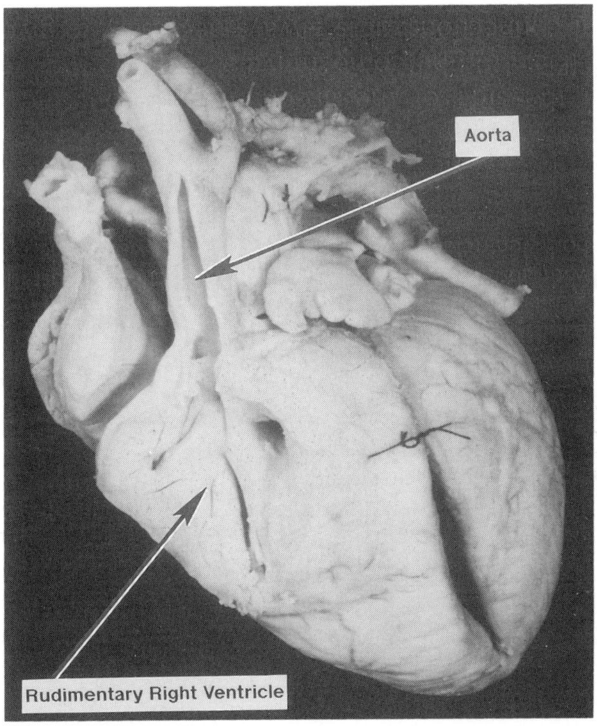

Fig. 32 This heart with tricuspid atresia also has a right-sided rudimentary right ventricle and discordant ventriculo-arterial connections, but cannot be distinguished from the heart shown in Fig. 31 on the basis of the structure of the small right ventricle.

Indeed, it is not possible when examining only the structure of the right ventricle to discern the precise junctional arrangements within the dominant left ventricle. Comparable morphology is also found when hearts with absence of the left-sided atrioventricular connection and the right atrium connected to a dominant left ventricle are compared with double inlet left ventricle, rudimentary right ventricle, and discordant ventriculo-arterial connections (Figs. 33, 34). In similar fashion, the rudimentary and incomplete left ventricle, found in postero-inferior position, is of comparable morphology irrespective of whether there is double inlet to the dominant right ventricle (Fig. 35) or absence of the right or left-sided atrioventricular connection with the other atrium joined to a dominant right ventricle (Fig. 36). In short, when there are univentricular atrioventricular connections, the nature of the myocardial morphologic characteristics of the ventricular mass is independent of the arrangements at the atrioventricular junctions. That is why, for full description, it is necessary to specify both the atrioventricular junctional arrangement and the ventricular morphology. Apart for those hearts having solitary ventricles, this can no longer be adequately achieved by using the terms "univentricular heart" or "single ventricle". It is recognition of the univentricular nature of the atrioventricular connection, however, which is the step which distinguishes those variants of atrioventricular valvar atresia which have affinities with double inlet from the others which, in morphologic terms, are akin to hearts having biventricular atrioventricular connections.

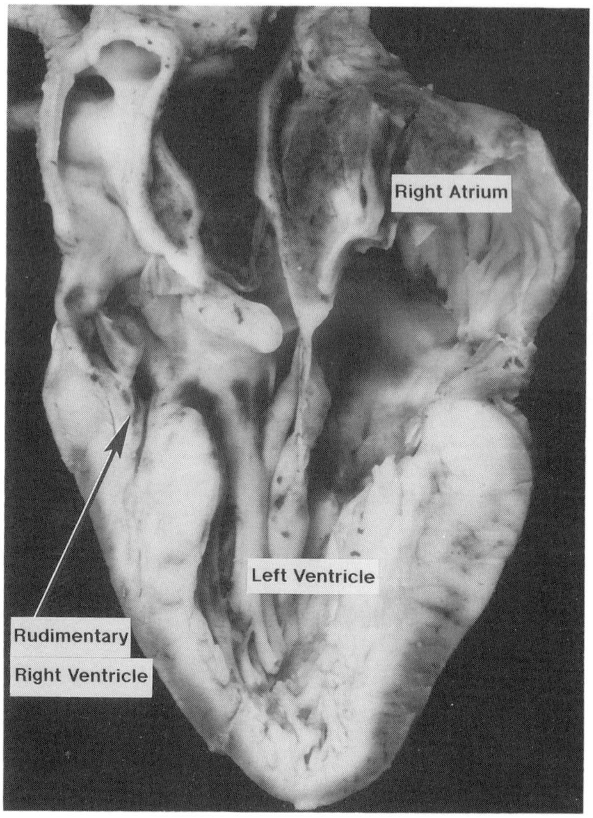

Fig. 33 This heart with a dominant left ventricle has absence of the left atrioventricular connection and an antero-superior rudimentary right ventricle.

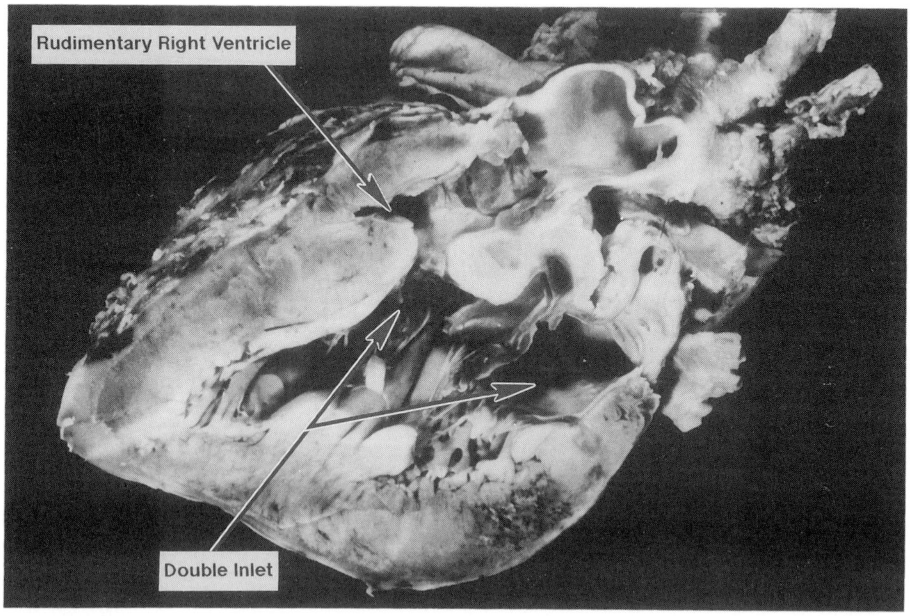

Fig. 34 This heart with double inlet left ventricle also has an antero-superior rudimentary right ventricle. The arrangement is directly comparable to that shown in Fig. 33.

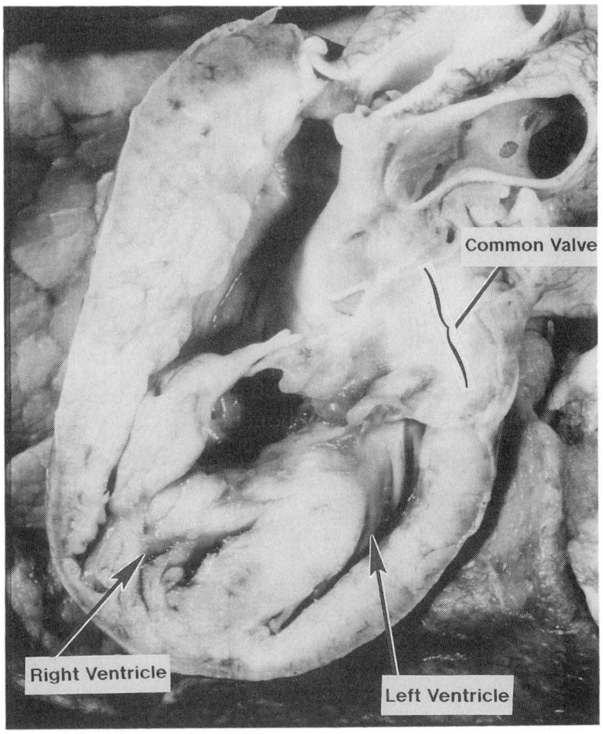

Fig. 35 In this heart, with double inlet right ventricle via a common atrioventricular valve and double outlet right ventricle, the rudimentary left ventricle is positioned postero-inferiorly.

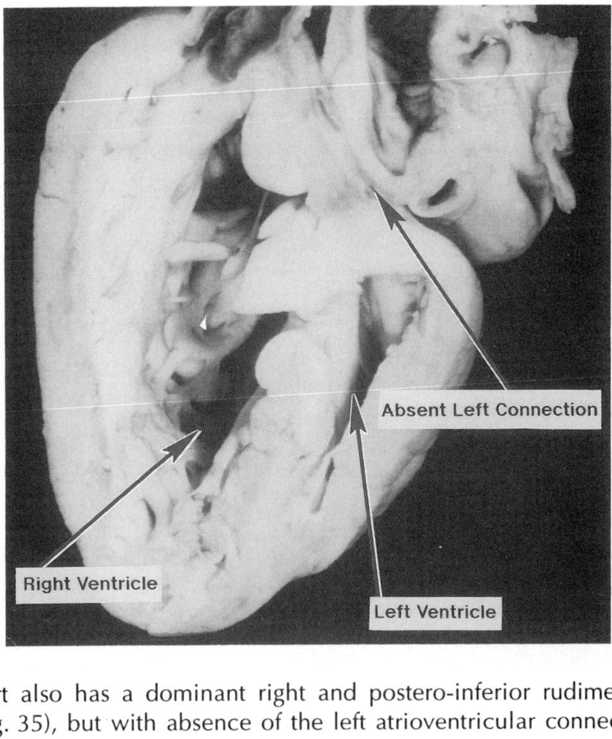

Fig. 36 This heart also has a dominant right and postero-inferior rudimentary left ventricle (compare with Fig. 35), but with absence of the left atrioventricular connection (mitral atresia with patent aortic root).

Having criticized so cogently the non-morphologic approach which we used when we described "univentricular hearts", it seems surprising to us that Van Praagh and his colleagues now espouse a system of classification which describes double inlet left ventricle as "single left ventricle"[(7)]. They claim that this approach is supported by the fact that the rudimentary and incomplete right ventricle is best considered an infundibulum. Their hypothesis, recently extended by Kumar and his colleagues to suggest that apical muscular defects open from the left ventricle to the infundibulum of the right ventricle,[18] fails to stand up to rigorous scrutiny. First, their suggestion that, in the normal heart, the ring formed between septomarginal trabeculation (septal band), moderator band, and supraventricular crest divides the apical component of the right ventricle into separate inlet and outlet trabeculated apexes, is not borne out by our examination of a large number of normal hearts. In most specimens, the normal right ventricular apical trabeculations form a loose meshwork of comparable character across the entirety of the trabecular component (Fig. 37). Second, the septum separating this extensive apical component from the left ventricle is the apical trabecular septum and not the outlet (infundibular) septum. Indeed, in the normal heart it is not possible to distinguish any part of the muscular septum as specifically separating the ventricular outlets. The axis responsible for atrioventricular conduction, however, branches on the crest of the muscular septum. Conduction tissue has never, in our experience, been found within the outlet (infundibular) septum when this is seen as a discrete muscular structure between the ventricular outlets. In hearts with dominant left and rudimentary and incomplete right ventricles, the muscular septum between them is almost always recognizable as having two discrete components (Figs. 33, 34). The conduction axis then branches on the more apical of these components,[19–21] providing strong evidence that this is the analogue of the apical muscular ventricular septum.

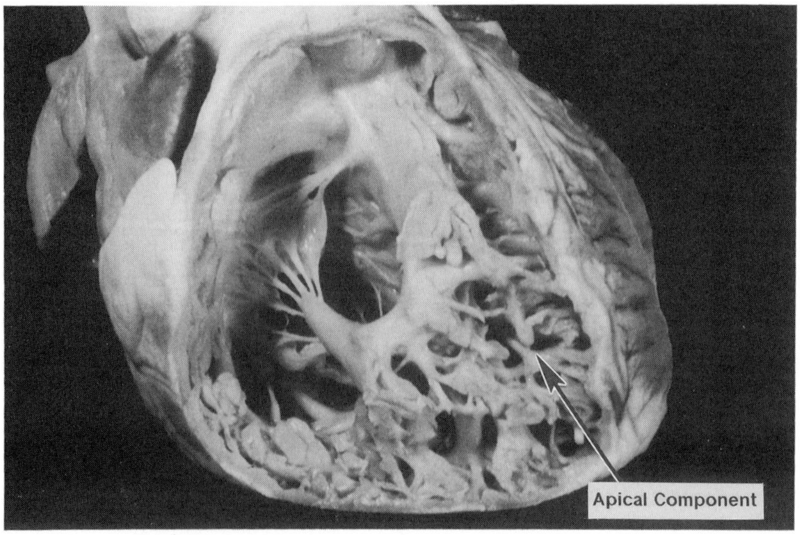

Fig. 37 This morphologically right ventricle, showing morphology typical of the normal heart, has coarse apical trabeculations throughout the apical component.

The distal component separates the ventricular outlets, and is the true outlet (or infundibular) septum. Furthermore, when the inlet of the right ventricle is sequestrated as a distinct entity (Fig. 38), then the apical trabeculations are found in an anterior ventricle (Fig. 39) which is directly comparable with the rudimentary and incomplete right ventricle seen in double inlet left ventricle or tricuspid atresia (compare Fig. 39 with Fig. 29). Of all these reasons, perhaps the most significant is that, when adjudicating on the basis of the nature of the apical trabeculations, there is no way of distinguishing between the inlet and outlet apical recesses of the right ventricle in those instances in which such an arrangement does exist in the normal heart (Fig. 40). The principle of myocardial morphologic characteristics[7] surely dictates that both parts are of right ventricular morphology? The rudimentary and incomplete ventricle seen in hearts with dominant left ventricle, therefore, is right ventricular in nature. Hearts containing such chambers of right ventricular morphology cannot logically be described as "single ventricles".[22]

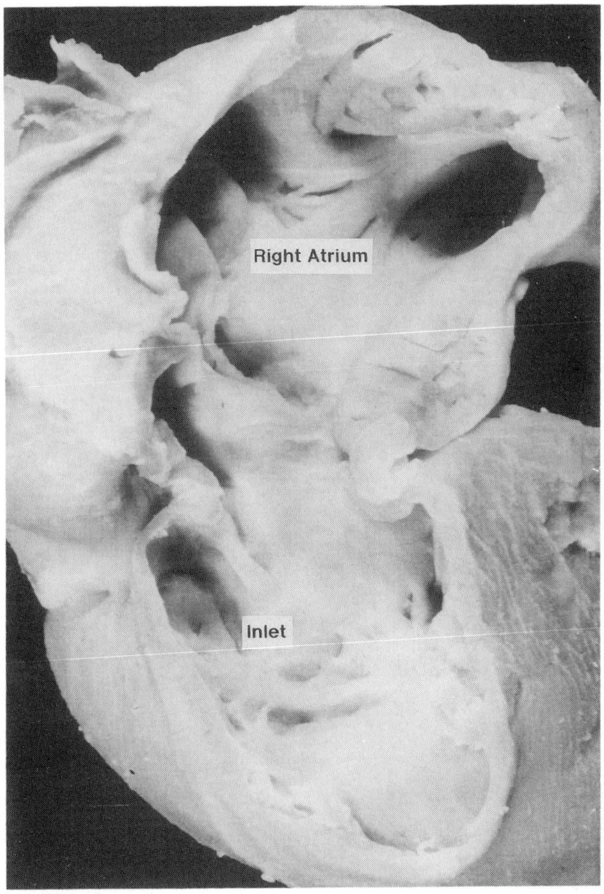

Fig. 38 In this heart, with a rare variant of tricuspid atresia, a muscular partition sequestrates the inlet component of the right ventricle (compare with Fig. 20). The minimal trabeculations present are not typical of the normal right ventricle (see Fig. 37).

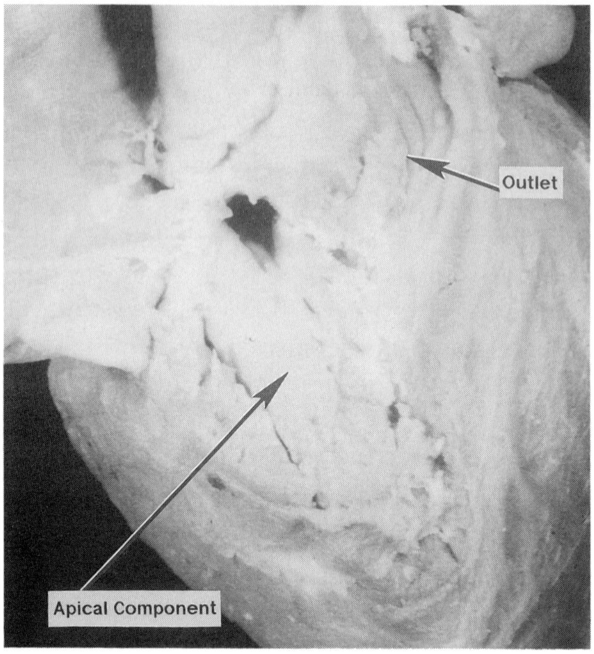

Fig. 39 This shows the apical and outlet components of the right ventricle from the heart shown in Fig. 38. The morphology is directly comparable with that seen in classical tricuspid atresia and double inlet left ventricle with concordant ventriculo-arterial connections (compare with Fig. 29).

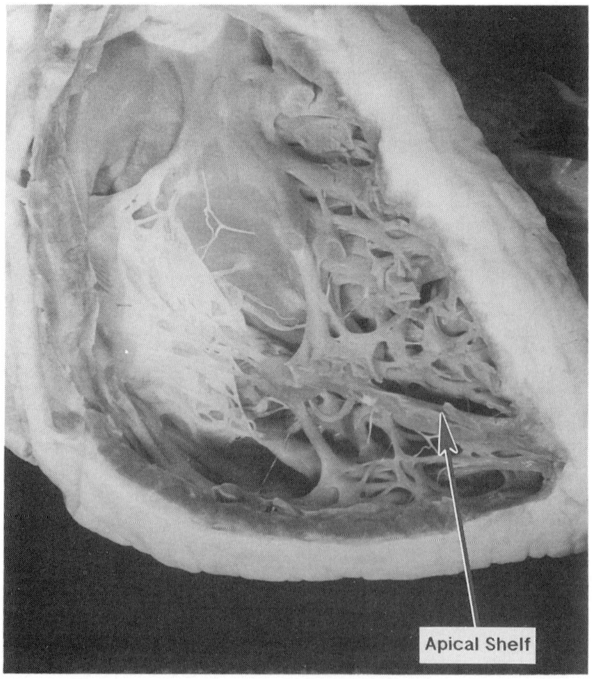

Fig 40 In this normal heart, the less common variant is seen in which a muscular shelf divides the apical trabecular component. The trabeculations are of typical right ventricular type, however, on both sides of the prominent apical trabeculation (arrowed). There is no way of distinguishing the two components on the basis of the myocardial morphologic method emphasized by Van Praagh and his colleagues.[7]

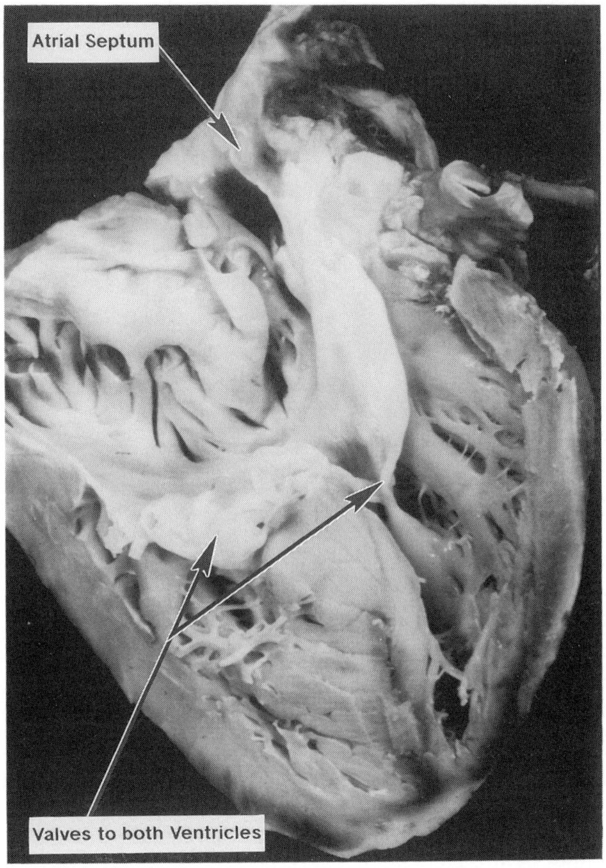

Fig. 41 In this heart with absent left atrioventricular connection, the atrial septum separates the left atrium from the right atrium, which is connected by its atrioventricular valve to both ventricles (uniatrial and biventricular connection).

THE UNIATRIAL BUT BIVENTRICULAR CONNECTION

This arrangement, as already discussed, is produced when a heart with absence of one atrioventricular connection is associated with straddling and overriding of the patent atrioventricular connection.[5] The effect is to produce double outlet from one atrium. This arrangement is also described in hearts with atrioventricular septal defect and common atrioventricular junction (see Chapter 2). The difference between the anomalies is that, in the setting of the atrioventricular septal defect, the valve which overrides the ventricular septum is a common valve, since it is hinged from both segments of atrial myocardium. In contrast, the valve found when one atrioventricular connection is absent is, of necessity, either a right-sided or a left-sided valve. It cannot be a common valve because the atrial septum walls off the valvar annulus from one of the atrial chambers (Fig. 42). Because the solitary atrioventricular junction is shared between the right and left ventricles, both of the ventricles are rudimentary and incomplete to greater or lesser degree. Usually one of the ventricles is dominant, but sometimes both ventricles can be comparable in size. So as to describe fully these hearts, it is necessary to

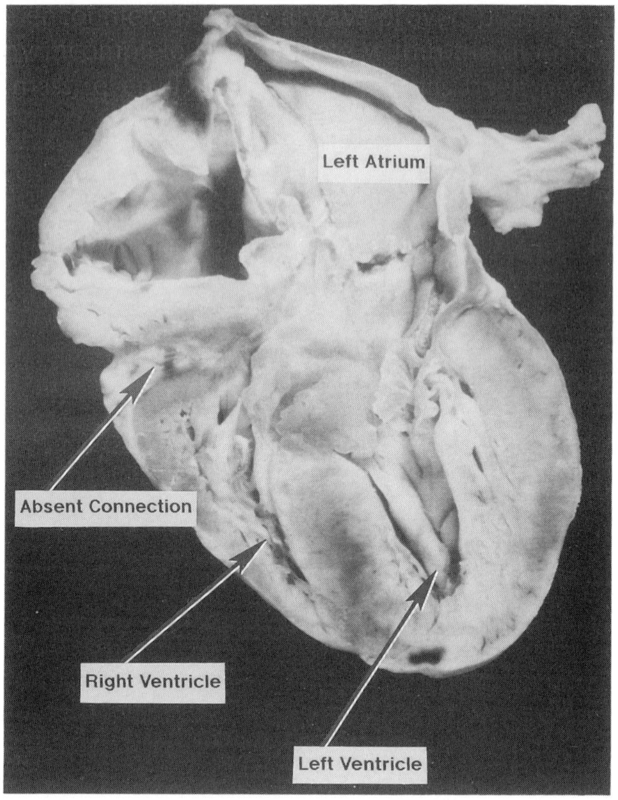

Fig. 42 This heart, with absent right atrioventricular connection (tricuspid atresia), has the left valve connected in both ventricles, which are of comparable size. The connection is uniatrial and biventricular.

take account of the side of the absent connection, the topology of the ventricular mass (Fig. 18), the comparative size of the two ventricles, and the ventriculo-arterial connections. It is always necessary to give a full catalogue of associated malformations.

THE OVERALL NATURE OF THE VENTRICULAR MASS

From the foregoing discussion, it will be evident that hearts with univentricular atrioventricular connection only rarely possess a truly solitary ventricle. When seen (Fig. 27), these hearts have characteristically coarse trabeculations which extend throughout the ventricular apex, along with multiple trabecular columns which support the tension apparatus of the atrioventricular valves. Doubt has been cast on the existence of the solitary and indeterminate ventricle.[3] On the basis of the myocardial morphologic characteristics, however, the solitary ventricles are of neither right nor left morphology. Furthermore, when apparently solitary ventricles of right morphology are encountered, it has always proved possible in our experience to discover a tiny incomplete left ventricle within the diaphragmatic surface of the ventricular mass, even if, on occasion, it has been necessary to resort to histology so as to discover the rudimentary cavity.[23] When discovered, the conduction tissue has always extended into the virtual cavity from an atrioventricular node located at the apex of the triangle of Koch. In the hearts diagnosed as having solitary and indeterminate ventricles, in contrast, the conduction axis has descended as a solitary strand from the lateral part of the atrioventricular junction (Fig. 43), or else has formed bizarre slings across the left-sided atrioventricular junction in hearts with isomeric right atrial appendages (Fig. 44).[24] All this evidence supports strongly the existence of an indeterminate ventricle as a morphological entity.

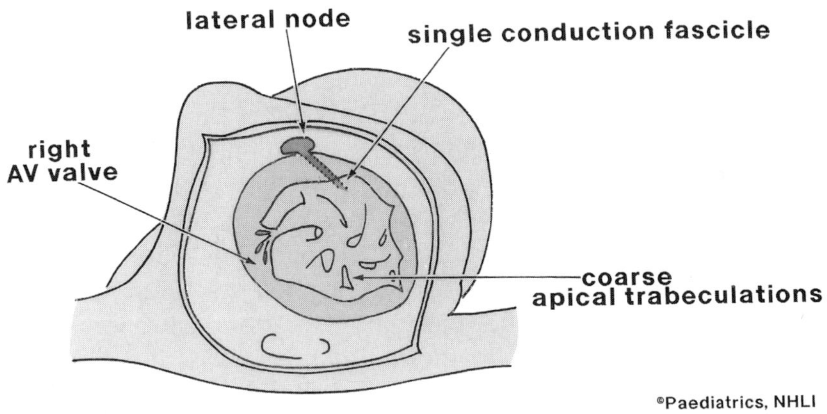

Fig. 43 The typical arrangement of the atrioventricular conduction axis as it would be viewed by the surgeon through a right atriotomy in double inlet via two atrioventricular valves to a solitary and indeterminate ventricle.

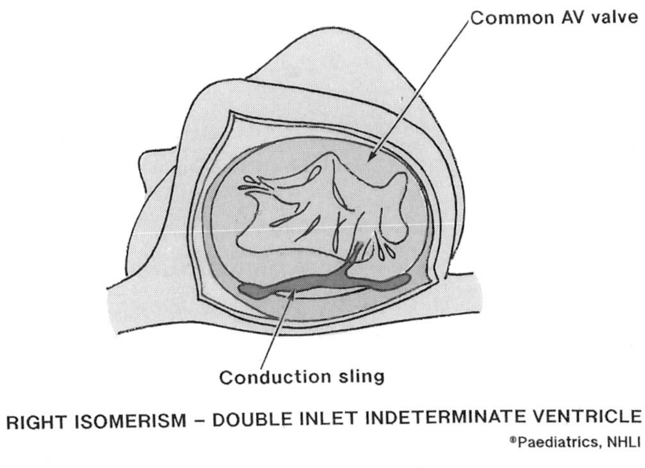

Fig. 44 The bizarre arrangement of a sling of conduction tissue between paired atrioventricular nodes in the postero-lateral wall of the common atrioventricular junction in a heart with double inlet through a common valve to a solitary and indeterminate ventricle.[24] The heart is shown as it would be seen by the surgeon in the operating room.

In the other variants of hearts with univentricular atrioventricular connection, the ventricular mass is dominated by either the right ventricle or the left ventricle. When the right ventricle is dominant, then two distinct patterns can be found which reflect the right-hand and left-hand topological arrangements, albeit with a rudimentary left ventricle positioned along the diaphragmatic surface of the ventricular mass. The right-hand pattern is the more frequent, and the rudimentary and incomplete left ventricle is then left-sided, be there usual atrial arrangement (Fig. 15), the mirror-image arrangement (Fig. 26), or isomeric atrial appendages. The conduction axis arises from a regular atrioventricular node in this setting (Fig. 45). When there is left-hand ventricular topology, then the rudimentary and incomplete left ventricle is right-sided, albeit still located postero-inferiorly in relation to the dominant right ventricle (Fig. 46). With this topological pattern, then the conduction axis either arises from an anterior atrioventricular node, or else a sling of conduction tissue is formed along the crest of the ventricular septum between anterior and posterior nodes (Fig. 47).[25]

Both the arrangement of the ventricular mass and the disposition of the atrioventricular conduction tissues point to the existence of right- and left-hand topological patterns when the right ventricle is dominant. The situation is not quite so clear cut when the left ventricle is dominant. The rudimentary and incomplete right ventricle is always carried on the antero-superior shoulder of the dominant left ventricle, and basically can be positioned to the right (Fig. 48) or to the left (Fig. 49). In these situations, it is not unreasonable to infer the presence of right-hand and left-hand topology respectively, particularly when the right-sided rudimentary right ventricle gives rise to the pulmonary trunk rather than to the aorta (see Fig. 29). In some circumstances, however, the rudimentary ventricle can be positioned directly anterior (Fig. 50). It is not then possible to say whether the ventricular mass shows right-hand or left-hand topology. Indeed, mere rotation of the heart in either direction would simulate either topologic arrangement. Furthermore, both of the atrioventricular valves when there is double inlet connection resemble morphologically mitral valves (Fig. 51), so this feature is also not universally of help, although in many cases one or other of the valves does have more "tricuspid"-like features.[26] The differences, nonetheless, are not sufficiently constant always to permit differentiation. Because of these difficulties, it is similarly not always possible to predict, when one atrioventricular connection is absent, the nature of the atrioventricular valve which would have been formed had the connection been present.[27] It is most accurate, therefore, to describe the position of the rudimentary right ventricle as being right-sided, directly anterior, or left-sided, and to account for either the right-sided or left-sided atrioventricular valves. Ventricular topology, and individual valvar morphology, can be inferred in many cases with univentricular connection to a dominant left ventricle, but certainly not in all.

It is the location of the apical trabecular septum which determines the location of the atrioventricular conduction axis in hearts with a dominant left ventricle. This is constant relative to the ventricular septal defect irrespective of the atrioventricular connection (Fig. 52), a feature which is particularly important when the ventricular septal defect is restrictive. It is

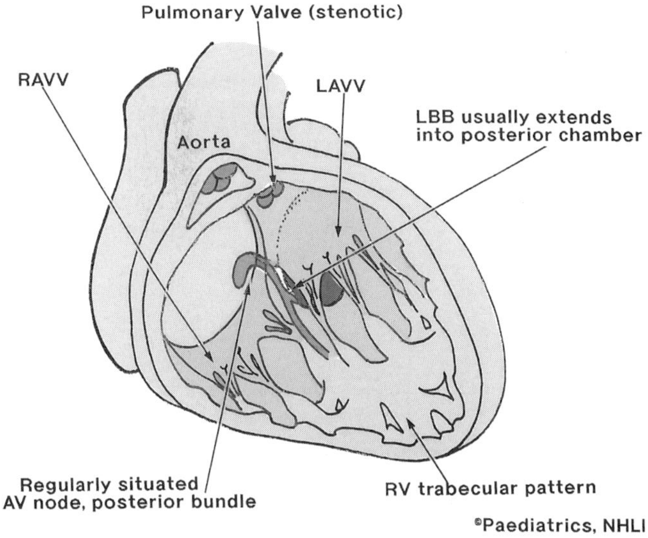

Fig. 45 The typical course of the atrioventricular conduction axis in hearts with double inlet right ventricle with right-hand ventricular topology as seen from the front of the dominant right ventricle (compare with Fig. 4).

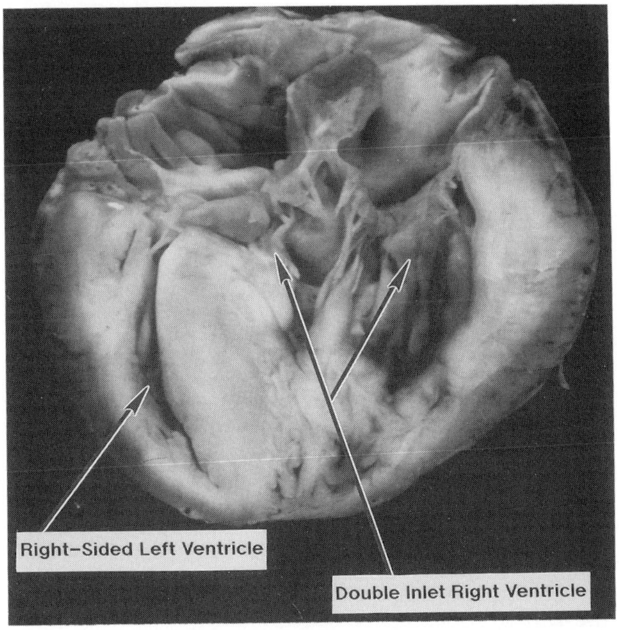

Fig. 46 This four-chamber section shows the junctional arrangement of double inlet right ventricle with right-sided rudimentary left ventricle (left-hand ventricular topology).

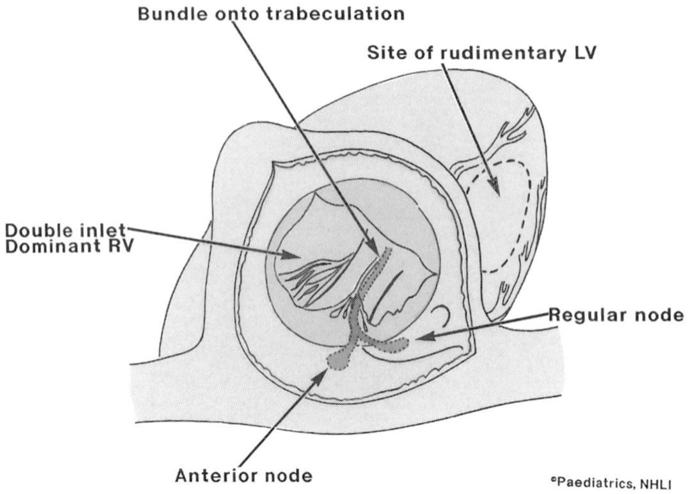

Fig. 47 The location of the atrioventricular conduction axis, shown as it would be seen by the surgeon in the operating room, in the case of double inlet right ventricle with right-sided rudimentary left ventricle studied by Essed and colleagues.[25]

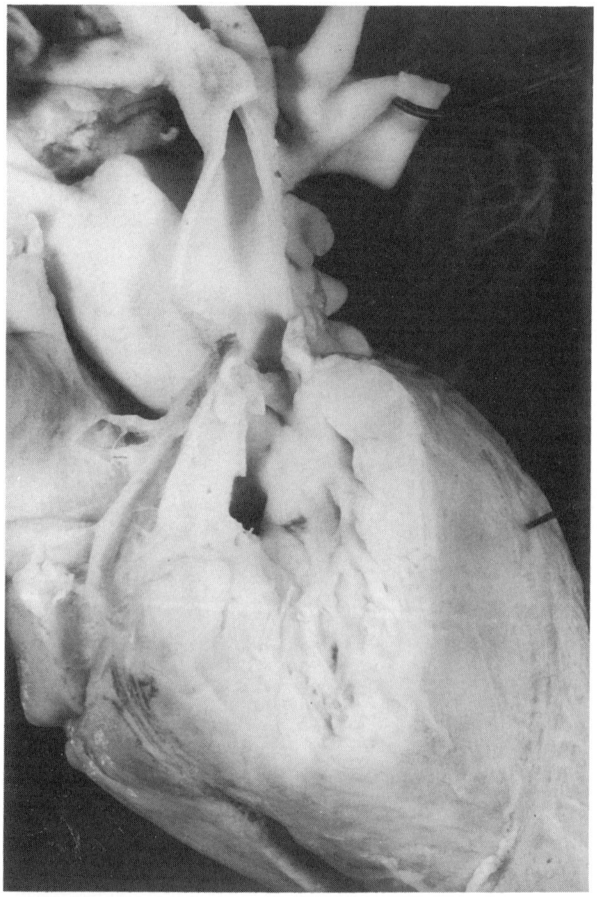

Fig. 48 This rudimentary right ventricle, from a heart with double inlet left ventricle, is positioned on the right shoulder of the ventricular mass.

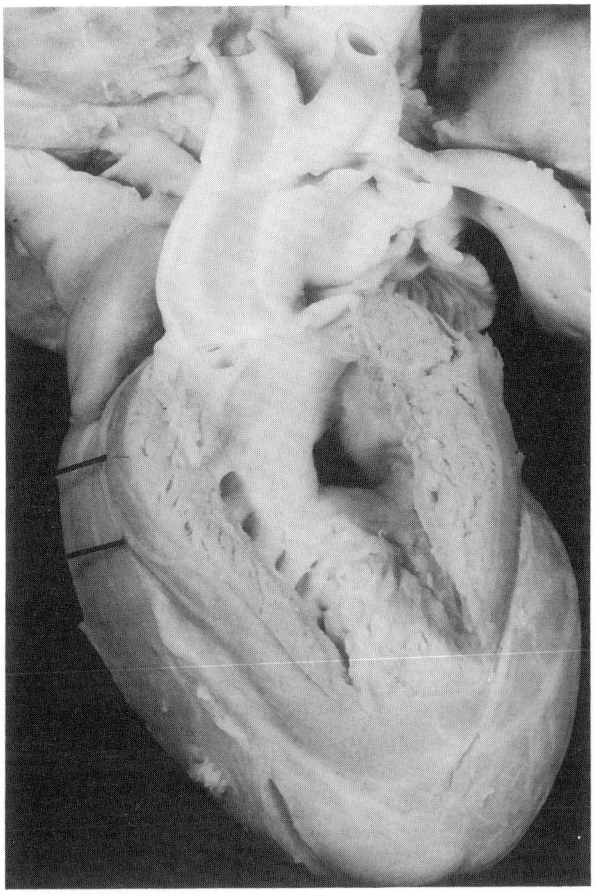

Fig. 49 In this example of double inlet left ventricle, the rudimentary left ventricle is found anteriorly and to the left.

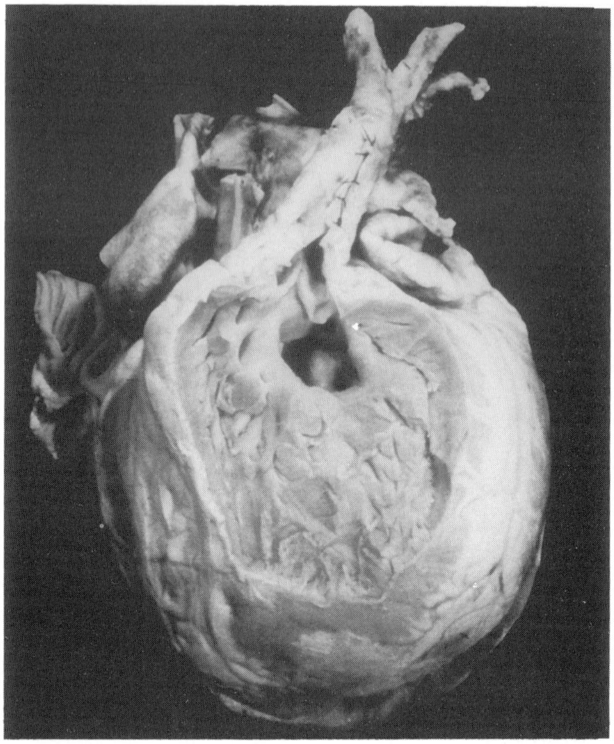

Fig. 50 The rudimentary right ventricle in this example of double inlet left ventricle is positioned directly anteriorly. Simple rotation of the ventricular mass could move the ventricle to right-sided (compare with Fig. 48) or left-sided (compare with Fig. 49) position.

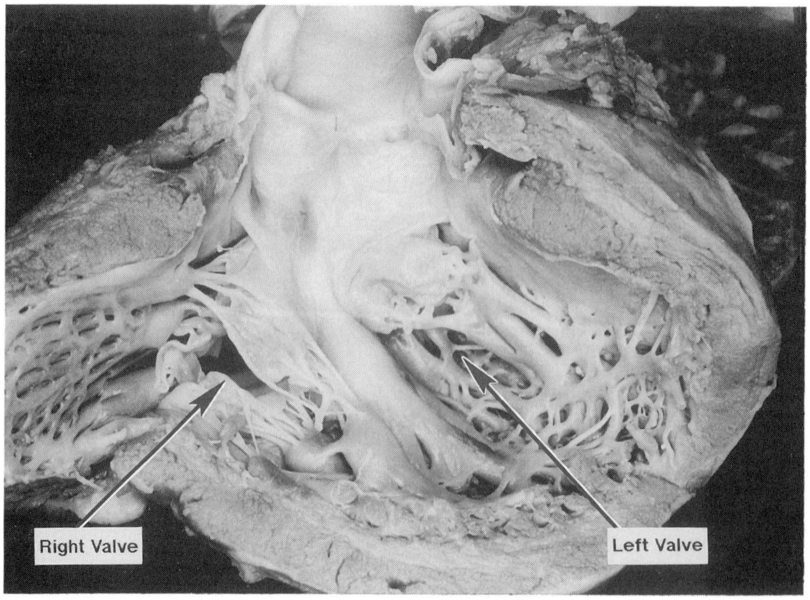

Fig. 51 The dominant left ventricle has been opened to show both atrioventricular valves. Both are of mitral morphology. In this heart, the rudimentary right ventricle was left-sided and supported the pulmonary trunk.

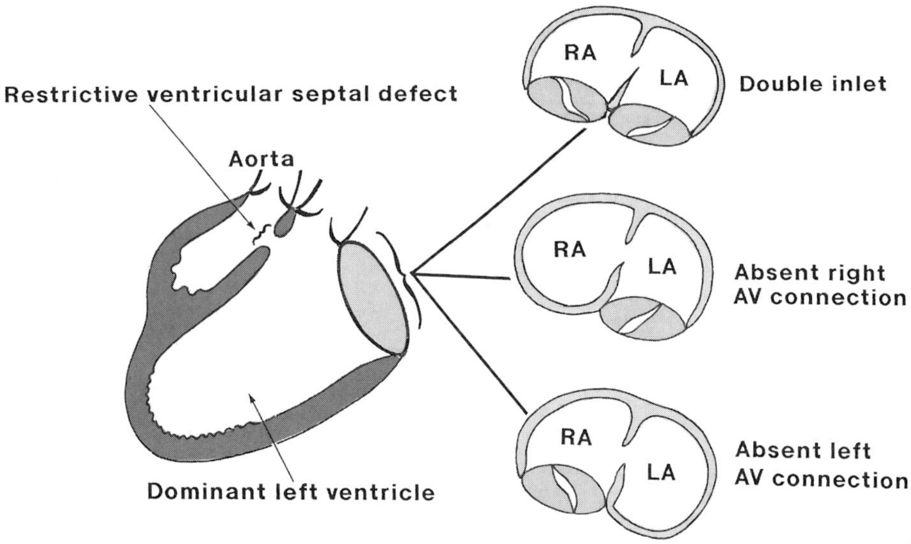

Fig. 52 Comparable ventricular morphology is found in hearts with dominant left ventricles irrespective of the presence of double inlet or absence of one or other atrioventricular connection. Similarly, the ventricular septal defect is in comparable location.

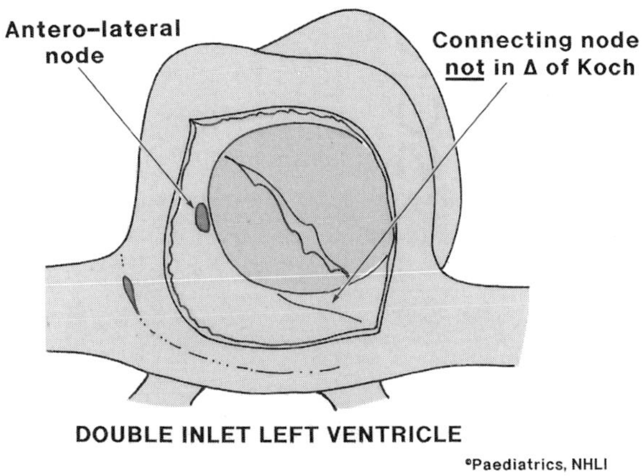

Fig. 53 The typical location of the atrioventricular node as it would be seen by the surgeon through a right atriotomy in hearts with double inlet left ventricle, irrespective of the location of the rudimentary right ventricle.

the apical trabecular septum which carries the ventricular component of the axis, and whenever there is usual atrial arrangement, this takes origin from an atrioventricular node located antero-laterally relative to the right atrioventricular valvar orifice (Fig. 53), or at the site of the dimple when the right atrioventricular connection is absent (Fig. 54). The dimple itself represents the atrioventricular component of the membranous septum (Fig. 6). The atrioventricular bundle descends directly from the anterior node to the ventricular septal crest when the rudimentary right ventricle is right-sided (Fig. 55) but encircles the outflow tract from the dominant left ventricle when the rudimentary ventricle is left-sided (Fig. 56). When viewed from the aspect of the rudimentary ventricle itself, however, the disposition of the axis is comparable irrespective of the location of the incomplete ventricle (Fig. 57). The surgeon is able, therefore, to remove a wedge of septal tissue closest to the obtuse margin of the ventricular mass so as to enlarge the ventricular septal defect without fear of damaging the conduction tissues (Fig. 58).

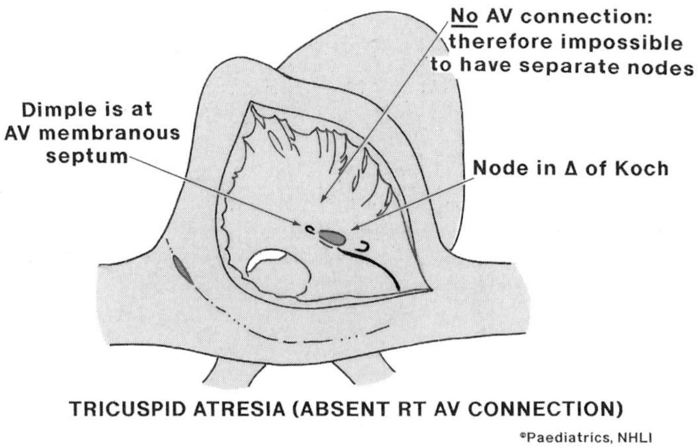

Fig. 54 When the right atrioventricular connection is absent, as in tricuspid atresia, then there is nothing to separate anterior and regular atrioventricular nodes. The extensive node is related to the dimple, shown in this diagram as it would be seen by a surgeon through a right atriotomy.

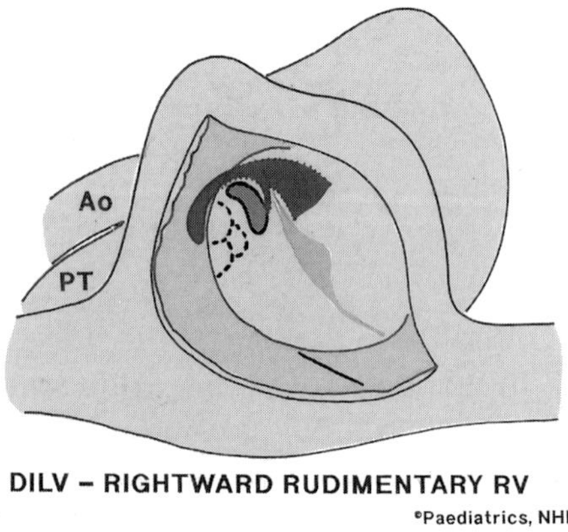

Fig. 55 The arrangement of the atrioventricular bundle in double inlet left ventricle (DILV) with right-sided rudimentary right ventricle (RV) as it would be seen by the surgeon operating through the right atrioventricular valve. The ventricular septal defect is shown in green. AO – aorta; PT – pulmonary trunk.

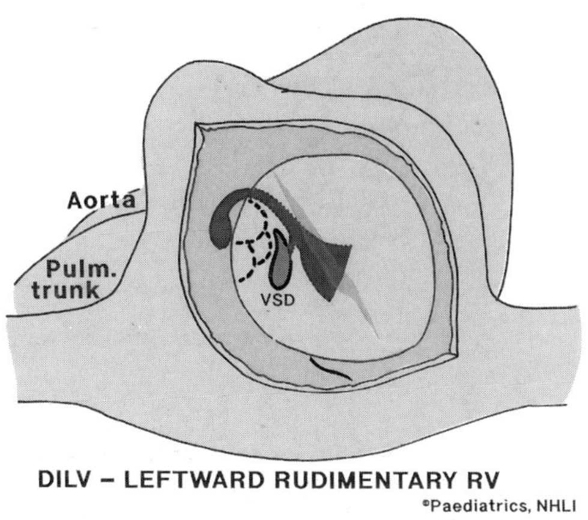

Fig. 56 When the rudimentary right ventricle (RV) is left-sided in double inlet left ventricle (DILV), the conduction axis (shown in red) encircles the pulmonary (pulm.) valve to reach the septum, descending antero-superior to the ventricular septal defect (VSD) as seen by the surgeon operating through the right atrioventricular valve (compare with Fig. 55).

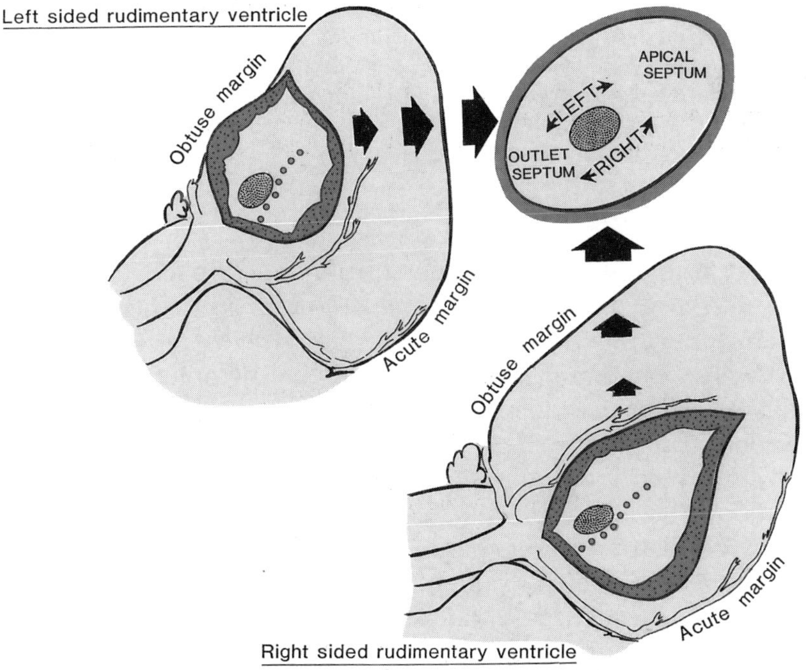

Fig. 57 When seen from the rudimentary right ventricle, shown here as it would be viewed in the operating room, the course of the conduction axis (dotted red line) is comparable relative to the ventricular septal defect (shown in blue).

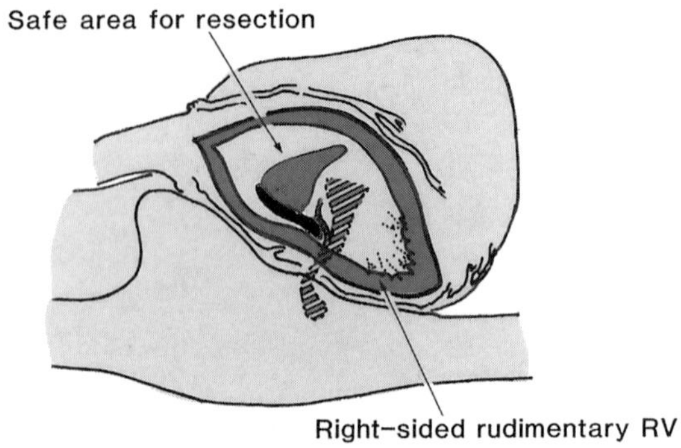

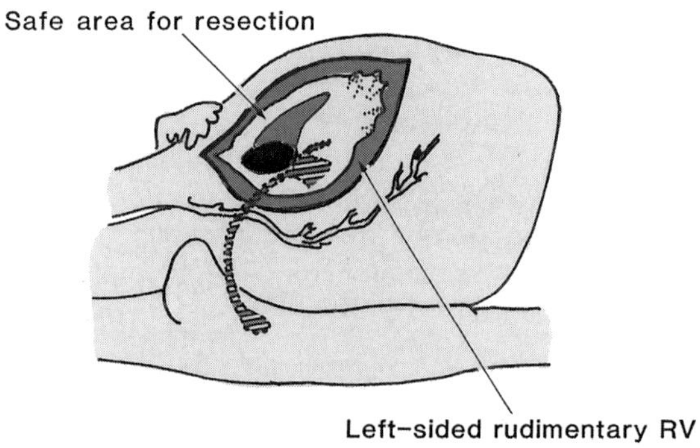

Fig. 58 This diagram, showing the rudimentary right ventricle as it would be seen by the surgeon in the operating room, indicates the wedge of apical septum (green) which can safely be removed without fear of damaging the atrioventricular conduction axis.

DEVELOPMENTAL CONSIDERATIONS

There are as many controversies surrounding the developmental origin of hearts with univentricular atrioventricular connection as there are disagreements concerning the best way to describe them. Almost all of these arguments were concerned with the origin of the inlet component of the morphologically right ventricle. Our own interpretations in this respect were initially wrong. Thus, we had argued that the inlet of the right ventricle was, most likely, derived from the descending limb, or inlet, of the primary ventricular loop (Figs. 59, 60). We then argued that, so as to unite this inlet component with the remainder of the right ventricle, which was recognized to develop from the ascending or outlet component of the ventricular loop, it was necessary to form an inlet muscular septum within the inlet part of the loop.[16] We presumed that this putative inlet septum fused with the muscular apical septum, which in turn was presumed to appear concomitant with the excavation of the apical components from the inlet and outlet segments of the loop. This hypothesis was strengthened by investigations of embryos which seemed to confirm the presence of a separate inlet septum.[28] It was confounded, however, by a study which demonstrated unequivocally that the muscular ventricular septum was derived exclusively from the structure separating the apical trabecular components.[29] This investigation was carried out on human embryos in which serial histological sections were processed with an antibody to the nodose ganglion of the chick. Serendipitously, this antibody marked the location of the developing atrioventricular conduction tissues (Fig. 61), which were disposed in a complete ring around the primary interventricular foramen (Fig. 62). Also of significance was that, at this early stage, the arrangement was reminiscent of a dominant left ventricle with absence of the right atrioventricular connection. Subsequent to the completion of cardiac septation, the ring of conduction tissue retained its positivity to the antibody, but was now disposed around the right atrioventricular junction and the subaortic outflow tract (Fig. 63). This showed conclusively that the entirety of the right ventricle, including its inlet component, was derived from the outlet component of the primary ventricular loop (Fig. 64). Univentricular connection to a dominant left ventricle, therefore, is well explained on the basis of failure of expansion of the atrioventricular junction into the outlet component of the ventricular loop. Balanced division of the atrioventricular junction in this setting will lead to double inlet left ventricle (Fig. 65), whereas sequestration of the junction by rightward or leftward deviation of the atrial septum will produce absent right or left atrioventricular connection, respectively. Excessive shift of the atrioventricular junction into the outlet segment of the ventricular loop will produce univentricular connection to a dominant right ventricle, with the specific atrioventricular connection again depending on the mode of division of the developing atrioventricular junction. Formation of a solitary and indeterminate ventricle is well explained on the basis of failure of excavation of separate trabecular components for

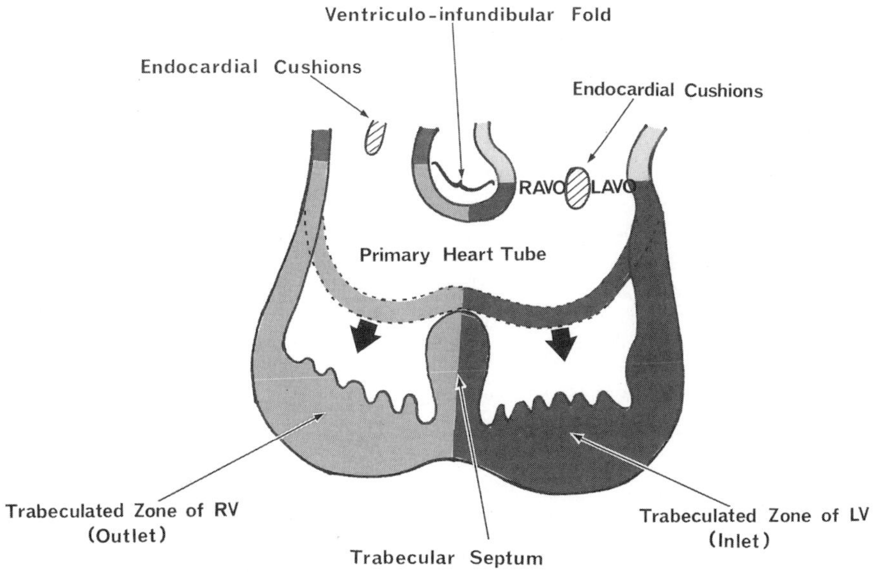

Fig. 59 It is the excavation of the apical trabecular components of left (LV) and right (RV) ventricles from the inlet (red) and outlet (green) components of the ventricular loop, respectively, which produces the apical trabecular septum. Note that, during early development, the right and left atrioventriuclar orifices (RAVO, LAVO) are both connected to the ventricular inlet.

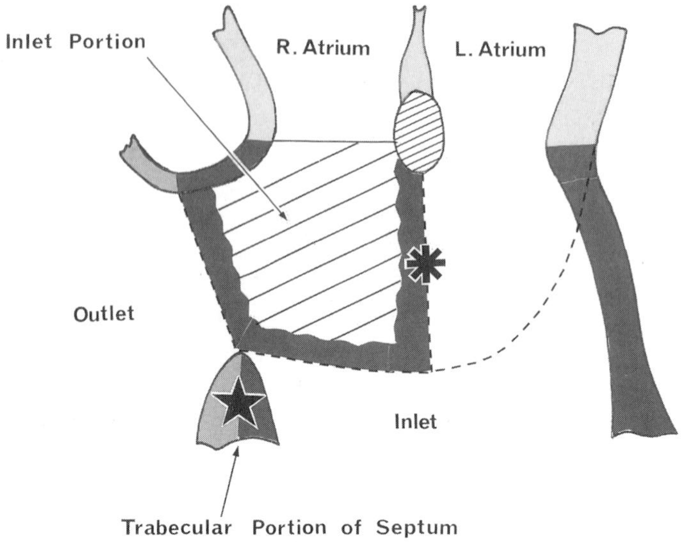

Fig. 60 Our initial concept of embryogenesis was that the inlet component of the right ventricle was derived from the inlet component of the ventricular loop (hatched area), meaning that a separate inlet septum (asterisk) was required to develop. We now know that this concept was wrong.

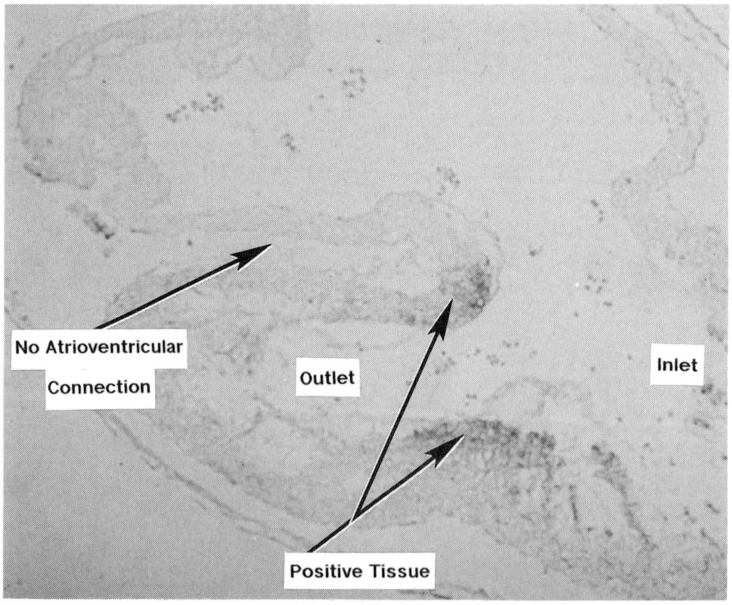

Fig. 61 This section through a developing human heart prior to expansion of the atrioventricular junction shows the tissue marked by an antibody to the nodose ganglion of the chick. The tissue surrounds completely the primary interventricular communication. Reproduced by kind permission of Prof. Wouter Lamers, University of Amsterdam. Note how the right junction resembles the arrangement seen in typical tricuspid atresia after formation of the atrial septum.[28]

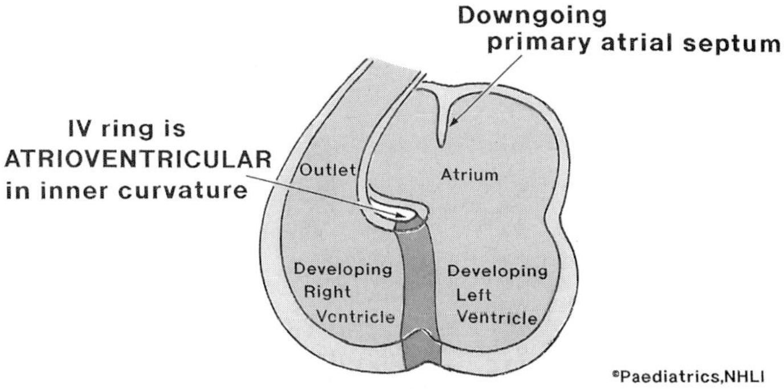

Fig. 62 The location of the ring of tissue in the developing heart marked by the antibody to the nodose ganglion of the chick. Note that the interventricular ring is already located in the right atrioventricular junction.

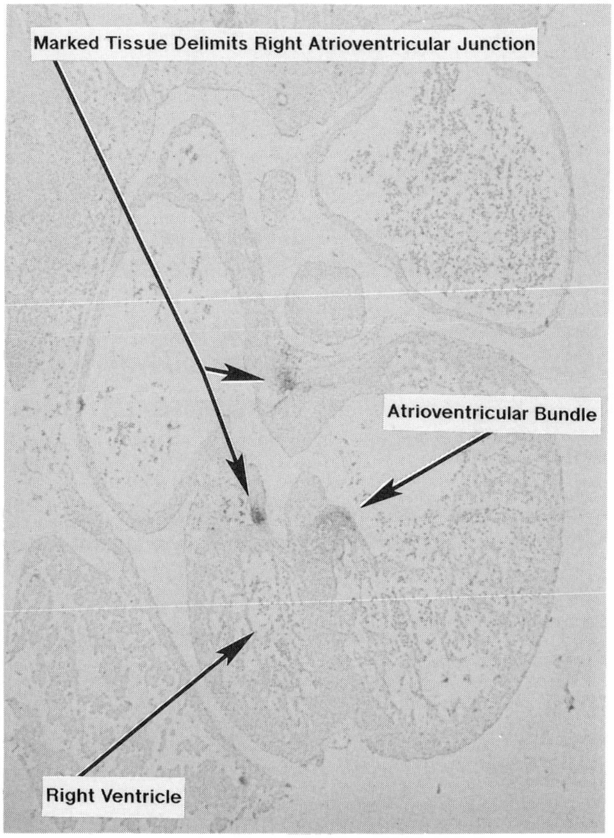

Fig. 63 At a later stage of development, when septation is complete, the ring marked by the antibody to the nodose ganglion is within the right atrioventricular junction and extends round the subaortic outflow tract, as well as forming the atrioventricular bundle. Reproduced by kind permission of Prof. Wouter Lamers, University of Amsterdam.[28]

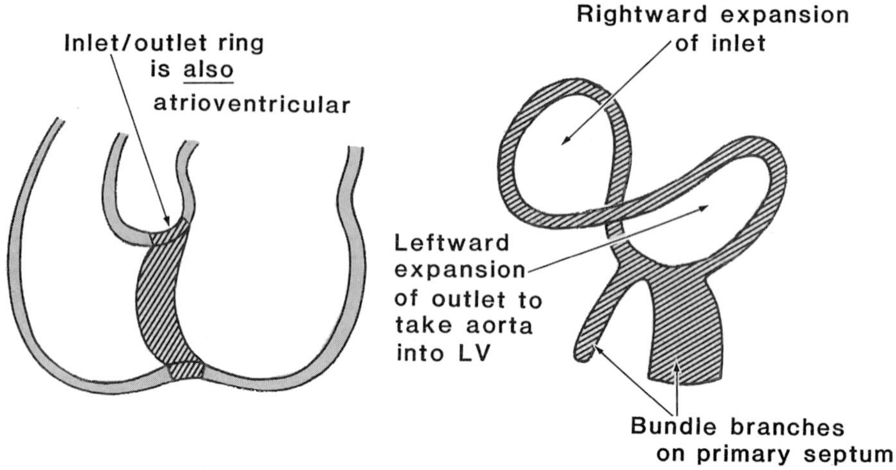

Fig. 64 The final location of the tissue marked by the antibody to the nodose ganglion of the chick shows the limits of the contribution of the distal limb of the ventricular loop. It has formed all of the right ventricle, along with the subaortic component of the left ventricle. The branching atrioventricular bundle marks the crest of the apical trabecular septum.

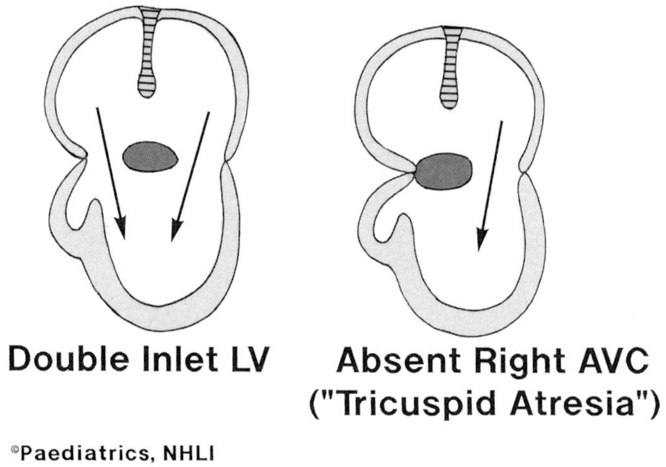

Fig. 65 It is the location of the tissues which divide the atrioventricular junction which determine whether, when the atrial chambers retain their connection to the proximal limb of the ventricular loop, there will be double inlet left ventricle (LV) or absence of the right atrioventricular connection (AVC).

the inlet and outlet parts of the ventricular loop. Again, the atrioventricular connections present will depend upon the mode of formation of the atrioventricular junctions. The mode of formation of the ventricular segment of the heart as revealed by the experiments with the antibody to the nodose ganglion offer no support to the hypothesis that the infundibulum of the right ventricle forms with its own apical component. On the contrary, the findings show that the apical trabeculations of right ventricular type are derived from the distal segment of the ventricular loop downstream to the developing muscular ventricular septum which carries on its crest the axis of atrioventricular conduction tissue. These findings support strongly the morphologic approach to the nomenclature of congenitally malformed hearts as outlined in this chapter.

REFERENCES

1. Anderson RH, Becker AE, Tynan M, Macartney FJ, Rigby ML, Wilkinson JL. The univentricular atrioventricular connection: getting to the root of a thorny problem. *Am J Cardiol* 1984;**54**:822–828.
2. Anderson RH, Macartney FJ, Tynan M, Becker AE, Freedom RM, Godman MJ, Hunter S, Quero Jiménez M, Rigby ML, Shinebourne EA, Sutherland GR, Smallhorn JF, Soto B, Thiene G, Wilkinson JL, Wilcox BR, Zuberbuhler JR. Univentricular atrioventricular connection: the single ventricle trap unsprung. *Pediatr Cardiol* 1983;**4**:273–280.
3. Van Praagh R, Plett JA, Van Praagh S. Single ventricle. Pathology, embryology, terminology and classification. *Herz* 1979;**4**:113–150.
4. Anderson RH, Becker AE. Historical review. In: Anderson RH, Crupi G, Parenzan L (eds). *Double Inlet Ventricle*. Tunbridge Wells: Castle House Publications. 1987: pp 29-35.
5. Anderson RH, Ho SY. Sequential segmental analysis — description and categorization for the millenium. *Cardiol Young* 1997;**7**:98–116.
6. Anderson RH, Becker AE, Freedom RM, Quero-Jimenez M, Macartney FJ, Shinebourne EA, Wilkinson JL, Tynan MJ. Problems in the nomenclature of the univentricular heart. *Herz* 1979;**4**:97–106.
7. Van Praagh R, Wise JRJ, Dahl BA, Van Praagh S. Single left ventricle with infundibular outlet chamber and tricuspid valve opening only into outlet chamber in 44-year-old man with thoracoabdominal ectopic cordis without diaphragmatic or pericardial defect: Importance of myocardial morphologic method of chamber identification in congenital heart disease. In: Van Praagh R, Takao A (eds). *Etiology and Morphogenesis of Congenital Heart Disease.* Mount Kisco, New York: Futura Publishing Company. 1980: pp 379–420.
8. Brandt PWT. Cineangiography of atrioventricular and ventriculo-arterial connexions. In: Godman MJ (ed). *Paediatric Cardiology Volume 4.* Edinburgh: Churchill Livingstone. 1981: pp 199–220.
9. Bharati S, Lev M. The concept of tricuspid atresia complex as distinct from that of the single ventricle complex. *Pediatr Cardiol* 1979;**1**:57–62.
10. Anderson RH, Shinebourne EA, Becker AE, Macartney FJ, Wilkinson JL, Tynan MJ. Tricuspid atresia and univentricular heart. *Pediatr Cardiol* 1979;**1**:165–166.
11. Rao PS. Is the term "tricuspid atresia" appropriate? *Am J Cardiol* 1990;**66**:1251–1254.
12. Orie JD, Anderson C, Ettedgui JA, Zuberbuhler JR, Anderson RH. Echocardiographic-anatomical correlations in tricuspid atresia. *J Am Coll Cardiol* 1995;**26**:750–758.
13. Van Praagh R, Ongley PA, Swan HJC. Anatomic types of single or common ventricle in man: morphologic and geometric aspects of sixty necropsied cases. *Am J Cardiol* 1964;**13**:367–386.
14. Lev M, Liberthson RR, Kirkpatrick JR, Eckner FAO, Arcilla RA. Single (primitive) ventricle. *Circulation* 1969;**39**:577–591.
15. Edwards JE. Discussion. In: Davila JC (ed). *2nd Henry Ford Hospital International Symposium on Cardiac Surgery.* New York: Appleton-Century-Crofts. 1977: p 242.

16. Anderson RH, Becker AE, Wilkinson JL, Gerlis LM. Morphogenesis of univentricular hearts. *Br Heart J* 1976;**38**:558–572.
17. Deanfield JE, Tommasini G, Anderson RH, Macartney FJ. Tricuspid atresia: analysis of coronary artery distribution and ventricular morphology. *Br Heart J* 1982;**48**:485-492.
18. Kumar K, Lock JE, Geva T. Apical muscular ventricular septal defects between the left ventricle and the right ventricular infundibulum: diagnostic and interventional considerations. *Circulation* 1997;**95**:1207–1213.
19. Anderson RH, Arnold R, Thaper MK, Jones RS, Hamilton DI. Cardiac specialized tissues in hearts with an apparently single ventricular chamber. (Double inlet left ventricle.) *Am J Cardiol* 1974;**33**:95–106.
20. Bharati S, Lev M. The course of the conduction system in single ventricle with inverted (L) loop and inverted (L) transposition. *Circulation* 1975;**51**:723–730.
21. Wenink ACG. The conduction tissues in primitive ventricle with outlet chamber: two different possibilities. *J Thorac Cardiovasc Surg* 1978;**75**:747–753.
22. Bevilacqua M, Sanders SP, Van Praagh S, Colan SD, Parness I. Double-inlet single left ventricle: echocardiographic anatomy with emphasis on the morphology of the atrioventricular valves and ventricular septal defect. *J Am Coll Cardiol* 1991;**18**:559–568.
23. Becker AE, Wilkinson JL, Anderson RH. Atrioventricular conduction tissues: A guide in understanding the morphogenesis of the univentricular heart. In: Van Praagh R, Takao A (eds). *Etiology and Morphogenesis of Congenital Heart Disease.* Mount Kisco, New York: Futura Publishing Company. 1980: pp 489-514.
24. Dickinson DF, Wilkinson JL, Anderson KR, Smith A, Ho SY, Anderson RH. The cardiac conduction system in situs ambiguus. *Circulation* 1979;**59**:879–885.
25. Essed CE, Ho SY, Hunter S, Anderson RH. Atrioventricular conduction system in univentricular heart of right ventricular type with right-sided rudimentary chamber. *Thorax* 1980;**35**:123–127.
26. Doherty A, Ho SY, Anderson RH, Rigby ML. The morphological nature of the atrioventricular valves in hearts with double inlet left ventricle. *Pediatr Pathol* 1989;**9**:521–529.
27. Restivo A, Ho SY, Anderson RH, Cameron H, Wilkinson JL. Absent left atrioventricular connection with right atrium connected to morphologically left ventricular chamber, rudimentary right ventricular chamber, and ventriculoarterial discordance. Problem of mitral versus tricuspid atresia. *Br Heart J* 1982;**48**:240–248.
28. Wenink ACG. Embryology of the ventricular septum: separate origin of its components. *Virchows Arch A Pathol Anat Histopathol* 1981;**390**:71–79.
29. Lamers WH, Wessels A, Verbeek FJ, Moorman AFM, Viràgh S, Wenink ACG, Gittenberger-de Groot AC, Anderson RH. New findings concerning ventricular septation in the human heart. Implications for maldevelopment. *Circulation* 1992;**86**:1194–1205.

Index

A

F

G

H

I

N

O

P

T

U

V

W

Z